Plate 2

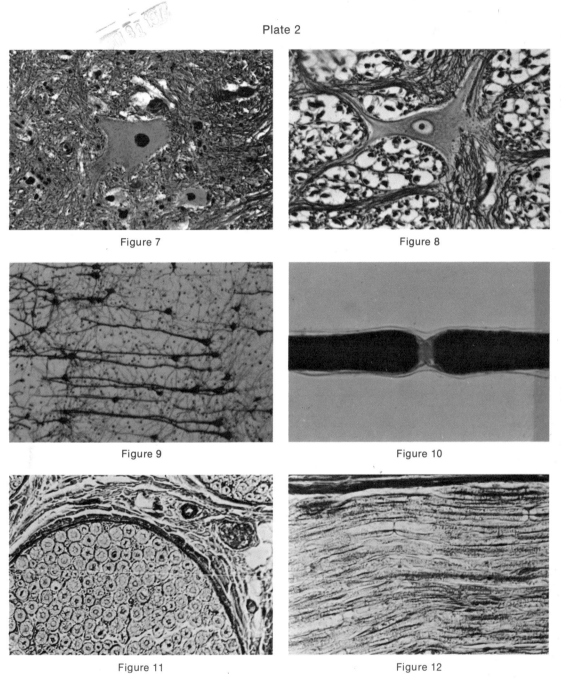

Figure 7

Figure 8

Figure 9

Figure 10

Figure 11

Figure 12

(7) Motor neuron, spinal cord. Silver method. ×100. (8) Neuron of a raphe nucleus, medulla. Probably a serotonin-synthesizing neuron. ×100. See Figure 3–20, p. 46 of text. (9) Pyramidal cells, cerebral cortex, rabbit. Cox-Golgi method. ×40. See Figure 3–4, p. 29 of text. (10) Single myelinated nerve fiber, frog sciatic nerve. Osmium tetroxide stain. ×250. See Figure 3–15, p. 42 of text. (11) Transverse section of peripheral nerve. Mallory trichrome stain.* (12) Longitudinal section of spinal nerve. Mallory trichrome stain.†

*From C. R. Leeson and T. S. Leeson: Histology. 2nd ed. W. B. Saunders Co., Philadelphia, 1970.
†From C. R. Leeson and T. S. Leeson: Practical Histology. W. B. Saunders Co., Philadelphia, 1973.

fundamentals of
NEUROLOGY
a psychophysiological approach

ERNEST GARDNER, M.D.

Department of Neurology,
University of California, Davis

SIXTH EDITION
ILLUSTRATED

W. B. SAUNDERS COMPANY
Philadelphia • London • Toronto

W. B. Saunders Company: West Washington Square
Philadelphia, Pa.   19105

1 St. Anne's Road
Eastbourne, East Sussex BN21 3UN, England

833 Oxford Street
Toronto, M8Z 5T9, Canada

Library of Congress Cataloging in Publication Data

Gardner, Ernest Dean, 1915–

Fundamentals of neurology.

Includes bibliographies.

1. Nervous system.   2. Neurology.   I. Title.   II. Title:
Neurology. [DNLM: 1. Nervous system—Anatomy and
histology.   2. Neurophysiology. WL102 G226f]

QP361.G36 1975   612'.8   74–6681

ISBN 0-7216-4002-8

Listed here are the latest translated editions of this
book together with the language of the translation
and the publisher.

Japanese (5th Edition)—Ishiyaku Publishers, Inc.,
Tokyo, Japan

Spanish (5th Edition)—Nueva Editorial Interamericana,
Mexico City, Mexico

Front cover illustration: Golgi type I cell, rat cerebral cortex.

Courtesy of Dr. Stanley Jacobson, Tufts University Medical School, Boston, Massachusetts.

Back cover illustration: Purkinje cell, cerebellum, rhesus monkey.

Fundamentals of Neurology   ISBN   0-7216-4002-8

Last digit is the print number: 9   8   7   6   5   4   3   2

To La Vearl Gardner

PREFACE TO THE
SIXTH EDITION

The purpose of this volume was expressed in the preface to the first edition and in each of the subsequent editions. It is to select from the available data those facts necessary to present neurology as concepts that can be the foundation for more detailed studies. The task of selection, however, has become increasingly difficult because of major advances in our knowledge of the nervous system. These advances are due in part to the application of elegant ultrastructural, biochemical, histochemical, and pharmacological methods. Moreover, research in developmental neurobiology is expanding rapidly, and increasingly sophisticated behavioral studies are proving of immense importance. The present edition, therefore, constitutes a major revision. Certain features, however, are relatively unchanged. The references cited are intended to provide the interested student with a starting point for further reading, and the short biographical sketches are of those men whose names are mentioned in the text.

I am particularly grateful to Professor Ronan O'Rahilly for his valuable advice and criticism. I wish to thank Anna Mary Griffin and Marleen Pibbs for their typing of the manuscript, Celeste Morrison and Sandra McMahon for the preparation of new illustrations, and Will Renner's Illustration Services for photographic materials. I also wish to thank the many teachers and students who have made valuable suggestions. Finally, I am indebted to the W. B. Saunders Company for the help and the many courtesies they extended me.

ERNEST GARDNER

CONTENTS

CHAPTER 4

EXCITATION, CONDUCTION, AND TRANSMISSION............................... 69

CHAPTER 5

BIOCHEMISTRY AND PHARMACOLOGY OF THE NERVOUS
SYSTEM.. 98

CHAPTER 6

SIMPLE NEURONAL CONNECTIONS AND REFLEX ARCS 115

Chapter 1

INTRODUCTION

The material in this volume is based upon data derived from dissection and microscopic study of the nervous system; from physiological, pharmacological, biochemical, and behavioral experiments; and from the study of neurological disorders. This knowledge has accumulated over many centuries, resulting from the efforts of countless investigators, working in many countries and using many different languages. Consequently an expanding and often confusing terminology has resulted. Names were often given to portions of the body because of shape or for other arbitrary reasons. For instance, an area of the brain which in general configuration was thought to resemble a sea horse was named the *hippocampus*. Often the name of the investigator who was the first (or was among the first) to describe a structure became associated with that structure, as occurred when the *vein of Galen* (p. 6) was identified.

The first attempt to clarify and simplify anatomical terminology was made in 1895 by a group consisting chiefly of German anatomists meeting at Basle. The terminology they adopted is the *Basle Nomina Anatomica* (B.N.A.). Later revisions were the *Birmingham Revision* (B.R., 1933) and the *Jena Nomina Anatomica* (I.N.A., 1936). In Paris in 1955, international agreement was reached on a Latin system of nomenclature based largely on the B.N.A. This *Nomina Anatomica,* as amended in 1960 and 1965, is used throughout this book where applicable, and translated into English where appropriate. (See citation on p. 7.)

The *Nomina Anatomica* was adopted with the following principles in mind: (1) Every term in the official list shall be in Latin, with each country at liberty to translate the official Latin terms into its own vernacular for teaching purposes. (2) With but few exceptions, each structure shall be designated by one term only. (3) Terms shall be primarily memory signs, but shall have some informative or descriptive value. (4) Eponyms shall not be used.

1

An important aspect of terminology has to do with the orientation of the body and its parts. For example, information about the position of any object, such as a house in a city, can be expressed in terms of direction, such as east and west, or right and left. When the human body is in the *anatomical position,* that is to say, when it is erect, with the head, eyes, and toes directed forward, and with the upper limbs at the sides and held so that the palms face forward, certain positions and directions may be defined (Fig. 1–1). These include three series or sets of primary planes.

Planes. The *median plane* is an imaginary vertical plane of section that passes longitudinally through the body and divides it into right and left halves. A *sagittal plane* (named after the sagittal suture of the skull, to which it is parallel) is any vertical plane through the body that is parallel to the median plane.

A *frontal plane* (or *coronal plane*) is any vertical plane that intersects the median plane at a right angle and separates the body into front and back parts. It is parallel to the coronal suture of the skull.

A *horizontal plane* is any plane at right angles to both the median and coronal planes which divides the body into upper and lower parts. The term *transverse* generally refers to any section that is at a right angle to the longitudinal axis of a structure. Thus,

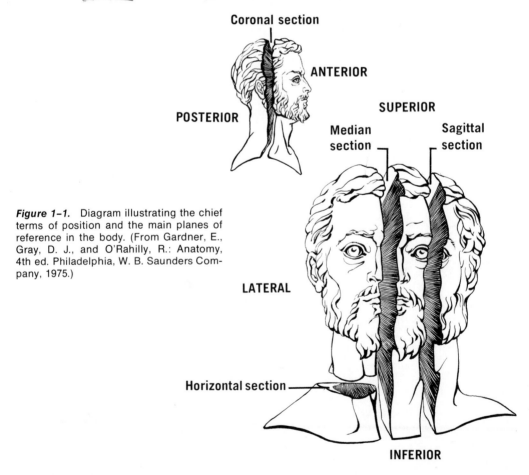

Figure 1–1. Diagram illustrating the chief terms of position and the main planes of reference in the body. (From Gardner, E., Gray, D. J., and O'Rahilly, R.: Anatomy, 4th ed. Philadelphia, W. B. Saunders Company, 1975.)

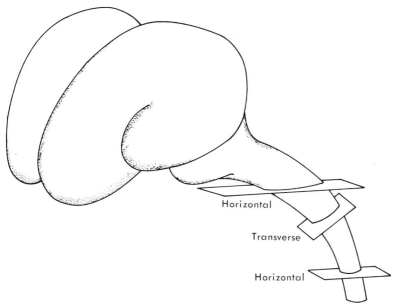

Figure 1-2. Diagram illustrating that the brain stem is at an angle with respect to the brain and that a section in a horizontal plane passes obliquely through most of the brain stem. Note that a transverse section through most of the brain stem is oblique with reference to a horizontal plane, but that more caudally a transverse section is in a horizontal plane.

a transverse section through the brain stem is not necessarily horizontal (although it is in the case of the spinal cord), and a horizontal section through the brain stem is not necessarily transverse (Fig. 1-2).

Directions and Positions. Structures toward the front of the body are *anterior;* toward the back, *posterior. Superior* refers to upper, and *inferior,* to lower, structures. In the trunk, *cranial* or *cephalic* is sometimes used instead of superior, and *caudal* instead of inferior. Another important term is *rostral,* which means nearer the head or front end (the hypophysial area in the early embryo and the region of the nose and mouth in postembryonic life).

Still other important terms are *medial,* nearer the median plane, and *lateral,* farther from that plane. *Proximal,* in referring to a limb, indicates a position nearer the trunk or central axis of the body; *distal,* a more peripheral position.

Comparative Anatomical Terms. The fact that humans stand upright has led to a difference from the terminology used in comparative anatomy. In lower forms, structures which in humans are toward the front of the body are *ventral,* those toward the back, *dorsal* (Fig. 1-3). Cranial and anterior become synonymous, as do caudal and posterior. In connection with the human nervous system, the comparative anatomical nomenclature is

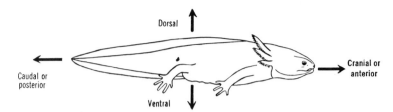

Figure 1–3. Diagram of an amphibian, illustrating a few features of comparative anatomical nomenclature.

often followed, particularly as regards "dorsal" and "ventral." For instance, the roots of the spinal cord usually are termed "dorsal" and "ventral" rather than "posterior" and "anterior." "Ventral" is sometimes used to indicate structures at the base of the human brain; the comparable surface in animals that walk on all fours is also "ventral."

METHODS OF STUDY

The following paragraphs contain examples of the methods of study. Many of the later chapters contain additional examples, as well as references that deal with methods.

GROSS AND MICROSCOPIC METHODS

Many important characteristics of the nervous system, such as size, shape, position, and surface markings, may be noted by ordinary inspection. Details may be revealed by dissection of the nervous system, that is, by separating it from other tissues or organs, or by cutting it in various ways so as to obtain access to structures not apparent on the surface. Comparative anatomical studies, both gross and microscopic, have been important in elucidating some features of the evolution of the vertebrate nervous system.

The minute anatomy of the nervous system can be examined under the microscope by methods developed for cells and tissues in general. There are a variety of methods for the direct observation of living tissues and cells. However, their usefulness is limited by the thickness of tissues and by their natural transparency. Therefore, special techniques are used to kill tissues and preserve them, and to cut them into thin slices called histological sections. These sections are stained with various dyes and are studied microscopically by transmitted light. It is important to note that many of the usual staining methods are not suitable for the nervous system, for which special methods have been developed that use, for example, special stains, histochemical and immunohistochemical techniques, and phase, interference, fluorescent, and electron microscopy. Transmission electron microscopy provides enormous magnification and very high resolution, thus enabling the study of details of structure that are beyond the resolution of the light microscope. Scanning electron microscopy provides high resolution at lower magnifications in a way that elegantly demonstrates topography and three-dimensional details. Investigations using the electron microscope have led to a substantial increase in our understanding of the *ultrastructure* (also called *fine structure*) of the nervous system. The most significant advances have been made in connection with the structure of cell membranes, and of myelin, synapses, receptors, and special sense organs.

PHYSIOLOGICAL, PHARMACOLOGICAL, BIOCHEMICAL, AND PSYCHOLOGICAL METHODS

These methods, singly or combined, are designed to study the living nervous system, directly or indirectly. Research based on these methods, and including ultrastructural and other microscopic techniques, probably constitutes the most active and significant field of biological research today. Indeed, the techniques being used and being developed are so numerous that only the major general categories are listed below. Specific examples are given in some detail throughout this text.

The function of a particular portion or structure in the nervous system may be adduced by stimulating it with an electric current and observing the results directly. A part of the nervous system may be removed surgically and any effect or loss of function noted. Habit formation, behavior, reactions to stimuli, and the like may be observed before and after surgical procedures in animals and in human beings. Drugs may be given which affect or stimulate certain elements of the nervous system and thereby alter their functions. The inception of function may be observed by correlating physiological and morphological development during embryonic, fetal, and infant life. Blood supply and cerebrospinal fluid formation, circulation, and absorption may be studied by a variety of methods. The electrical activity of living tissue can be studied and recorded by special electronic equipment. These methods allow one to examine a variety of phenomena, among which are the electrical activity of single nerve cells, nerve conduction, the localization of active nerve centers, and the tracing of pathways in the central nervous system. The effect of various drugs, such as anesthetics, on electrical activity can also be included.

General biochemical investigations, histochemical studies that combine microscopic and biochemical procedures, special cytochemical techniques, and the rapidly developing and increasingly important field of neuropharmacology have yielded important information about membrane functions, chemical composition and general and intermediary metabolism of brain and nerve, and specific neurological functions. Experimental techniques have been devised of so elegant and precise a nature that they permit the study of single nerve cells. All of these approaches, combined with studies of ultrastructure and the use of radioisotopes, have led to major advances in our understanding of neural functions and disorders.

Psychological studies constitute a field of such scope and importance that for the techniques employed reference must be made to the works cited in various chapters of this text.

CLINICAL METHODS

A disease or injury of the nervous system usually causes a loss of function or may give rise to an abnormal condition. If a patient with a neurological disorder dies, the signs and symptoms which that patient displayed during life may be correlated with pathological changes found after death. Over many years the study of great numbers of such cases has yielded considerable information. Data may also be obtained when operations are necessary, and from special diagnostic procedures such as angiography, ventriculography, and electroencephalography, and other procedures involving blood and cerebrospinal fluid. Diagnostic biochemical tests, especially those for inborn errors of metabolism, are becoming increasingly important, as are associated genetic studies. Disturbances of behavior and of such higher level functions as language afford an opportunity for psychological studies.

HISTORICAL ASPECTS

It is beyond the scope of this text to deal with the history of neurology. Some inkling of the contributions that have been made is provided by **NAMES IN NEUROLOGY.** These are short biographical sketches of people whose names are mentioned in the text (usually as eponyms). The chief sources of information are given below in **REFERENCES**. Sometimes additional information has been obtained from a specific article or book; this is then cited with the biographical sketch.

NAMES IN NEUROLOGY

GALEN OF PERGAMUM (OR PERGAMON) (c. 129–199)

Galen was a Greek physician who, after many years of study, settled in Rome. As the founder of experimental physiology, his knowledge being acquired from surgery and from the dissection of animals, he knew of the effects of cutting the spinal cord, and described the cerebral aqueduct and several of the cranial nerves.

Probably his most outstanding contribution to medicine was his insistence upon the importance of experimental studies, as well as the necessity of relating form to function. Although his findings and concepts were accepted dogmatically for many centuries, attempts to minimize his contributions are unjustified; he must be recognized as one of the great scientific figures. (Galen: On the Usefulness of the Parts of the Body. Translated from the Greek by May, M. T.: Ithaca, Cornell University Press, 1968.)

REFERENCES

For further details on anatomical terminology, see the anatomical textbooks cited on p. 159. A list of internationally accepted anatomical terms is provided in the following publication.

Nomina Anatomica. 3rd ed. Amsterdam, Excerpta Medica Foundation, 1966.

The following references provide information about methods of study. Many of the references cited in other chapters also contain information about methods, techniques, and experimental approaches.

Bloom, W., and Fawcett, D. W.: A Textbook of Histology. 10th ed. Philadelphia, W. B. Saunders Company, 1975. The first chapter is an excellent general description of the methods of histology and cytology.
Koehler, J. K. (editor): Advanced Techniques in Biological Electron Microscopy. New York, Springer-Verlag, 1973. Detailed accounts of those techniques that have been essential to research in ultrastructure.
Myers, R. D. (editor): Methods in Psychology. New York, Academic Press, 1971. Two volumes that bring together information about the basic laboratory methods used in experiments relating the brain to behavior.
Nauta, W. J. H., and Ebbesson, S. O. E. (editors): Contemporary Research Methods in Neuroanatomy. New York, Springer-Verlag, 1970. Detailed accounts of some of the important special techniques necessary for the microscopic study of the nervous system.

The first two of the following five references are the chief sources of information for the biographical sketches.

Clarke, E., and O'Malley, C. D.: The Human Brain and Spinal Cord. Berkeley, University of California Press, 1968.
Haymaker, W., and Schiller, F. (editors): The Founders of Neurology. 2nd ed. Springfield, Ill., Charles C Thomas, 1970.
Brazier, M. A. B.: The historical development of neurophysiology. Chapter 1, pp. 1–58, vol. 1, in Field, J. Magoun, H. W., and Hall, V. E. (editors): Handbook of Physiology. Washington, D.C., American Physiological Society, 1959.
McHenry, L. C.: Garrison's History of Neurology. Springfield, Ill., Charles C Thomas, 1969.
Meyer, A.: Historical Aspects of Cerebral Anatomy. London, Oxford University Press, 1971.

Chapter 2

THE GENERAL FEATURES OF THE VERTEBRATE NERVOUS SYSTEM

The nervous system of vertebrates is characterized by a hollow, dorsal nerve cord which ends in the head region as an enlargement, the brain. Even in its most primitive form this cord and its attached nerves are the result of evolutionary specialization, and their further evolution from lower to higher vertebrate classes is a process which is far from fully understood. Nevertheless, the basic arrangements are similar in all vertebrates, and the study of lower animals gives insight into the form and structure of the nervous system of higher animals. Moreover, for any species, the study of the embryological development of the nervous system is indispensable for an understanding of adult morphology.

In any vertebrate two chief parts of the nervous system may be distinguished. These are the *central nervous system* (the nerve cord mentioned above), consisting of the *brain* and *spinal cord,* and the *peripheral nervous system,* consisting of the *cranial, spinal,* and *peripheral nerves,* together with their motor and sensory endings. The term *autonomic nervous system* refers to the parts of the central and peripheral systems that supply and regulate the activity of cardiac muscle, smooth muscle, and many glands.

The nervous system is composed of many millions of nerve and glial cells, together with blood vessels and a small amount of connective tissue. The nerve cells or *neurons* are characterized by many processes and are specialized in that they exhibit to a great degree the phenomena of irritability and conductivity. The glial cells of the central nervous system are supporting cells collectively termed *neuroglia.* They are characterized by short processes that have special relationships to neurons, blood vessels, and connective tissue. The comparable cells in the peripheral nervous system are termed *neurilemmal cells.*

CENTRAL NERVOUS SYSTEM

The central nervous system lies dorsal to the digestive system and is surrounded by more or less strong skeletal structures that compose the vertebral column and most of the skull. In all vertebrates, freshly cut sections of brain or spinal cord exhibit characteristic arrangements of *gray matter* and *white matter.* Gray matter (p. 44) consists mostly of the bodies of neurons and neuroglial cells and their local processes. In many parts of the central nervous system, neurons form well-defined groups that are usually termed *nuclei* (similar collections in the peripheral nervous system are termed *ganglia*). White matter consists largely of the distant or projecting processes of nerve cells, together with neuroglial cells; the whitish appearance results from lipid insulating material that surrounds many of the long neuronal processes. In some regions of the brain and spinal cord, diffuse mixtures of gray and white matter form what is termed *reticular formation.*

Within the white matter, the processes (fibers) of nerve cells serving similar or comparable functions are often collected into bundles termed *tracts.* Tracts are usually named according to origin and destination, but sometimes by position also. Thus, a corticospinal tract is a collection of nerve fibers that originates from neurons in the cortex (surface) of the brain and ends in the spinal cord. By contrast, the nerve cell processes that leave the central nervous system are collected into bundles that form the various nerves.

SPINAL CORD

The spinal cord is a long mass of nervous tissue, usually oval or rounded in transverse section, which occupies a variable extent of the vertebral canal. In many species, for example fishes, the spinal cord extends throughout the entire length of the vertebral canal. In many higher forms, however, the spinal cord is shorter than the vertebral column.

Gray matter is present in the interior of the spinal cord and is arranged into longitudinal columns or *horns* (Fig. 2–1) that surround the lumen (*central canal*) of the cord. The white matter, which surrounds the gray matter, is arranged into *funiculi* (Fig. 7–20, p. 143). The neurons of the gray matter include those that have processes which leave the spinal cord, enter nerves, and supply skeletal muscle or end in certain autonomic ganglia. Many other neurons in the gray matter are concerned with sensory and reflex mechanisms. The white matter consists chiefly of tracts, some of which ascend to or descend from the brain, whereas others interconnect various levels of the spinal cord. In those vertebrates having well-developed limbs, the cervical and lumbosacral regions of the spinal cord, to which the nerves of the limbs are attached, are thicker than the rest of the cord, owing to the greater number of neurons in these two enlargements.

In all vertebrates each lateral half of the spinal cord has attached to it the roots of the peripheral nerves, each root being associated with a segment of the body. The roots consist of a *dorsal root,* attached to the dorsal aspect of the spinal cord, and a *ventral root,* attached to the ventral aspect of the spinal cord. Each dorsal root is formed by nerve cell processes that enter the spinal cord and which arise from sensory neurons that are collected together to form an enlargement termed a *spinal ganglion.* Each ventral root is formed by nerve-cell processes that arise from neurons within the spinal cord.

In the lowest vertebrates (cyclostomes), the dorsal and ventral roots of the same side alternate with one another along the spinal cord (Fig. 2–1). The muscles supplied by the ventral roots are arranged in simple transverse segments, and the roots are therefore segmental in position. The dorsal roots, however, are intersegmental in position. Their spinal ganglia lie close to the spinal cord, and many of the sensory cells lie within the spinal cord (this intraspinal position is characteristic of the spinal cord of the prevertebrate animal, amphioxus). The peripheral processes of the ganglion cells are distributed to skin by way of *dorsal rami* and *ventral rami,* as are the fibers of the ventral roots.

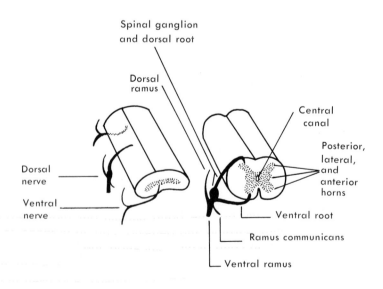

Figure 2–1. Schematic outline of the spinal cord in A, a cyclostome (the lamprey, Petromyzon), and in B, a mammal. (After Johnston, J.: Nervous System of Vertebrates. Philadelphia, P. Blakiston's Son & Co., 1906.)

In true fishes and in all higher vertebrates the dorsal and ventral roots of a given segment lie in nearly the same transverse plane, and the two roots join at or just beyond the spinal ganglion to form a *spinal nerve* (Fig. 2–1), which in turn divides into a dorsal and a ventral ramus. The *ramus communicans* is a branch of either the spinal nerve or the ventral ramus; it provides a connection to autonomic ganglia. The number of spinal nerves varies according to species, and is closely related to the number of vertebral segments.

The spinal cord is similar in structure and function in all vertebrates. It is segmental in arrangement and it exhibits little of the diversification and specialization so characteristic of the brain, and it carries out sensory, integrative, and motor functions. These may be categorized as follows: (1) Reflex: A stimulus is followed by a coordinated motor response. (2) Reciprocal activity: As one activity starts, another stops (excitation and inhibition). (3) Monitoring and modulating: Incoming sensory impulses are controlled, coded, and transmitted; these impulses monitor and influence motor activities and themselves are monitored and influenced by motor cells and tracts. (4) Transmission: The white matter of the cord transmits impulses to and from the brain.

BRAIN

The brain (*cerebrum* or *encephalon*) is the enlarged head end of the central nervous system; it occupies the cranium or brain case. The enlargement is the result of *encephalization,* a great expansion in size and function of the head end of the vertebrate nervous system. The brain has few segmental arrangements, and exhibits an extraordinary diversity and specialization within classes and even from one species to another. These features are related to the functions of the brain: (1) The brain has additional (with respect to the spinal cord) association mechanisms for the integration of motor and sensory functions. Hence, a given class of functions is the property of several neurological levels; the higher the level the more complicated and recently evolved the function. (2) There are general structural and functional features relative to the special senses and the pharyngeal arches. (3) There are specific adaptations in structure and function, especially with regard to the special senses and the pharyngeal arches. (4) The brain carries out higher level functions dealing with learning and behavior and, in humans, language.

In spite of diversification and specialization, and in spite of an extraordinary range in weight (from a few grams in lower forms to 1200 to 1400 grams in humans, and even more in certain larger mammals), the brain in all vertebrates presents three divisions each of which has certain relatively constant components and subdivisions. The three parts are *hindbrain (rhombencephalon), mid-*

brain (mesencephalon), and forebrain (prosencephalon). The forebrain in turn has two subdivisions, telencephalon (endbrain) and diencephalon (interbrain). The hindbrain likewise has two subdivisions, metencephalon (afterbrain) and myelencephalon (marrowbrain). Also, in all vertebrates, the lumen of the brain forms fluid-filled cavities termed ventricles.

The various parts of a relatively simple vertebrate brain are shown in Figure 2–2. Comparative features and specialization in several vertebrate brains are shown in Figure 2–3.

Hindbrain

The Medulla Oblongata.   This is the common name for the portion of the hindbrain otherwise known as the myelencephalon. In some respects, the medulla oblongata is the rostral continuation of the spinal cord, and there is no sharp separation between them. As the cord merges into the medulla oblongata, the dorsal parts

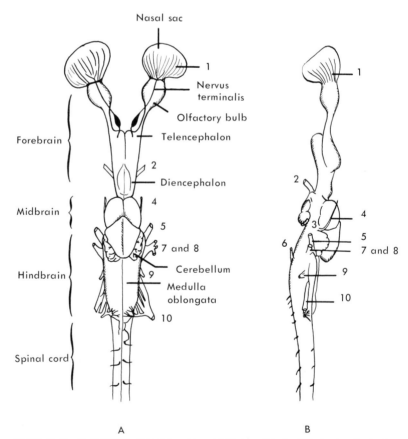

A   B

Figure 2–2.   Schematic diagrams of a relatively simple fish brain, that of a selachian. A, dorsal view; B, lateral view. The cranial nerves are numbered. (After Johnston, J.: The Nervous System of Vertebrates. Philadelphia, P. Blakiston's Son & Co., 1906.)

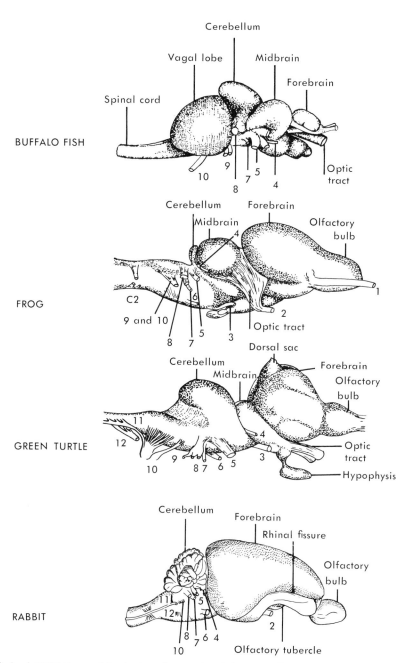

Figure 2-3. Lateral views of the brains of several vertebrates to illustrate differences and specialization: buffalo fish (from Herrick, C. J., and Herrick, C. L.); Frog, green turtle, and rabbit (from Papez, J.: Comparative Neurology. New York, Hafner Publishing Company, Inc., 1967.) The brains are drawn at different scales, and the cranial nerves are numbered.

of the latter spread apart, and the central canal becomes enlarged and continues into the *fourth ventricle.*

The metencephalon (a term which is seldom used) is the upper part of the hindbrain. It consists of a ventral portion that is essentially a rostral continuation of the medulla oblongata, and a dorsal portion, the *cerebellum,* which covers the upper part of the fourth ventricle. In mammals, the ventral part of the metencephalon is enlarged to form the *pons,* which is a bridge between the two halves of the cerebellum.

The cerebellum varies greatly in size according to class of vertebrate. Arising from the lateral edge of the ventral portion of the metencephalon, it is highly fissured and often is arranged into a median portion and two lateral portions or hemispheres. It is large in all true fishes, is small in amphibians, and becomes larger and progressively more important in reptiles, birds, and mammals. It has major functions concerned with the automatic regulation of movement and posture. Its surface is composed of gray matter termed cortex, and its interior is formed of white matter and nuclei of gray matter.

Midbrain

The midbrain is characterized by thick lateral and ventral walls, and by a roof (*tectum*) which is divided by a longitudinal groove into two *optic lobes.* In mammals, these lobes are divided by transverse furrows into rostral and caudal parts. The four eminences thus formed are termed *colliculi.* The narrow cavity of the midbrain is the *cerebral aqueduct;* it is continuous caudally with the fourth ventricle and rostrally with the third ventricle.

Forebrain

Diencephalon. The diencephalon, whose lumen is the *third ventricle,* is characterized by a roof that is largely membranous, by thick lateral walls formed on each side by the *thalamus* dorsally and the *hypothalamus* ventrally, and by a floor formed by the hypothalamus. The floor is connected with the *hypophysis (pituitary gland),* part of which is embryologically derived from the hypothalamus.

The diencephalon is the upper part of what is generally called the *brain stem.* This comprises, from rostral to caudal, the diencephalon, mesencephalon, ventral portion of the metencephalon (pons), and medulla oblongata. This unpaired stalk contains nuclei and diffuse masses of gray matter. In all vertebrates it contains, in addition to tracts that descend and ascend through it, collections of nerve cells that (1) comprise major integrating centers for sensory and motor functions; (2) form the nuclei of most cranial nerves (all the cranial nerves except the first are attached to the brain stem); (3) form centers concerned with the regulation of a variety of visceral, endocrinological, behavioral, and other activities; (4) are associated with most of the special senses; (5) control muscular activity in the head and part of the neck; (6) supply pharyngeal arch and lateral line structures; and (7) are connected with the cerebellum.

Telencephalon. The telencephalon is relatively small in fishes, is larger in amphibians and reptiles, and is the largest subdivision of the central nervous system in birds and mammals. These features are shown to some extent in Figure 2–3 but can be appreciated more fully by reference to the human brain (Figs. 7–3 to 7–11, pp. 130 to 136).

In the cyclostomes, the most primitive vertebrates, the brain consists of a median structure, the *telencephalon medium,* with two lateral evaginations. Each evagination is divided into two parts: a rostral portion, the *olfactory bulb,* which receives the olfactory nerve filaments; and a caudal portion, the *olfactory lobe.* The latter is the forerunner of the *cerebral hemispheres* of higher forms. The third ventricle extends into the telencephalon medium and has two extensions, the *lateral ventricles,* one into each lateral evagination.

In fishes, the brain remains in large part a median structure with two lateral evaginations. Each contains a complex central mass of gray matter which is surrounded by incomplete layers of neurons that form a covering or *pallium.* The central complex in each evagination suggests the earliest indication of basal ganglia, which in higher forms are major centers for the integration of motor activities.

It is traditionally supposed that the brains of lower forms, in particular the central telencephalic gray matter, are largely concerned with olfactory and gustatory functions. Hence, the term olfactory is applied to many structures and nuclei. It must be emphasized, however, that homologies thought to exist because of studies of normal morphological material are now being called into question. Moreover homologous structures often have quite different functions. The importance of experimental studies in comparative neurology is illustrated by the fact that experimental studies of the shark telencephalon have shown that its central gray matter receives a major, nonolfactory input from the thalamus which is visual in nature. It should further be emphasized that comparative studies are not necessarily relevant to evolutionary lines, that most such studies deal with adaptation and specialization, and that our understanding of nonmammalian brains is still quite limited.

In the brains of amphibians, the cerebral hemispheres are larger, and the telencephalon medium is relatively reduced in size. The hemispheres are separated to a greater degree, and the gray matter in each exhibits an organization into regions that are present, in one form or another, in all higher vertebrates. As shown In Figure 2–4, these are: (1) basal ganglia (corpus striatum); (2)

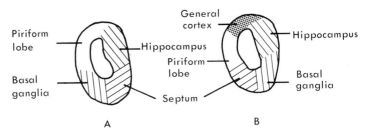

Figure 2-4. Highly schematic representation of the rostral part of a cerebral hemisphere of A, an amphibian, and B, a reptile, to show the basic
regions and the location of the general cortex. Note that as the general
cortex is replaced by a much larger neocortex in mammals (Fig. 2–5), the
limbic system (hippocampus) will be crowded medially and ventrally and
the piriform lobe ventrally.

piriform lobe; (3) hippocampus (limbic system); and (4) septum.
Since piriform lobe and septum are chiefly olfactory structures, an
even simpler grouping is possible, namely into (1) corpus striatum,
(2) limbic system, and (3) olfactory structures.

The brains of reptiles appear to forecast the characteristic
neocortex of mammalian brains by the presence of a general
cortex between the piriform lobe *(paleocortex)* laterally and the
limbic system or hippocampus *(allocortex* or *archicortex)* medially
(Fig. 2–4). However, reptilian brains are also characterized by
highly specialized basal ganglia, one portion of which, the external
striatum, is thought to be the major forerunner of neocortex.

The transition from reptilian brains to those of birds is distinct,
but not abrupt. Avian brains are relatively comparable to those of
modern reptiles, and are characterized by large, complex, highly
organized basal ganglia.

The transition from reptilian to mammalian brains is marked,
to such a degree that they cannot be readily compared by the usual
methods of study. The outstanding feature of the mammalian brain
is the replacement of general cortex by a new type of cortex, a
multilayered (usually six layers) *neocortex* or *isocortex*. As a consequence the simpler allocortex of the limbic system or hippocampus is crowded medially, and the paleocortex, which is separated from the neocortex by the *rhinal fissure,* moves ventrally.
The external striatum of birds and reptiles is absent in mammals,
and is thought to be the major source of neocortex (Fig. 2–5).

The elaboration of the neocortex is such that in many mammals, especially in primates, the surface area and volume of gray
matter is increased enormously by a folding and fissuring of the
surfaces of the cerebral hemispheres. The increasing prominence
of the neocortex in higher mammals is related to an increasingly
complex control and integration of motor and sensory functions,
and especially to those higher level primate functions dealing with
intelligence, behavior, and, in humans, language.

There is little doubt that the larger brains of higher vertebrates
contain more neurons, for the brain as a whole and also per unit

of volume. However, it should be emphasized that an increase in numbers of neurons, and therefore an increase in brain weight, is not sufficient to explain the evolution of behavior. There is substantial evidence that the circuitry of the forebrain has also undergone reorganization during evolution.

The fundamental morphological relationships of the other major components of the telencephalon are present in mammals, but they are obscured by the relatively enormous cerebral expansion. Moreover, in most primates, there is an angle between the long axis of the brain stem and the horizontal axis of the hemispheres which is due to the characteristic position of the head on the vertebral column. This hemisphere—brain-stem angle introduces additional topographical changes.

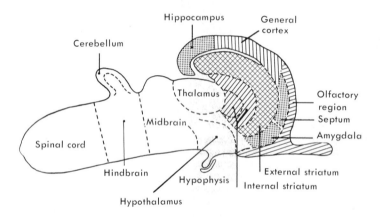

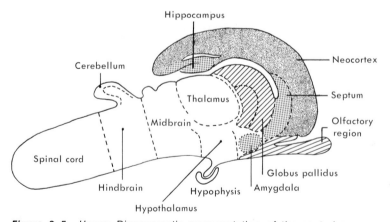

Figure 2–5. Upper: Diagrammatic representation of the central nervous system of a nonmammalian brain (chiefly reptiles and birds) in longitudinal view. *Lower:* Schematic representation of the mammalian brain. Note the shift in forebrain parts and the presence of neocortex. (From Nauta, W., and Karten, H.: A general profile of the vertebrate brain, with sidelights on the ancestry of cerebral cortex. In F. Schmitt, editor: The Neurosciences. New York, Rockefeller University Press, 1970. By permission of authors and publisher.)

CEREBROSPINAL FLUID

In all vertebrates, the cavity of the embryonic neural tube persists in the adult brain as fluid-filled cavities. In the brain these are termed ventricles (Fig. 2–6); they are four in number; (1) and (2) a lateral ventricle in each cerebral hemisphere, each connecting with (3) the third ventricle in the telencephalon medium and the diencephalon. This connects, by means of the cerebral aqueduct in the mesencephalon, with (4) the fourth ventricle behind the pons and medulla oblongata. The fourth ventricle continues below into a narrow channel, the central canal, which is present in the lower part of the medulla oblongata and throughout the length of the spinal cord.

The ventricles of the brain are lined by neuroglial cells collectively termed *ependyma.* In certain parts of the ventricles, specialized ependymal cells and blood vessels form *choroid plexuses,* which are major sources of the almost protein-free cerebrospinal fluid that circulates through the ventricles (it also fills the central canal). In the higher vertebrates, it leaves the fourth ventricle, circulates around the brain and spinal cord, and eventually filters back into the venous system. Further details about the cerebrospinal fluid are given on p. 152.

MENINGES

The brain and spinal cord are surrounded and protected by layers of non-nervous tissue collectively termed *meninges* (p. 126). In mammals these layers, from without inward, are the *dura mater,* the *arachnoid,* and the *pia mater.* The space between the arachnoid and the pia mater, the *subarachnoid space,* contains cerebrospinal

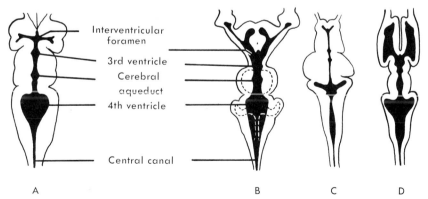

Interventricular
foramen

3rd ventricle

Cerebral

aqueduct

4th ventricle

Central canal

A B C D

Figure 2-6. The outlines of the brains, ventricles, and central canals of several vertebrates as seen from above, to show variation in the ventricular system. Compare with the human ventricular system (p. 134). The brains are drawn at different scales. A, brain of a cyclostome; B, brain of a selachian (the outlines of the ventricles in the optic lobe and cerebellum are drawn in dotted lines); C, brain of a bony fish; D, brain of a tailed amphibian. (From Johnston, J.: The Nervous System of Vertebrates. Philadelphia. P. Blakiston's Son & Co., 1906.)

fluid which enters it from the fourth ventricle. The pia mater itself is closely applied to the surface of the brain and spinal cord and, together with neuroglial processes, forms a strong limiting membrane.

BLOOD SUPPLY

The pattern of blood supply to the brain is extremely variable. In mammals, the chief supply to the cerebral hemispheres is by way of the internal carotid arteries or by the vertebral arteries, depending on species. In human beings, the brain is supplied by branches of both. The spinal cord, spinal roots, and spinal meninges are supplied by the vertebral arteries and by the segmental arteries.

The capillaries of the brain and spinal cord differ from those in other tissues and organs. Their cells are tightly coupled in such a way that they form a *blood-brain barrier,* which is selectively permeable to substances in the blood.

PERIPHERAL NERVOUS SYSTEM

The peripheral nervous system includes the cranial nerves, the spinal nerves with their dorsal and ventral roots and peripheral branches and endings, and the peripheral components of the autonomic nervous system. Strictly speaking, the term peripheral nerve includes the cranial nerves, but it is ordinarily used to refer to those nerves arising from the spinal nerves, either directly or from plexuses.

A nerve is a collection of nerve fibers the constituent fibers of which are bound together by connective tissue. Each fiber is microscopic in size, and hundreds or thousands of fibers are present in each nerve. Thus, according to the number of constituent fibers, a nerve may be visible only under the microscope, or it may be quite thick.

FUNCTIONAL CLASSIFICATION OF NERVE FIBERS

A number of classifications of nerve fibers have been proposed, based on their various morphological and functional properties. One classification that is in common use is that of Herrick; it is based chiefly on comparative studies and describes seven kinds of fibers or functional components, of which only the first four are present in spinal nerves.

1. Somatic efferent. Motor to skeletal muscle; present in ventral roots and in cranial nerves 3, 4, 6, and 12.

2. General visceral efferent. Autonomic fibers present in most ventral roots and in cranial nerves 3, 7, 9, 10, and 11.

3. General somatic afferent. Sensory from skin, muscles, joints, and deep tissues; present in dorsal roots and cranial nerves 5, 7, 9, and 10.

4. General visceral afferent. Sensory from viscera; present in dorsal roots and in cranial nerves 9 and 10.

5. Special visceral efferent. Motor to striated muscle of the pharyngeal arches; present in cranial nerves 5, 7, 9, 10, and 11.

6. Special visceral afferent. Sensation from special sense receptors in pharyngeal arches, that is, taste and smell; present in cranial nerves 1, 7, 9, and 10.

7. Special somatic afferent. Sensation from special sense receptors of placodal origin; present in cranial nerves 2 and 8.

The preceding classification is useful in clarifying nerve distribution as well as the nuclei of origin and termination, but, like all classifications, it is somewhat arbitrary and should not be followed too rigorously.

SPINAL AND PERIPHERAL NERVES

Spinal nerves are formed by the union of dorsal and ventral roots (Fig. 2–1). Each divides into a dorsal and a ventral ramus. The ventral rami that supply limbs usually first intermingle to form plexuses out of which major peripheral nerves emerge. As a result, the fibers in spinal nerves are distributed through two kinds of patterns: dermatomal (or segmental) and peripheral (p. 168).

Whatever the pattern of distribution, major peripheral nerves and some cranial nerves usually have five kinds of branches: (1) muscular (containing motor, sensory, and autonomic fibers); (2) cutaneous or mucosal (containing sensory and autonomic fibers); (3) articular (containing sensory and autonomic fibers); (4) vascular (containing sensory and autonomic fibers); (5) terminal (containing one, several, or all of the foregoing).

CRANIAL NERVES

Cranial nerves differ significantly from spinal nerves, especially in their mode of embryological development and their relation to the special senses, and also because some cranial nerves supply pharyngeal arch structures. They are attached to the brain at irregular rather than regular intervals; they are not formed of dorsal and ventral roots; some have more than one ganglion, whereas others have none; and the optic nerve is a central nervous system tract and not a true peripheral nerve. Cranial nerves also vary in the number of functional components present; some cranial nerves are composed of only one type, whereas others have several.

The number of cranial nerves in mammals is traditionally set at twelve. They are (1) *olfactory,* (2) *optic,* (3) *oculomotor,* (4) *trochlear,* (5) *trigeminal,* (6) *abducent,* (7) *facial,* (8) *vestibulo-*

cochlear, (9) *glossopharyngeal,* (10) *vagus,* (11) *accessory,* and (12) *hypoglossal.*

The origin, distribution, central connections, functions, and evolutionary significance of these nerves are complicated. Moreover, the number twelve is arbitrary because some of the nerves comprise parts that could readily be considered separately. Also, an additional nerve, the *nervus terminalis,* is present in all vertebrates so far studied, and still another, the *vomeronasal nerve,* is present in many vertebrates.

The cranial nerves of reptiles and birds are twelve in number and are similar to those of mammals. In amphibians, the hypoglossal is a part of the second cervical ventral root (the first cervical nerve being absent in the adult), and the accessory nerve is the most caudal rootlet of the vagus. In fishes, as in amphibians, the hypoglossal and accessory nerves are not present as separate nerves. Moreover, in many amphibians and in fishes a variety of lateral line nerves is present, derived from several of the caudal cranial nerves.

DEVELOPMENT

Development begins with fertilization, a process that is initiated when a spermatozoan makes contact with an oocyte and ends with the intermingling of maternal and paternal chromosomes. A series of cell divisions then follows. As the mass of cells increases, certain areas grow at different rates, so that metabolic or physiological gradients are said to exist. Moreover, the cells come to be arranged in layers. Those cells on the dorsal portion of the embryo form a layer called *ectoderm.* The more ventrally placed cells form a layer termed *endoderm,* and the cells which are diffusely distributed between ectoderm and endoderm form the *mesoderm.*

In the ectoderm, the cells in the median plane differentiate more rapidly and soon form a *neural plate.* This deepens and forms a *neural groove,* which then closes to form a *neural tube.* In spite of subsequent complex morphological changes, the brain and spinal cord remain as tubular structures. In all vertebrates, the brain and spinal cord, with the exception of blood vessels and certain neuroglial cells, are formed from the neural tube. Ectodermal cells lateral to the neural tube differentiate to form *neural crest cells.* These cells form spinal ganglia, and, therefore, dorsal roots and sensory fibers. They also contribute to cranial ganglia, and they form certain autonomic ganglia, all neurilemmal cells, the medullae of adrenal glands, a number of skeletal and muscular structures, and pigment cells of the skin. In the cranial region, additional ectodermal cells form *placodes;* these form portions of the special sense organs and contribute to some of the cranial ganglia.

The chapter on the development of the human nervous system (p. 177) illustrates how the neural tube, neural crest cells, and placodes form an adult nervous system.

SUMMARY

The basic arrangements and patterns of organization of the nervous system are similar in all vertebrates. It consists of the central nervous system (brain and spinal cord), and the peripheral nervous system (cranial, spinal, and peripheral nerves). The nervous system is composed of neurons, which are specialized for irritability and conductivity, and supporting cells (termed neuroglia in the central nervous system and neurilemma in the peripheral nervous system). The cell bodies of neurons form gray matter, and their processes white matter.

The spinal cord is a long cord of nervous tissue that is arranged into segments to which dorsal and ventral roots are attached. The cord has a similar structure throughout, its interior gray matter being arranged into columns and its white matter into funiculi. In all vertebrates, the spinal cord carries out sensory, associational, and motor functions.

The brain, which occupies the brain case or cranium, has developed as a result of encephalization, has few segmental arrangements, and exhibits diversity and specialization. It superimposes upon the spinal cord additional association mechanisms; it has major structural and functional features related to the special senses and the pharyngeal arches; it controls and integrates visceral, endocrinological, and behavioral mechanisms; and it carries out higher level functions.

In all vertebrates, the brain is composed of the forebrain (telencephalon and diencephalon), midbrain, and hindbrain (ventral metencephalon, cerebellum, and medulla oblongata).

The diencephalon, midbrain, ventral metencephalon, and medulla oblongata comprise a median stalk, the brain stem, to which all but the first cranial nerves are attached. The brain stem is concerned with the integration of motor and sensory functions; special senses; pharyngeal arch and lateral line structures; and visceral, endocrinological, and behavioral mechanisms.

The cerebellum, a fissured structure attached to the back of the brain stem, has important functions concerned with the automatic regulation of movement and posture.

The telencephalon consists of a median portion from which two laterally placed cerebral hemispheres evaginate. The hemispheres become progressively larger in the higher vertebrates, and in primates are convoluted and fissured, and enlarged to such a degree that they form most of the brain. The gray matter of the telencephalon forms masses comprising olfactory structures, limbic system, and basal ganglia. A pallial layer or cortex becomes more prominent in reptiles, but in mammals is replaced by the multilayered neocortex, which is thought to be chiefly derived from the external striatum of reptiles.

In all vertebrates, the lumen of the embryonic neural tube becomes a series of cavities filled with cerebrospinal fluid. These are two lateral ventricles, a cerebral aqueduct, a fourth ventricle, and a central canal.

The peripheral nervous system includes the cranial nerves, the spinal nerves with their dorsal and ventral roots and peripheral branches and endings, and the peripheral components of the autonomic nervous system. The constituent fibers of these nerves may be classified according to the functions they subserve.

Cranial nerves differ significantly from spinal nerves, especially in terms of embryological development, relation to special senses, topography, and functional components. Twelve cranial nerves are present in mammals, birds, and reptiles. Ten are present in amphibians and fishes, together with a variable number of lateral line nerves. None of the above enumerations takes into account the nervus terminalis and the vomeronasal nerve.

In all vertebrates, the tubular nervous system develops from ectodermal cells, some of which form a neural plate, then a groove, and then a tube; others form more laterally placed neural crest cells and placodes which also contribute to the formation of the nervous system.

NAMES IN NEUROLOGY

C. J. HERRICK (1869–1960)

C. J. Herrick's lifetime spanned comparative neurology from its origin to our current understanding of the vertebrate nervous system and its evolution. His doctoral dissertation, which analyzed the cranial nerves of bony fishes, is considered to have been the major impetus to the establishment of the "American School," which interpreted the structure of the nervous system in terms of its functions. Turning then to the nervous system of the more generalized tailed amphibians, which occupied him for decades, Herrick coupled meticulous researches with perceptive generalizations and analyses of vertebrate brains in general. He must be considered the major founder and a major developer of comparative neurology. (Bartelmez, G. W.: Charles Judson Herrick, Neurologist. Science *131*:1654–1655, 1960. O'Leary, J. L., and Bishop, G. H.: C. J. Herrick and the founding of comparative neurology. Arch. Neurol. *3*:725–731, 1960.)

REFERENCES

The following are major texts wholly or partially on comparative neurology, including evolutionary aspects. They contain the references to the classical papers in this field.

Ariëns Kappers, C. U., Huber, G. C. and Crosby, E. C.: The Comparative Anatomy of the Nervous System of Vertebrates, Including Man. Originally published in 1936. Reprinted New York, Hafner Publishing Company, Inc., 1967.

Herrick, C. J.: Neurological Foundations of Animal Behavior. New York, Henry Holt and Company, 1924. Reprinted New York, Hafner Publishing Company, Inc., 1962.

Johnston, J. B.: The Nervous System of Vertebrates. Philadelphia, P. Blakiston's Son & Co., 1906.

Papez, J. W.: Comparative Neurology. Originally published in 1929. Reprinted New York, Hafner Publishing Company, Inc., 1967.

Romer, A. S.: The Vertebrate Body. 4th ed. Philadelphia, W. B. Saunders Company, 1970.

Sarnat, H. B., and Netsky, M. G.: Evolution of the Nervous System. New York, Oxford University Press, 1974.

The following book contains brief but excellent accounts of various types of nervous systems and their evolution.

Dethièr, V. G., and Stellar, E.: Animal Behavior. 3rd ed. Englewood Cliffs, Prentice-Hall, Inc., 1970.

The following papers provide examples of the importance of experimental work in comparative neurology and point up problems inherent in studying evolution and in determining homologies.

Cohen, D. H., Duff, T. A., and Ebbesson, S. O. E.: Electrophysiological identification of a visual area in shark telencephalon. Science, *182*:492–494, 1973.

de Beer, G.: Homology, an Unsolved Problem. London, Oxford University Press, 1971.

Ebbesson, S. O. E., and Schroeder, D. M.: Connections of the nurse shark's telencephalon. Science, *173*:254–256, 1971.

Holloway, R. L., Jr.: The evolution of the primate brain: some aspects of quantitative relations. Brain Research, *7*:121–172, 1968.

Nauta, W. J. H., and Karten, H. J.: A general profile of the vertebrate brain, with sidelights on the ancestry of cerebral cortex. In F. O. Schmitt (editor): The Neurosciences. Second Study Program. New York, Rockefeller University Press, 1970.

Riss, W., Halpern, M., and Scalia, F.: The quest for clues to forebrain evolution—the study of reptiles. Brain Behav. Evol., *2*:1–50, 1969.

Chapter 3

MICROSCOPIC ANATOMY OF THE NERVOUS SYSTEM

GENERAL CHARACTERISTICS

The tissues of the body are composed of cells and intercellular material, the latter including formed elements, such as fibers, and an amorphous "ground substance" or matrix. Cells are the functional units; they vary in size, structure, and appearance according to the tissue they compose and the functions they carry out; and even within a specific tissue they may show great diversity. Nevertheless, cells have certain common characteristics. Many of these were known from classical cytological studies using the light microscope (Fig. 3–1), but our current knowledge of cellular structure and organization is based chiefly upon studies using the electron microscope.

Cells consist of *protoplasm* bounded by a membrane termed a *plasma membrane* or *plasmalemma.* This is a triple-layered structure about 75 to 100 Å (Ångström units) thick, the outer aspect of which is covered by a mucopolysaccharide layer termed the *glycocalyx.* Membranes are composed of lipids, protein (including glycoproteins), and water; their electron microscopic appearance is commonly thought to result from an arrangement into two protein layers separated by a lipid layer. The interchange of materials between a cell and its environment is regulated in large part by the surface membrane, which is also chiefly responsible for the presence of a potential difference (voltage difference) between the interior of a cell and the exterior. Cell membranes may show a variety of specializations, for example, cilia, contacts with other cells (the glycocalyx may be absent at such contacts), features associated with transport, and a variety of localized mechanisms termed *receptors* which interact with hormones, transmitters, and

25

other compounds. Finally, membranes are a feature of most intra-cellular structures.

In mammalian cells, the protoplasm consists of the *cytoplasm* and the *nucleus.* The cytoplasm is the site of most of the bio-chemical processes of the protoplasm, whereas the nucleus con-tains the genetic material in the form of nucleic acids, especially *deoxyribonucleic acid (DNA).* Under the light microscope, when basic dyes are used, DNA is evident as a substance termed *chromatin.* In the interphase period, the nucleus controls the metabolic acitivities of the cell, i.e., the information encoded in the DNA of the chromosomes is translated into specific amino acid sequences in *messenger RNA (ribonucleic acid).* This RNA leaves the nucleus and goes to specific sites or structures where the in-structions it carries then initiate and direct the synthetic activities of the cytoplasm. Nuclei usually contain one or more basophilic bodies termed *nucleoli.* These are composed chiefly of *ribosomal RNA.* Nuclei are surrounded by a membrane which exhibits pores, and which is closely associated with or is derived from the endo-plasmic reticulum.

Within the cytoplasm are a number of structures with specific functions. These *organelles* include *mitochondria, endoplasmic reticulum, ribosomes, Golgi apparatus, lysosomes, centrioles,* and *fibrils* (tubules and filaments). Additional structures, sometimes termed *inclusions,* include pigment granules, secretory granules, stored lipids and carbohydrates, and crystals.

Mitochondria are small, self-replicating structures of variable

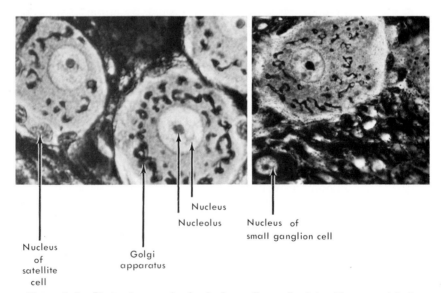

Nucleus

Nucleolus

Nucleus of small ganglion cell

Nucleus of satellite cell

Golgi apparatus

Figure 3-1. Photomicrograph of spinal ganglion cells stained by a special silver method to demonstrate a part of the Golgi apparatus. The arrow in the figure on the right points to a small ganglion cell whose cytoplasm is densely stained. Compare with other silver methods (Figs. 3-7, 3-8). Magnification about 200×.

size and shape that are bounded by double membranes. They are the principal site of the oxidative reactions by which energy is made available for the metabolic activities of cells.

The endoplasmic reticulum is a network of membrane-bound cavities, vesicles, and tubules that ramify throughout the cytoplasm. Associated with parts of the reticulum are the ribosomes, which consist chiefly of RNA, and which are the sites of protein synthesis. Reticulum with ribosomes is termed *granular (rough-surfaced) endoplasmic reticulum.* That which lacks ribosomes is termed *agranular (smooth-surfaced) endoplasmic reticulum.* Ribosomes may also occur free in the cytoplasm. The Golgi apparatus is a complex of broad, flattened cisternae with many small vesicles.

These various organelles (endoplasmic reticulum, ribosomes, and Golgi apparatus) comprise a system that is concerned with synthesis and transport. For example, secretory products in the form of enzymes are synthesized on ribosomes and transported to the Golgi complex where they are concentrated into droplets or granules. These are then incorporated into the plasmalemma in such a way that they can be discharged from the cell. Other synthesized products, such as transmitters and hormones (or their precursors), may be transported over very long distances, e.g., over axons, before being discharged. The Golgi apparatus is chiefly responsible for forming glycoproteins, including the mucopolysaccharides of the glycocalyx. It also packages hydrolytic enzymes in vesicles that become lysosomes. These enzymes, which are released by a variety of processes, including cell injury, can bring about the extracellular digestion of cells, and autolysis, that is, the intracellular hydrolysis of various compounds and structures.

Centrioles are self-replicating organelles located near the nucleus. They are involved in cell division, and are the source of the cilia.

Fibrils of various kinds are common and important cellular constituents. Composed chiefly of structural proteins, they vary in size, shape, and structural features.

NEURONS

The adult nervous system consists chiefly of two different classes of cells, neurons and neuroglia. The latter are described on p. 56. Neurons are specialized in that they exhibit to a great degree the general phenomena of membrane excitability and conductivity, as well as transmission and secretion; these features are discussed later in this chapter and also in Chapter 4. Moreover, they are characterized by processes that extend varying distances from the cell body (Fig. 3–2), and which make possible the func-

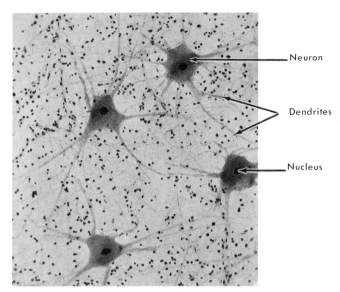

Neuron

Dendrites

Nucleus

Figure 3–2. Photomicrograph of motor neurons teased out of fresh spinal cord and stained. Note the extent of neural processes. The numerous small dots are nuclei of neuroglial cells. Magnification about 60×.

tional connections between different nerve cells or between nerve cells and receptor or effector organs (also, some neurons are ciliated). There are two types of processes, the types differing according to structure or to direction of conduction, or some combination of these. One type comprises processes known as *dendrites* which are afferent in nature and conduct impulses toward the cell body, or, in the case of most central nervous system neurons, are cytoplasmic extensions of the cell body. Other processes are efferent and conduct impulses away from the cell body. These are known as *axons,* and there is usually but one axon to a nerve cell. Some neurons (e.g., the amacrine cells of the retina, p. 254) have no axon.

Direction of conduction is imposed, not necessarily because of structural features but because the nerve impulse normally is initiated only at certain locations, and has only one direction in which to go. Moreover, the nerve impulse can be transmitted from one nerve cell to another in one direction only, the direction being determined by the structural and functional features of synapses (p. 45). The site at which impulses normally originate provides a basic classification of neurons (Fig. 3–3).

Additional classifications are in common use. For example, nerve cells vary greatly in size. The cell bodies of some neurons may have a diameter of 50 to 100 μm or more, and thus are almost visible to the naked eye. These large neurons, which have axons that extend for long distances, up to a meter or more, are often called *Golgi type 1* (Figs. 3–4, 3–5). A large number of neurons in the brain, and to some extent in the spinal cord, are quite small

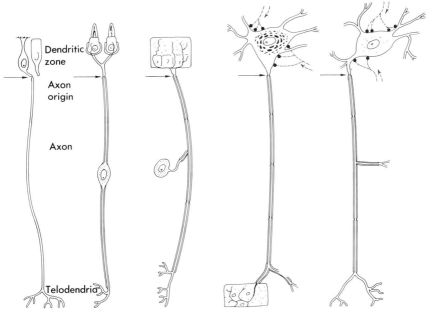

Dendritic zone

Axon origin

Axon

Telodendria

Figure 3-3. Schematic representation of generalized vertebrate neurons to show how impulse origin, rather than location of cell body, may be taken as the focal point in defining dendrites and axons. From left to right, olfactory receptor neuron, auditory receptor neuron, cutaneous receptor neuron, motor neuron, and interneuron. (Modified from Bodian, D., in Science, *137*:323–326, 1962.)

Apical dendrite

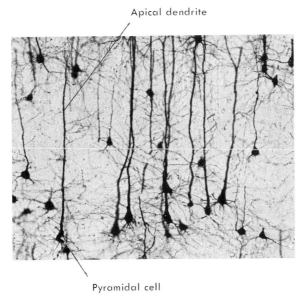

Pyramidal cell

Figure 3-4. Photomicrograph of a section of cerebral cortex (rabbit) showing neurons and their processes. Cox-Golgi stain. Magnification about 18×.

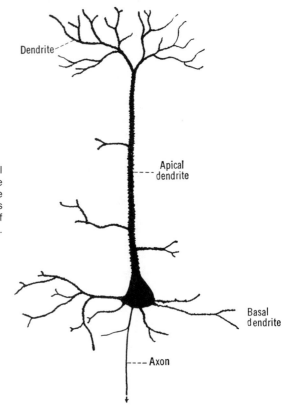

Figure 3-5. Drawing of a pyramidal cell from the rabbit cortex illustrated in Figure 3-4. This is a Golgi type 1 neuron. Note the surface irregularities of the dendrites (dendritic spines). The axon of this type of cell in man may be a meter in length. Magnification about 100×.

(4 to 5 μm in diameter), with short processes. Such *microneurons* are often called *Golgi type 2* (Fig. 3-6).

Neurons may also be classified according to the number of processes. Most nerve cells are *multipolar;* each of them has many dendrites and one axon. These cells comprise nearly all the neurons in the central nervous system and in the peripheral autonomic ganglia. By contrast, the cells in the spinal ganglia and in most of the cranial ganglia are *unipolar* (Fig. 3-7). The single process of each cell divides into two branches; one projects toward the central nervous system and the other to the periphery. The peripheral process conducts impulses from receptors (where the nerve impulse originates) toward the cell body and is therefore a dendrite. The central process conducts toward the central nervous system and is therefore an axon. Nevertheless, both processes are structurally identical to the axons described below. Certain ganglion cells are *bipolar,* that is, have two processes, one central (an axon) and one peripheral (a dendrite). Like those of unipolar cells, the processes are structurally identical. Bipolar cells comprise the spiral and vestibular ganglia (p. 269), the receptors of the olfactory epithelium (p. 281), and one of the layers of the retina (p. 250).

Neurons may also be classified as projection neurons (those

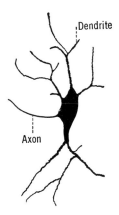

Dendrite

Axon

Figure 3-6. A spindle-shaped neuron from rabbit cortex (Fig. 3–4), about 10 μm in diameter. This is a Golgi type 2 neuron. Only the first part of the axon is shown. Magnification about 500×.

whose axons project relatively long distances), interneurons (connecting different neurons), motor neurons (their axons supplying effectors), and sensory neurons (composing the spinal and cranial ganglia).

Finally, there are biochemical classifications, which are based on the type of transmitter synthesized by a particular class of neurons.

No single technical method is adequate to demonstrate the various features of nerve cells. Figures 3–8 and 3–9 illustrate

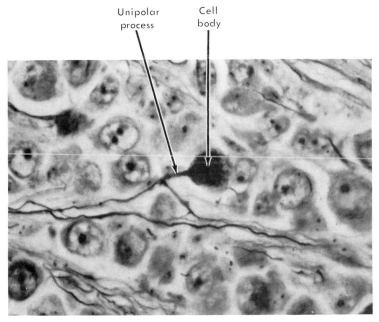

Unipolar process

Cell body

Figure 3-7. Photomicrograph of a unipolar nerve cell in a dorsal root ganglion of a three month human fetus. Silver method. The nucleus of this cell was not included in the section. Note how the single process divides a short distance from the cell body.

that several staining methods are required to demonstrate some of the major arrangements and organelles.

The space between the cell bodies of neurons and neuroglia consists almost entirely of a complex entanglement of neuronal and neuroglial processes known as *neuropil*. Hence, there is relatively little intercellular space. Nevertheless, this space is of vital importance in the transport of materials from the blood vessels of the nervous system to its constituent cells. It is also a matter of some importance that the endothelial cells of the capillaries form a *blood-brain barrier* which is relatively impermeable to many large

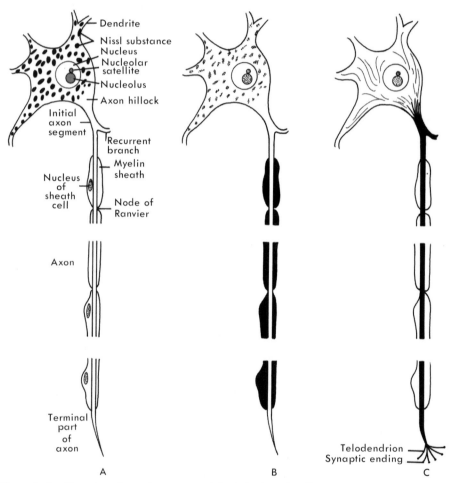

Figure 3–8. Diagrams of a motor neuron of the spinal cord to illustrate that no single staining method is sufficient to demonstrate the various neuronal features. Moreover, the total extent of a nerve cell cannot be seen in a single, thin microscopic section. A, staining with a basic aniline dye or with hematoxylin demonstrates Nissl substance, nuclei, and nucleoli; the myelinated axon is unstained. See also Figure 3–11. B, a number of methods stain the myelin sheath blue or black, leaving nuclei and Nissl substance faintly stained, if at all. See also Figure 3–9. C, a number of silver methods deposit silver grains around fibrils, so that the axon (but not the myelin sheath) appears black.

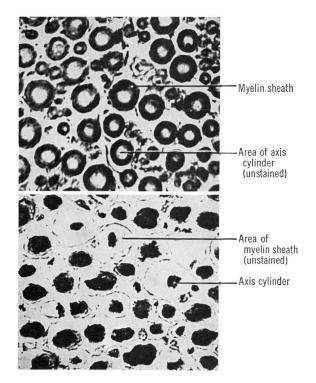

Myelin sheath

Area of axis cylinder (unstained)

Area of myelin sheath (unstained)

Axis cylinder

Figure 3–9. Photomicrographs of cross sections of dorsal roots (rabbit). The fibers in the upper half of the figure are stained by the Weigert method to show myelin sheaths. The method involves treatment with a compound such as potassium dichromate or iron alum; the myelin sheaths then stain blue or black with the dye hematoxylin. The largest fibers may reach 20 μm in diameter, including the myelin sheath. The fibers in the lower half of the figure have been stained by a silver method that demonstrates axons but not myelin sheaths.

molecules that would otherwise enter the intercellular space (p. 149).

STRUCTURE OF THE CELL BODY (SOMA)

The surface membrane and the organelles of nerve cells, although specialized, are similar to those of other cells (Fig. 3–10). The nuclei are usually prominent. In large cells, especially in motor neurons and in pyramidal cells of the cerebral cortex and Purkinje cells of the cerebellum, they are rounded and light staining. In other neurons they show great diversity in size, shape, position, and amount of chromatin. Nerve cells, once formed, can no longer divide mitotically. Hence, their nuclei are always interkinetic, and most of their chromatin is in a dispersed or extended form. Since neurons cannot divide, they cannot be a source of tumors. Primary tumors of the central nervous system, exclusive of those originating from the meninges, arise from neuroglial cells.

The nucleolus of a large neuron is usually single, and is always prominent. Smaller neurons may have more than one nucleolus. In the females of many species, the heterochromatic X chromosome forms a small, spherical mass, the *nucleolar satellite,* on the surface of the nucleolus. In primates the satellite is attached to the inner aspect of the nuclear membrane.

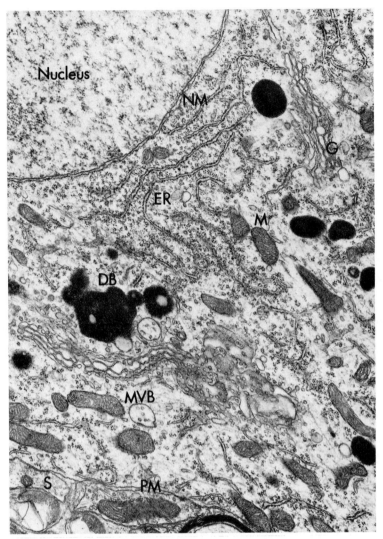

Figure 3-10. Electron photomicrograph of a portion of a neuron showing many of the structures and organelles normally present. NM, nuclear membrane; G, Golgi complex; ER, rough endoplasmic reticulum (Nissl substance); M, mitochrondrion; DB, dense body (probably a lipofuscin granule); MVB, multivesicular body; PM, plasma membrane; S, synaptic ending. Magnification 18,260×. (From Andrews, J. M., and Vernaud, R. L., in Bull. L.A. Neurol. Soc., 36:131–155, 1971. By courtesy of the authors and publisher.)

Owing to the intense synthetic activity of nerve cells, the granular endoplasmic reticulum is especially prominent, as are the Golgi complex, the smooth endoplasmic reticulum, and lysosomes. The granular endoplasmic reticulum is basophilic and stains with aniline dyes. Under the light microscope it usually appears as granules or clumps termed *Nissl substance.* This substance is large and abundant in motor neurons (Figs. 3–8, 3–11). In many other large neurons, however, and in most small ones, it is dispersed as dust-like particles or appears as small granules. Electron microscopic studies indicate that differences which have been observed in the structural features of the granular endoplasmic reticulum may be related to the production of proteins that are specific for cell types.

In large multipolar neurons, the region from which the axon arises (the *axon hillock,* Fig. 3–11) either lacks Nissl substance or it is present in small amounts. In other neurons, however, the distinction between the axon hillock and the rest of the cell body is not so apparent.

Many different classes of proteins and other compounds are synthesized by nerve cells. Some are necessary for the secretory functions of nerve cells, and include transmitters, hormones, surface membrane receptors, and enzymes, the nature and presence or absence of each depending upon the neuron and its function. The products are then transported toward adjacent plasmalemma or into the neuronal processes. In those neurons that synthesize hormones, the axons have special relationships with blood capillaries so that the hormone can be discharged into the blood stream. Many of the proteins that are synthesized are necessary for the structural integrity of the cell and its processes. It is

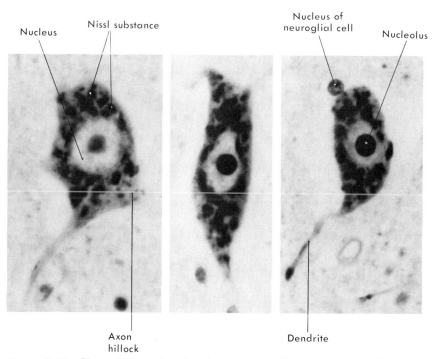

Figure 3–11. Photomicrographs of motor neurons of human spinal cord. Note the abundant Nissl substance, prominent nucleoli, and relative clearness of the nuclei. The sections do not show axons, and include the axon hillock in but one of the cells. Cresyl violet stain. Magnification about 270×.

clear, therefore, that the cell body is necessary for the maintenance of its processes.

The mitochondria of neurons are variable in size and shape. They are present in axons and dendrites as well as in cell bodies, and are numerous in synaptic endings.

The fibrils in the cytoplasm can be seen in living cells by phase microscopy, and also in histological sections studied by light microscopy after special staining methods have been used. A number of such methods have been devised; in each, solutions of a silver salt are used and the fibrils are made visible because silver grains are deposited on the proteins which form the fibrils. Electron microscopy reveals two types of fibrils, *microtubules* and *neurofilaments.* Microtubules are long tubular elements about 200–260 Å in width, whereas neurofilaments are more slender, being about 100 Å in width. Both types tend to run in parallel fashion, to occupy most of the intracellular space not occupied by organelles, and to extend into and throughout dendrites and axons.

A variety of inclusions occur in nerve cells. Some are secretory granules, or precursors of hormones. Others are pigment granules. For example, in certain areas of the brain, such as the substantia nigra (p. 139), the cells normally contain large amounts of melanin. The presence of this melanin is related to the catecholamine metabolism that occurs in these cells. Many neurons contain a yellow pigment termed lipofuscin which tends to increase in amount with age. No pathological significance has been attached to such an increase. Rather the pigment seems to result from lysosomal degradation products, and the pigment masses are also known as secondary lysosomes.

STRUCTURE OF DENDRITES

The dendrites of multipolar cells are relatively short, branched, tapering extensions of the cell body; they contain the same organelles, including both types of endoplasmic reticulum, and they lack myelin. In many neurons, the dendrites have an irregular contour, owing to the presence of thorns or spines (Fig. 3–5). The microtubules and neurofilaments usually do not enter the spines. The pattern of branching of dendrites,which is sometimes termed the dendritic tree, varies greatly according to class of neuron. The extent of branching is such as to provide an enormous increase in the surface area of neurons. The dendrites of a given class of neuron may arise from only one region of the cell body rather than from all parts.

The dendrites of unipolar and bipolar cells form sensory endings termed *receptors* in relation to, or in combination with, non-nervous tissues (p. 221). In some instances the neuron and its dendrite are so greatly modified as to lose all resemblance to a typical nerve cell. Examples are the rods and cones of the retina (p. 252) and the hair cells of the cochlea and vestibule (pp. 268 to 278).

STRUCTURE OF AXONS

An axon is a relatively long single neuronal process of smooth contour and relatively uniform diameter; it conducts impulses away from the dendritic or receptor portion of a neuron. It is sometimes termed an *axis cylinder,* but the more common synonym is *nerve fiber.* Axons conduct for considerable distances, they may be myelinated, they lack Nissl substance, and their terminal branches or *telodendria* exhibit specializations that are related either to synaptic transmission or to neurosecretion. Like the rest of the neuron, the axon has a delicate surface membrane (plasmalemma or *axolemma*) about 70 to 80 Å thick, and cytoplasm (also known as *axoplasm*) with organelles and inclusions.

The initial segment of the axon of multipolar cells is specialized in that bundles of microtubules from the cell body come together and form bands or fascicles. A layer of dense material is attached to the inner aspect of the plasmalemma, and small, membrane-bound dense bodies are present, as are a few ribosomes. These various special features usually disappear before the myelin sheath or neurilemmal cell sheath begins. Branches may arise from the initial axon segment and synaptic junctions are common along it.

From the initial segment to terminal branches, axons are relatively uniform in structure, as are the processes of unipolar and bipolar neurons. Nissl substance is absent, as are free ribosomes. However, smooth endoplasmic reticulum is present, as are mitochondria and large numbers of neurofilaments (but relatively few microtubules).

The proteins and other compounds that are necessary for the maintenance of neuronal processes and that also comprise hormones and the enzymes that synthesize transmitters are synthesized chiefly in the cell body and then migrate peripherally in the neuronal processes (some synthesis may also occur in processes). This migration, which depends upon energy derived from oxidative metabolism, is evidenced as a peripheral movement termed *axoplasmic flow.* It can be demonstrated in a variety of ways, for example, by tying a ligature around a nerve. The axons then swell as axoplasm piles up against the obstruction. The rate of migration varies according to the nature of the migrating compound. For example, there is a slow migration, about 1 to 2 mm a day, which probably represents the migration of structural proteins (or polypeptides). A fast migration at 100 mm or more a day (much faster for neurohormones) probably represents the migration of compounds such as transmitters. Moreover, there is significant evidence for migration in the reverse direction, that is, toward the cell body. For example, axoplasm piles up on both sides of a ligature. Migration toward the cell body probably represents the movement of proteins that enable the periphery to influence the metabolism of the neuron.

Cellular Sheaths–Peripheral Nervous System. All axons and dendrites in the peripheral nervous system, as well as the cell

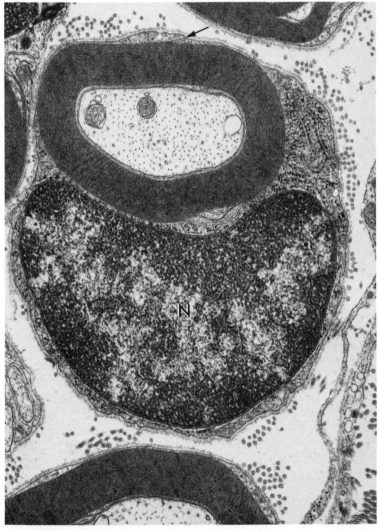

Figure 3–12A. An adult rat trigeminal nerve fiber sectioned at the level of a nucleus of a neurilemmal cell, N. The arrow indicates the external mesaxon of the myelin sheath. Note the two mitochondria and the neurofilaments and microtubules in the axoplasm. Magnification 29,300×. (From Peters, A., and Vaughn, J. E., in Davison, A. N., and Peters, A.: Myelination. Springfield, Ill., Charles C Thomas, 1970. Courtesy of the authors and publisher.)

bodies of sensory ganglion cells, are surrounded by specialized cellular sheaths. The cells that form the sheaths around axons are known as *neurilemmal cells* or *cells of Schwann.* Those that surround ganglion cells are termed *satellite cells.* Both types of cells are discussed on p. 58.

Axons that are larger than 1 or 2 μm in diameter are surrounded by spiraling cytoplasmic processes of neurilemmal cells that form a series of membrane lamellae. These layers, between which little cytoplasm remains, compose the *myelin sheath* (Figs. 3-12, 3-13). An axon and its myelin sheath are known, therefore, as a *myelinated fiber,* and the manner in which it forms is shown in Figure 3-14. Only the outermost layer of the myelin sheath (the layer with cytoplasm) can be readily identified under the light microscope as being a part of a neurilemmal cell, and it is to this

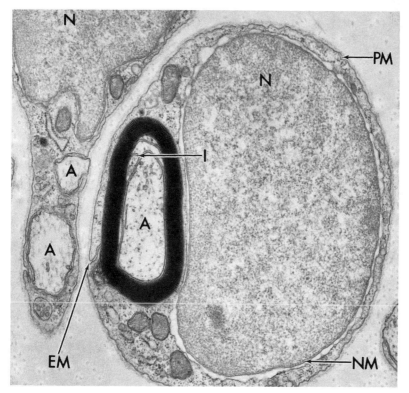

Figure 3-12B. Electron micrography of a small myelinated fiber from rat spinal ganglion cell matured in tissue culture. The infolding plasma membrane (PM) of the neurilemmal cell forms an external mesaxon (EM) continuous with the outermost lamella of the myelin sheath. An internal mesaxon (I) surrounds the axon (A) and is continuous with the most internal lamella of the myelin sheath. At the left are two nonmyelinated axons (A) associated with another neurilemmal cell. N, nucleus of neurilemmal cell; NM, nuclear membrane. Magnification 25,400×. (From Truex, R. C., and Carpenter, M. B.: Human Neuroanatomy. 6th ed. Baltimore, The Williams and Wilkins Company, 1969. Courtesy of M. B. Bunge and R. P. Bunge and the publisher.)

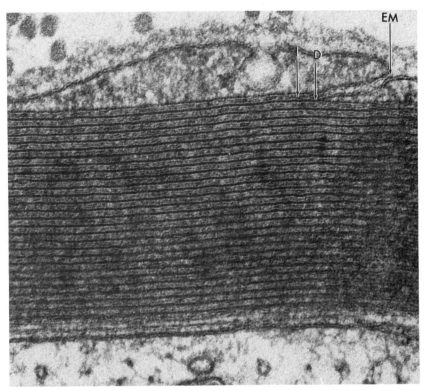

Figure 3-13. The region of the external mesaxon of Figure 3–12A. Note that the extracellular space between the two plasma membranes of the external mesaxon (EM) continues into the intraperiod line (I) in which the outer portions of the membranes are separated by the basal laminae. This separation is less pronounced in central nervous system myelin, in which the intraperiod line is more pronounced. The major dense line (D) is formed by the apposition of the inner or cytoplasmic aspects of plasma membranes. Magnification 257,500×. (From Peters, A., and Vaughn, J. E., in Davison, A. N., and Peters, A.: Myelination. Springfield, Illinois, Charles C Thomas, 1970. Courtesy of the authors and publisher.)

layer that the terms neurilemma and neurilemmal sheath have been applied (Fig. 3–15).

The myelin sheath formed by each neurilemmal cell extends for several hundred μm, and successive cells are separated by short gaps from which myelin is absent and which are known as *nodes of Ranvier* (Figs. 3–15 to 3–17). At the nodes, a layer of dense material is attached to the inner aspect of the axolemma (just as in the initial segment). As the myelin sheath approaches a node, the lamellae begin to end in a manner that is shown in Figure 3–17. Immediately external to the neurilemmal cells is a protein-muco-polysaccharide layer termed the *basal lamina,* and external to this are the delicate collagenous and reticular fibers of the endoneurium (p. 162).

The nodes of Ranvier serve to increase the speed of conduction of nerve impulses by a mechanism which is known as saltatory

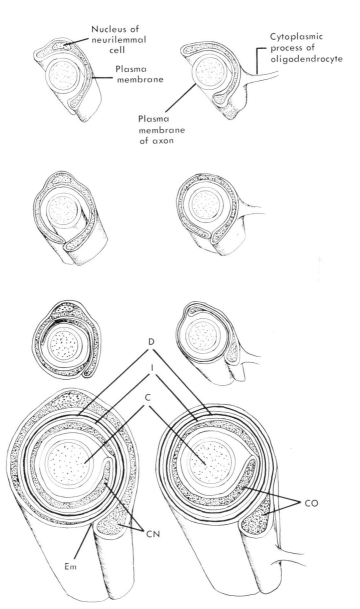

Figure 3–14. The formation of myelin.
    Left column of diagrams: peripheral nerve fiber. Note that the myelin lamellae are formed as the ensheathing cell grows spirally around the axon. Where the neurilemmal cytoplasm disappears, the inner (cytoplasmic) aspect of the plasma membrane comes into apposition and forms the dense line (D). The intraperiod line (I) is formed by the apposition of the outer aspect of the plasma membrane. Note also that neurilemmal cytoplasm persists in the innermost and outermost myelin lamellae. C, cytoplasm of axon; CN, cytoplasm of neurilemmal cell; Em, external mesaxon.
    Right column of diagrams: central nervous system fiber whose myelin sheath is formed by an oligodendrocyte (see Figure 3–17). Note the almost complete absence of cytoplasm (CO) in the final outermost lamella. In both types of fibers, the beginning and the ending of the lamellae are at the external and internal mesaxons, respectively, and that these, together with the intraperiod line, comprise a channel of extracellular space.

Node of Ranvier

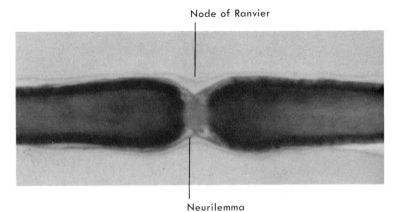

Neurilemma

Figure 3-15. Photomicrograph of a single myelinated fiber about 15 μm in diameter, from frog sciatic nerve, stained with osmium tetroxide. The myelin stains black and is interrupted at the node. The thin membrane external to the neurilemma represents a combination of basal lamina and endoneurium. The axis cylinder (stained grayish) continues through the node.

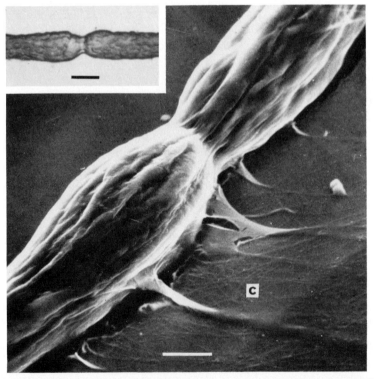

Figure 3-16. A scanning electron micrograph of a normal myelinated nerve fiber at the level of a node of Ranvier. Longitudinal paranodal flutings are prominent. C, collagen fiber. Scale = 10 μm. *Inset*: Photomicrograph of a node of Ranvier of a teased, osmicated peripheral nerve fiber (rat). Scale = 10 μm. (From Spencer, P. S., and Lieberman, A. R., in Z. Zellf., *119*:534–551, 1971. Courtesy of the authors and publisher.)

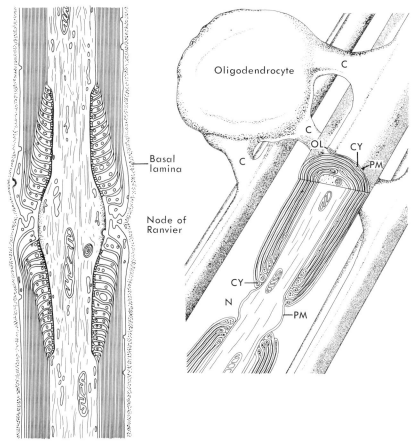

Figure 3–17. Left diagram: The nodal region of a myelinated peripheral nerve fiber. (Based on Andres, K. H., and Düring, M. v.: Handbook of Sensory Physiology. Berlin, Springer-Verlag.) *Right diagram:* Myelinated fiber of central nervous system. C, cytoplasmic processes to several fibers; CY, cytoplasm; N, node of Ranvier; OL, outer lamella; PM, plasma membrane. (Based on Bunge, M. B., Bunge, R. P., and Ris, H., in J. Biophys. Biochem. Cytol., *10*:67–94, 1961. Courtesy of the authors and publisher.)

conduction (p. 84). The speed is directly related to the total diameter of a myelinated fiber, which ranges up to 20 or more μm.

Axons that are less than 1 or 2 μm in diameter have a different relationship with neurilemmal cells. As shown in Figure 3–18, an axon indents a neurilemmal cell and is partially enclosed by its cytoplasm. Myelin is not formed and the fiber is known as a *nonmyelinated fiber.* In many instances, a single neurilemmal cell may partially enclose numbers of axons (Fig. 3–24A). The speed of conduction of nonmyelinated fibers is very much less than that of myelinated fibers.

The unipolar neurons of cranial and spinal ganglia are surrounded by satellite cells which form a layer that is continuous

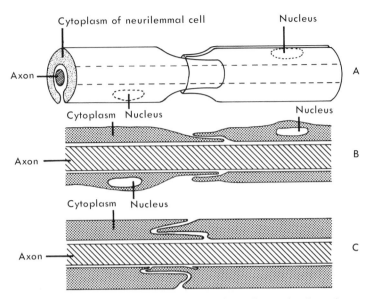

Figure 3-18. Schematic representations of neurilemmal cells and non-myelinated axons. A: A single axon is partially ensheathed by a neurilem-mal cell, which is overlapped by an adjacent neurilemmal cell. B: A schematic longitudinal section of A. C: An example of more common complex overlapping, with interdigitations of neurilemmal cells. (From Eames, R. A., and Gamble, H. J., in J. Anat., *106*:417–435, 1970. By permission of the authors and publisher.)

with that formed by neurilemmal cells. The satellite cells around bipolar neurons may form myelin.

In the peripheral nervous system, myelinated and nonmyelinated fibers are bound together by connective tissue to form nerves (Fig. 3–19). The manner in which this occurs, the arrangement of the connective tissue, and certain classifications of the fibers are described in Chapter 8.

Cellular Sheaths—Central Nervous System.   Axons in the central nervous system are structurally similar to those of the peripheral nervous system and comprise myelinated and non-myelinated types. The myelin sheaths are formed by oligodendrocytes (Fig. 3–14), and nodes of Ranvier are present. However, a single oligodendrocyte usually forms myelin around a number of axons (Fig. 3–17), and a basal lamina and endoneurium are absent.

The white matter of the central nervous system is white because it contains large numbers of myelinated fibers (unstained myelin, especially in gross slices of brain and spinal cord, is whitish in appearance). Gray matter is gray by contrast because it is composed mainly of cell bodies as well as fibers which, for the most part, lack myelin.

Axon Terminals.   The axons of multipolar cells end in relation to other neurons by means of *synapses,* or in relation to effectors by means of *neuroeffector junctions,* or in relation to blood vessels for the discharge of neurohormones. The axons (central processes) of unipolar and bipolar cells also end by forming synapses.

SYNAPSES

A synapse is a functional contact between an axon terminal and a neuronal cell body or process. Synapses are present in the central nervous system (Figs. 3–20, 3–21), and in peripheral autonomic ganglia, and are formed as follows. As the terminal part of an axon approaches another neuron, it decreases in diameter, loses its myelin (if a myelinated fiber), and divides repeatedly, forming small branches termed *telodendria.* Each branch makes contact with the surface of a dendrite *(axodendritic synapse),* the cell body *(axosomatic synapse),* or an axon *(axo-axonal synapse).* The last may be in relation to the terminal part of another axon, or to the initial segment of an axon. In each of the above types, the telodendria often form synapses by side-to-side contact during their course *(bouton de passage).* The terminal synapse, wherever it may be, is known as a *bouton terminal.* In certain regions of the brain, synapses occur between dendrites *(dendro-dendritic),* and *dendosomatic* and *somatosomatic* synapses have also been described.

The synapses outlined above present an extraordinary diversity in size, shape, and arrangement. Nevertheless, they also present certain fundamental structural and functional features (Fig. 3–22). These are related to the fact that when a nerve impulse reaches the synaptic region, a transmitter substance is released. This compound crosses the *presynaptic membrane* (which shows

Vein

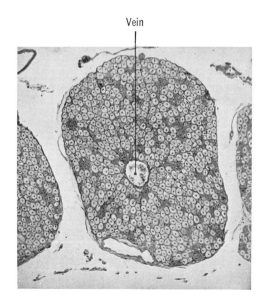

Figure 3–19. Photomicrograph of a cross section of a human ventral root. Each fiber is seen as a round, clear area, in the center of which is a dot. The clear area is myelin; the dot, an axis cylinder. The largest fibers in the root are about 20 μm in diameter.

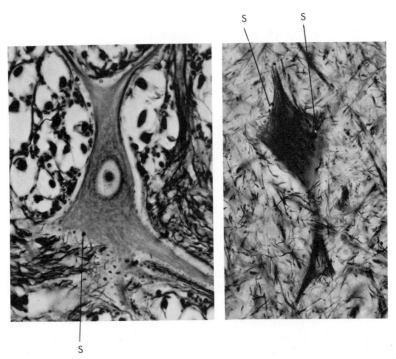

Figure 3–20. Photomicrographs of nerve cells stained with silver. That at the left is from medulla oblongata and shows synaptic endings, S, at the edge of the cell body and dendrites. The cell on the right, from spinal cord, is cut near its surface, hence the nucleus is not included. Synaptic endings, S, occur on its surface. The left-hand leader ends between two synaptic endings. Magnification about 400×.

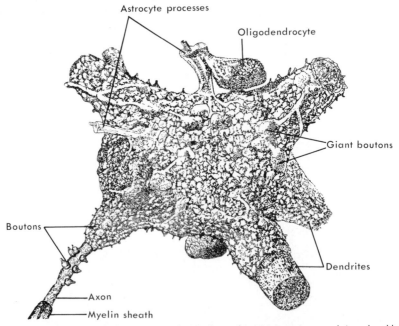

Figure 3–21. Synaptic boutons on the surface of a motor neuron as determined by reconstruction from electron micrograms. (Based on Poritsky, R., in J. Comp. Neurol., 135:423–452, 1969. By permission of author and publisher.)

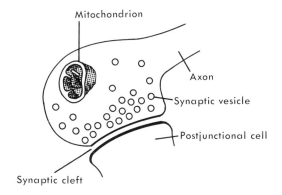

Mitochondrion

Axon

Synaptic vesicle

Postjunctional cell

Synaptic cleft

Figure 3–22. Schematic diagram of some of the key morphological features of a single synapse as demonstrated by electron microscopy. Note that the pre- and postsynaptic membranes are thickened.

a specialized thickening), the *synaptic cleft* (about 200 to 300 Å wide), and, by acting upon the specialized *postsynaptic membrane,* brings about either excitation or inhibition of the postsynaptic neuron. For a variety of reasons, particularly because the transmitter is located only on the presynaptic side, a synapse is said to be unidirectional or polarized, i.e., it can transmit in only one direction.

Synapses that depend upon a transmitter are known as *chemical synapses* or *chemically transmitting synapses.*

The presynaptic part of a synapse, that is, the terminal part of the telodendron, contains a number of structures, in particular mitochondria and synaptic vesicles (Fig. 3–23). The vesicles contain some or all of the neurotransmitter substance and vary in shape and density, according to the nature of the transmitter (e.g., whether acetylcholine or norepinephrine), and whether the transmitter is excitatory or inhibitory. Synaptic vesicles are usually about 400 to 500 Å in diameter. Those that contain norepinephrine or other catecholamines often have an electron-dense core (Fig. 3–27, p. 52). Those that contain acetylcholine are clear. Other differences in synaptic vesicles have been reported. At inhibitory synapses (e.g., on the bodies of neurons in cerebral cortex) the vesicles may be flattened or elongated, whereas those at excitatory synapses (e.g., on dendritic spines) tend to be rounded. Still other differences have been reported. For example, neurofilaments may enter synaptic endings. Because neurofilaments can be demonstrated by silver methods, these synapses are the ones which have been studied by light microscopy (Fig. 3–20). In many synapses, however (e.g., in the cerebral cortex), the neurofilaments do not continue into the synaptic ending, which therefore cannot be readily stained. Hence, the nature of cortical synapses eluded light microscopic studies. It remained for electron microscopic methods to demonstrate the abundance of synaptic endings in cerebral cortex.

The diversity and complexity of synaptic arrangements is further illustrated by the fact that neurilemmal and glial cells are closely associated with synaptic endings in a variety of ways (Fig.

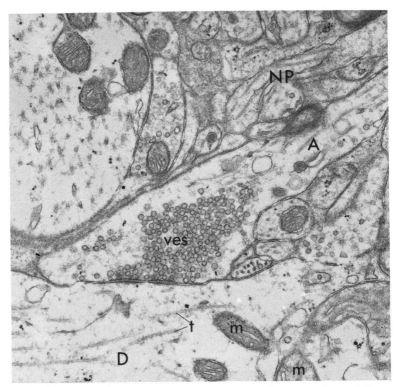

Figure 3-23. An axodendritic synapse in the oculomotor nucleus of the cat. Numerous synaptic vesicles (ves) are clustered near the presynaptic membrane, which is separated from the postsynaptic membrane by a synaptic cleft. A, axon. D, dendrite. NP, adjacent neuropil. m, mitochondrion. t, microtubules. Magnification 39,850×. (From Pappas, G. D., and Waxman, S. G., in Pappas, G. D., and Purpura, D., editors: Structure and Function of Synapses. New York, Hoeber, 1970. By courtesy of the authors and publisher.)

3-24). It is likely that they serve to insulate or isolate groups of endings.

Finally, it should be emphasized that there may be thousands of synapses on the surface of a single neuron and its processes. When one considers that there are billions of neurons, the complexity of circuitry is beyond comprehension.

In certain parts of the adult nervous system, and commonly in embryonic brains and in many invertebrate nervous systems, *electrical synapses (gap junctions)* are present. These are characterized by close apposition of the plasma membranes of the two neurons, with a median gap of about 20Å. Few, if any, synaptic vesicles are present. These gap junctions comprise a pathway of low electrical resistance. Hence, current flow from one neuron can act upon the succeeding neuron (p. 91).

Tight junctions, which seem to consist of an actual adherence by two apposed plasma membranes, also occur in the nervous system. They are usually restricted to endothelial cells, ependymal cells, and myelin sheaths.

NEUROEFFECTOR JUNCTIONS

Effectors are muscle cells and gland cells, and are the structures that carry out all aspects of the outward manifestations of
behavior. Neuroeffector junctions are functional contacts between

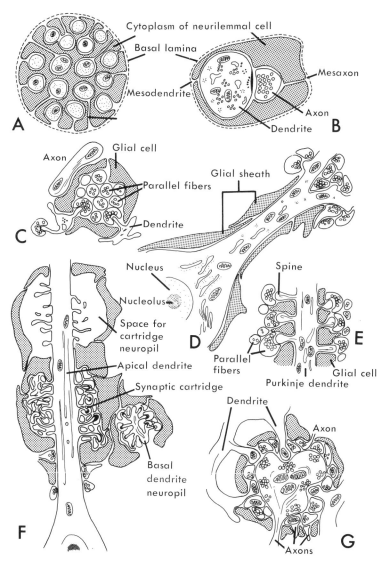

Figure 3–24. Glial, neuronal, and synaptic relationships. A, peripheral nonmyelinated fibers and neurilemmal cell. B, neurilemmal cell and synapse in sympathetic
ganglion. C, group of nonmyelinated parallel fibers in cerebellum (p. 362). D, a cell
body and dendrite with glial capsule excluding synapses. E, part of a Purkinje cell
dendrite with glial cells limiting contact to heads of spines. F, apical dendrite of
pyramidal cell of cerebral cortex with glial cells separating synapses into "synaptic
cartilages." G, glial cells and synapses arranged into a "synaptic glomerulus."
(From Szentágothai, J., in Andersen, P., and Jansen, J. K. S. editors: Excitatory
Synaptic Mechanisms. Oslo, Universitetsforlaget, 1970. By permission of the author
and publisher.)

axon terminals and effector cells. These are synapses, but the post-synaptic structure is not a nerve cell.

Skeletal (Striated) Muscle. Skeletal muscle fibers are multi-nucleated cells, whose cell membrane is known as *sarcolemma* and its cytoplasm as *sarcoplasm.* Each fiber contains myofibrils that exhibit alternating light and dark segments. Because the segments of adjacent myofibrils are aligned, the fibers appear to be cross-striated (Figs. 3–25, 3–26).

Those axons that supply skeletal muscle arise from motor neurons in the brain stem and spinal cord. They leave the central nervous system and then enter a muscle where they divide into a number of branches. Each branch approaches a muscle fiber, loses its myelin sheath, and divides into a number of telodendria which form a complex ending on the surface of the muscle fiber. This ending or junction is known as a *motor end plate* (or *myoneural junction* or *neuromuscular ending*). The end of each telodendron contains synaptic vesicles, and the postsynaptic membrane (sarcolemma) shows specialized features and relationships. The synaptic cleft is wide, about 1200 Å. The neuromuscular junction is a chemical excitatory synapse, with properties similar to those present in the central nervous system. Release of the transmitter (acetylcholine) across the synaptic cleft results in excitation of the postsynaptic membrane. Under the appropriate conditions,

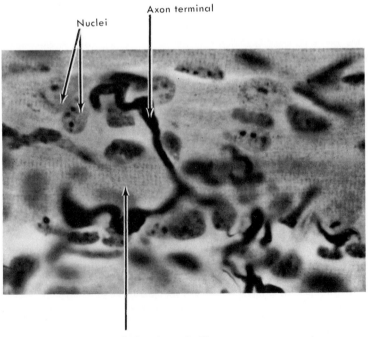

Nuclei

Axon terminal

Striated muscle fiber

Figure 3–25. Photomicrograph of motor endings in skeletal muscle of a newborn mouse. Silver method. Note the clusters of nuclei in relation to the expanded tips of the axon terminals.

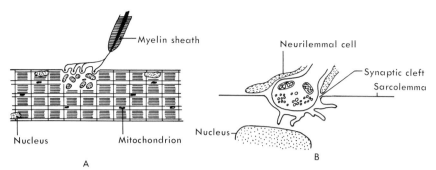

Figure 3–26. A: Schematic representation of a skeletal muscle fiber and a motor nerve ending (*alpha* type fiber, p. 20). Note the division of the single axon into multiple terminal fibers, each of which forms a synaptic ending in a sarcolemmal "gutter." B: The synaptic region in a single gutter (the one on the right in A) at higher magnification, as demonstrated by electron microscopy.

this excitation leads to a conducted impulse along the muscle fiber and a mechanical contraction of the fiber.

Further structural and functional details are considered in Chapters 4 and 10.

Cardiac (Striated) Muscle. The muscle fibers of the heart are also cross-striated, but the individual fibers are connected by specialized gap junctions known as *intercalated discs.* Special arrangements exist for the nerve supply of the heart, which is supplied by the autonomic nervous system (see Chapter 15). The right atrium contains a group of specialized muscle fibers termed the *sinu-atrial node.* At the base of the interatrial septum is another group termed the *atrioventricular node.* The muscle fibers in both nodes are specialized for conduction. They are activated by nerve impulses reaching them over autonomic fibers, and in turn, by virtue of their extensions into the walls of the heart, they activate the muscle fibers in these walls. Presumably the spread of excitation from one cardiac muscle fiber to another is across the intercalated discs, which undoubtedly have a low electrical resistance.

Smooth Muscle. The unit of smooth muscle is a small, spindle-shaped cell which contains but a single nucleus; its myofibrils lack cross-striations. Smooth muscle fibers are often arranged in bundles in which gap junctions between muscle fibers are common.

Smooth muscle is present in most organs, in the walls of blood vessels, and around hair follicles. Smooth muscle is supplied by the autonomic nervous system. The motor nerve fibers are non-myelinated, and on approaching a bundle of smooth muscle cells break up into thin filaments (0.1 to 0.2 μm in diameter) that either singly or in groups course for long distances between the muscle cells. Each filament exhibits small swellings or "varicosities" that are up to 2 μm in diameter (Fig. 3–27). The filaments are also known as "beaded" fibers. The varicosities make close contact with muscle cells, and some of these contacts comprise synapses,

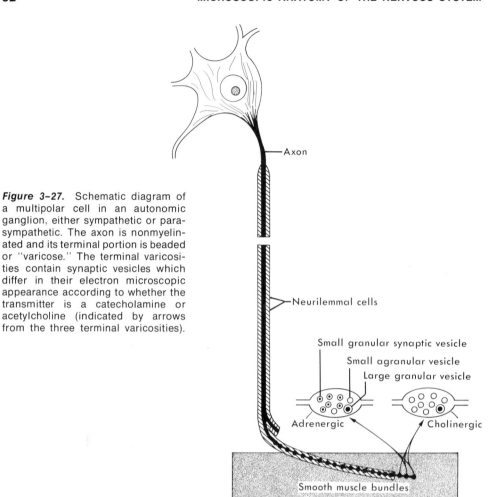

Figure 3–27. Schematic diagram of a multipolar cell in an autonomic ganglion, either sympathetic or parasympathetic. The axon is nonmyelinated and its terminal portion is beaded or "varicose." The terminal varicosities contain synaptic vesicles which differ in their electron microscopic appearance according to whether the transmitter is a catecholamine or acetylcholine (indicated by arrows from the three terminal varicosities).

with pre- and postsynaptic membranes, vesicles, and a synaptic cleft. The number of synapses and the density of innervation vary according to the structure or organ supplied. In some structures, such as the ductus deferens, each smooth muscle cell is innervated. In other organs (uterus, colon, arteries) the innervation is sparse. In such instances, the excitation from those muscle cells that are activated by chemical synapses spreads to other muscle cells across gap junctions. The details of smooth muscle innervation are considered further on p. 94 and also in Chapter 15.

Glandular Cells.   Glands may be unicellular or multicellular, and secrete substances such as enzymes, hormones, and mucus. If they discharge these substances onto a surface or into a cavity, they are termed *exocrine glands,* or glands of external secretion. Certain glands, however, discharge their secretions (hormones) into the blood stream, and are known as *endocrine glands,* or glands of internal secretion.

Many details of the nerve supply of glands remain obscure. The cells of most endocrine glands are not activated by nerve impulses but instead are stimulated or inhibited by substances reaching them by way of the blood stream. However, many exocrine glands and some endocrine cells do receive a nerve supply from the autonomic nervous system. As in the case of smooth muscle, the autonomic fibers branch and become varicose. These varicosities form junctions with gland cells that have now been described in a number of glands (e.g., salivary, lacrimal, and pancreatic islets). In some glands, such as the lacrimal, the density of innervation is high. The suprarenal medulla, the cells of which are developmentally akin to neurons (p. 190), is likewise heavily innervated by the autonomic nervous system.

Neurosecretion. Certain nerve cells, especially in the hypothalamus, synthesize hormones and other factors that act upon the endocrine system (p. 347). These compounds form granules that migrate to the axonal endings. These endings abut blood vessels and the hormones are released from the endings into the blood stream, which then carries them to the target organs. It is also possible that some hormones are first released into the cerebrospinal fluid and then transported to special vascular areas where they are absorbed into the blood.

RECEPTORS

Receptors are specialized structures that detect changes in the environment, that is, changes in energy. The change in energy initiates processes that result in the activation of a nerve fiber, with nerve impulses being transmitted to the central nervous system. These nerve impulses comprise the only information that the nervous system receives from the external world.

Receptors are arrangements of dendrites (or neurons) and non-nervous tissue, so specialized as to be particularly sensitive (but not necessarily exclusively sensitive) to one kind of stimulus (the term receptor is also applied to specialized portions of cell membranes). The stimulating energy change may be mechanical, electrical, or some part of the electromagnetic spectrum, and these energy changes form the basis for one of the many classifications of receptors. Other receptors are outlined below, and more detailed discussions of structure and function are provided in Chapters 11 and 12.

Some receptors consist almost entirely of a neuron soma with a modified dendrite (e.g., bipolar neurons of olfactory epithelium, p. 281), or may be very highly specialized cells (e.g., rods and cones of the retina, p. 252). Still other neurons are receptors in the sense of being activated by substances circulating in the blood, or by physical conditions of blood and extracellular fluid (p. 334). Most receptors, however, are formed by the dendrites of unipolar cells. Each dendrite, which, as mentioned previously, is structurally like an axon, ends in a specialized relationship with non-nervous tissue. This specialized relationship may consist of a pattern of branching within connective tissue or epithelium, the so-called free nerve endings. It may also consist of a termination within complex arrangements of connective tissue or muscle fibers. Such endings are sometimes termed encapsulated. Examples are shown in Figs. 3–28 and 3–29. In all instances, myelinated fibers lose their myelin before entering a receptor, whether free or encapsulated.

Another categorization groups receptors according to whether they deal with the general or special senses (Chapters 11 and 12). Still another classification categorizes receptors according to location, that is, whether they are located in skin (exteroceptive), in muscles and joints (proprioceptive), or in viscera (interoceptive). Finally, receptors may be defined according to the sensory perception involved, e.g., light touch, pressure, or pain.

A receptor responds to a stimulus by undergoing an electrical change which then initiates a nerve impulse or a series of nerve impulses. These impulses are "triggered off" in the terminal portion of the nerve fiber or in a portion immediately adjacent to or within the receptor (as indicated in Figure 3–3, the site of impulse origin is the basis for a general classification of vertebrate neurons). The mechanisms and characteristic features of receptor activation are discussed in Chapter 4.

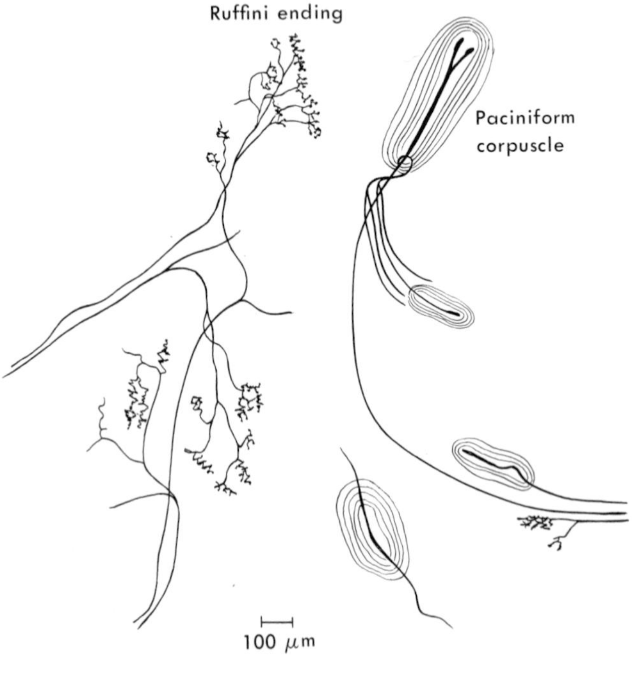

Figure 3–28. Drawings of Ruffini and paciniform endings in capsule of monkey knee joint. Methylene blue stain. Both types of endings are mechanoreceptors; the Ruffini ending is the more common. (Based on Gardner, E., in Anat. Rec., 124:293, 1956.)

Ruffini ending

Paciniform corpuscle

100 μm

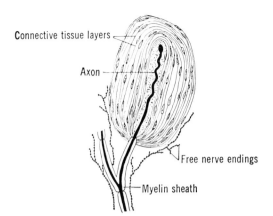

Connective tissue layers

Axon

Free nerve endings

Myelin sheath

Figure 3-29. Simplified representation of a pacinian corpuscle. Note that the connective tissue layers are separated from the axon by a central space. Note also the accessory nonmyelinated fibers forming free endings. The myelin may extend a short distance into the central space, but usually disappears. No neurilemmal cells are present in the central space; the axon is directly exposed to extracellular fluid.

DEPENDENCE OF EFFECTORS AND RECEPTORS ON NERVE SUPPLY

Skeletal muscle cannot function without a motor nerve supply. Denervated fibers lose tone and eventually atrophy (p. 216). But other effectors are not so dependent. Cardiac muscle fibers contract rhythmically in the embryo before they receive their nerve supply. In the adult they do not lose their contractility when denervated. The autonomic nervous system appears rather to coordinate or time the contractions of various parts of the heart. Smooth muscle and glands may be even more striking in their independence of nerve supply, sometimes being able to function in an almost normal manner when nerve connections are completely severed. This is particularly true of glands, since their secretory activity may be initiated by other means, as, for example, by hormones.

When afferent fibers are severed, the peripheral receptors ultimately degenerate, but the effect on associated non-nervous tissue is variable. Skeletal muscle, for instance, undergoes relatively little morphological change as long as its motor supply is intact. Denervated skin, on the other hand, is susceptible to infections and may become the site of persistent ulcers.

NEUROGLIA, EPENDYMA, AND NEURILEMMA

These are categories of non-nervous cells which form a major portion of both central and peripheral nervous systems. In fact, glial cells comprise half or more of the bulk of the brain. These various cells do not form synapses and they do not conduct impulses, but they all present the picture of metabolically active cells, with, for example, mitochondria, endoplasmic reticulum, ribosomes, and lysosomes.

NEUROGLIA

Neuroglial cells occur only in the central nervous system and in the optic nerves and retinae. They consist of two categories, the *macroglia* and the *microglia.* The macroglia in turn consist of *astrocytes* and *oligodendrocytes,* both of which arise from ectoderm (p. 180).

In contrast to neurons, neuroglial cells can divide throughout life and, together with ependymal and meningeal cells, are the source of primary tumors of the central nervous system. All neuroglial cells can respond to injury of nervous tissue by dividing and becoming phagocytes which ingest and destroy injured and dead tissue and cells.

Macroglia.   Astrocytes consist of two types, *protoplasmic* and *fibrous.* These terms are based on the nature of the processes that each type of astrocyte possesses. Astrocytes and their processes are often difficult to distinguish in sections stained by the usual histological methods and require special staining methods for their demonstration (Fig. 3–30).

On the basis of both light and electron microscopic studies,

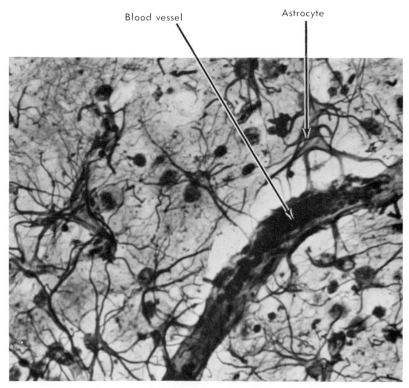

Figure 3-30.   Photomicrograph of a section of human cerebral cortex stained for astrocytes. The cortex had been involved by an infection which had caused astrocytes to increase in number. The leader to the indicated astrocyte ends on the nucleus. Note how the extensions of this cell attach to the adjacent blood vessel.

it is known that astrocytes are "star-shaped" cells that are covered by glycocalyx and which have many cytoplasmic fibrils and branching processes. Each astrocyte has at least one process that forms an expansion termed an "end-foot" which is applied either to the surface of a capillary (Fig. 3–30), or to the basal lamina just beneath the pia mater. Those processes that end on blood vessels form, together with the basal lamina of the capillary, a cellular sheath for the capillary endothelium. The processes that end in the subpial basal lamina form what is termed the glial limiting membrane. Most astrocytic processes, however, extend into the neuropil, where they form gap junctions with each other. These processes have intimate arrangements with synaptic endings (Fig. 3–24). It is now known that the space between neurons is occupied almost entirely by macroglia and their processes. Hence, the amount of extracellular space is limited.

Fibrous astrocytes are found mostly in white matter and have abundant fibrils. Protoplasmic astrocytes are present chiefly in gray matter and have fewer processes and fibrils. These astrocytes may be arranged around a neuron, like satellite cells around a sensory ganglion cell.

Special arrangements of astrocytes (or astrocyte-like cells) occur in the cerebellum (p. 361) and in the retina (p. 251), and the pituicytes of the neurohypophysis (p. 351) resemble astrocytes.

Oligodendrocytes are smaller than astrocytes. They have few if any fibrils, their processes are shorter and fewer in number, they stain more darkly, they lack a glycocalyx, and they are often difficult to distinguish from small nerve cells. Oligodendrocytes are found in white matter where they are often arranged in rows along nerve fibers (*interfascicular oligodendrocytes*). They are also present in gray matter where, together with protoplasmic astrocytes, they are often arranged around neuronal cell bodies (*perineuronal satellites*).

Oligodendrocytes are the myelin-forming cells of the central nervous system. The process of myelin formation is similar to that of the formation of peripheral nerve fibers and is shown in Figure 3–14. Oligodendrocytes do not form sheaths for non-myelinated fibers; these have no sheath comparable to that formed for non-myelinated fibers by neurilemmal cells.

Microglia. As their name indicates, microglial cells are smaller than macroglial cells. They stain more darkly with the usual histological stains, have a few very short processes, and are present in both gray and white matter. They readily divide and become phagocytes in response to injury. The general functions of microglia otherwise remain largely unknown, and the identification of these cells in normal material still poses problems. Microglia consist mostly of monocytes that leave the blood and migrate into adjacent tissues to become macrophages.

Functions of Neuroglia. It seems likely that neuroglial cells, at least the macroglia, provide structural support for neurons. In addition, as mentioned previously, all neuroglial cells can become phagocytes. Moreover, after injured and dead tissues are removed, proliferating astrocytes remain and occupy the area of injury. The astrocytic response may be pronounced enough to warrant the term glial scar.

The role of oligodendrocytes in myelin formation is a critically important process. Still other functions have been ascribed to or considered for the various macroglial cells. One of the most important is undoubtedly the separation and isolation of synaptic endings by astrocytic end-feet. This arrangement constitutes a mechanism whereby the effects of impulses arriving over one axon and its telodendria can be insulated from the effects of impulses arriving over another axon. It is also likely that the occupation of most of the interneuronal space by neuroglia provides an arrangement whereby extracellular diffusion is channeled directly toward neurons.

Among the important but unsolved problems are those related to communication between neuroglial cells and neurons. Some kind of signaling very likely exists, as evidenced by the neurilemmal and neuroglial response to injury of nerve cells and fibers, and by the subsequent roles they may play in remyelination. It is known that glial cells can respond (by changes in membrane polarization) to liberation of potassium by neurons. The specific functional roles, if any, of such responses remain unknown.

EPENDYMA

Ependymal cells, which are sometimes classified as a form of neuroglia, form a layer one-cell thick which lines the ventricles and the central canal. Each cell has a free ventricular surface that is often ciliated, lateral surfaces joined by gap junctions, and a basal aspect with a process extending toward a basal lamina. Ependymal cells are involved in the formation of cerebrospinal fluid (p. 152), especially in the choroid plexuses where the ependymal cells are highly specialized (Fig. 7–27, p. 153).

NEURILEMMA

The cell bodies and processes of neurons in the peripheral nervous system are surrounded by or enclosed in cellular sheaths, as described previously. The neurilemmal and satellite cells that form the cellular sheaths are metabolically active. Perhaps the most important functions of neurilemmal cells are the formation of myelin and the regeneration of injured nerve fibers. Other functions have been postulated, including biochemical relationships with neurons, phagocytic properties, and the formation of collagen fibers, but none of these potential functions has been satisfactorily demonstrated to exist.

DEGENERATION AND REGENERATION IN THE NERVOUS SYSTEM

Adult nerve cells cannot divide mitotically and cannot, therefore, replace any that happen to be destroyed. For unknown reasons, some nerve cells die during the normal lifetime of an individual. It has been estimated that up to a fourth of all the nerve cells in the brain, spinal cord, and peripheral ganglia may be lost by the eighth or ninth decade. This loss is a major factor in the sensory changes that are common with advancing age, e.g., diminishing sensitivity to touch and in taste and vision.

If the axon of a nerve cell is destroyed, the cell body may survive, although it usually undergoes characteristic changes. For example, if an axon of a motor cell in the spinal cord is severed, protein synthesis stops (a response in some way to the stopping of axoplasmic flow). This is evidenced microscopically by *chromatolysis,* the gradual disappearance of Nissl substance (Fig. 3–31). The cell body, nucleus, and nucleolus increase in size, and the

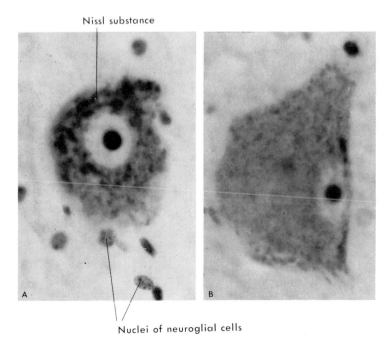

Figure 3–31. Photomicrographs of giant pyramidal cells of human cerebral cortex. The cell on the left is normal. That on the right is undergoing chromatolysis. Note the swelling, the shifting of the nucleus, and loss of Nissl substance. The magnification is the same as that of Figure 3–11 (p. 35) which allows a comparison of relative sizes.

nucleus shifts toward the periphery of the cell. After several days or weeks the cell gradually reconstitutes itself. The chromatolysis and the changes in volume probably represent redistribution of nucleoproteins and also the synthesis of new axonal material. The various changes are more noticeable in large cells with abundant Nissl substance, and their severity is related to the distance of axonal section from the cell body, being increasingly severe the closer the division.

Recovery is not invariable. Some cells die when axons are severed, and this is more likely to happen if the injury is near the cell body. Cells confined entirely to the central nervous system may not survive axonal section.

Cellular changes after axonal injury may be used to locate the cells of origin of axons in a peripheral nerve or in a pathway of the central nervous system. If a nerve or pathway is cut, and an appropriate interval allowed, the nervous system can be studied microscopically. Cells whose axons contribute to the nerve or tract which was sectioned undergo chromatolysis. Such experiments must be carefully controlled by examination of similar areas in normal material because, in certain regions of the brain and spinal cord, there are cells that normally appear as if they were undergoing chromatolysis. Furthermore, if the tissues being examined are not fixed promptly after death, postmortem disintegration causes cellular changes that may, in their early stages, resemble chromatolysis.

An axon that has been severed from its cell body undergoes irreversible changes that collectively constitute *wallerian degeneration* (Fig. 3-32). Within a short time, a few hours to a few days (the time probably depends upon the amount of protein synthesis that occurs in the axon itself), the axon begins to disintegrate. This fragmentation seems to progress in a proximodistal direction, from site of injury to terminal parts. The latter are often more resistant. If the fiber is myelinated, changes in the cytoplasm of neurilemmal cells are evident soon after injury, and are followed by disintegration of the myelin sheath. Neurilemmal cells divide and hypertrophy, and connective tissue cells proliferate and begin to phagocytize the disintegrating fibers (it is likely that many phagocytic cells migrate from the blood stream). Eventually, all remains of axis cylinder and myelin are removed and only cords of neurilemmal cells are left. Similar changes may extend for a short distance proximal to the point of axon section (*retrograde degeneration*).

Similar axonal changes are found in the central nervous system except that neuroglial cells proliferate (gliosis) and act as phagocytes. Also, if the affected neuron is located entirely within the central nervous system, the cell body may die after axonal section. The subsequent breakdown and phagocytosis extend toward the cell body from the point of section, as well as away from it, and the entire nerve cell disappears. In human beings, phagocytosis may not be completed for several months or longer.

If many nerve fibers are severed, the proliferating glial cells that replace the nerve fibers and cells form a dense glial scar.

Degenerating myelin differs chemically from normal myelin. Degenerating myelin, after chemical treatment with a compound such as potassium dichromate, will stain black with osmium tetrox-

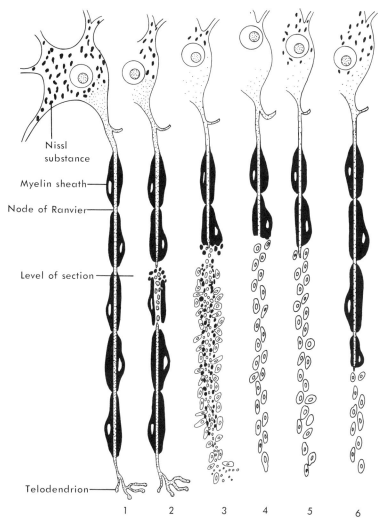

Figure 3–32. Schematic representation of degeneration of a peripheral (motor) nerve fiber after section of its axon at the level shown in the first diagram. 1: The degenerative processes are similar in the central nervous system. 2: The axon and myelin begin to disintegrate in the region of the section. 3: Nissl substance begins to disappear (chromatolysis) and the nucleus begins to shift toward the periphery of the cell. The disintegration proceeds distally, and adjacent neurilemmal and other cells proliferate and become phagocytes. 4, 5, and 6: The axon begins to grow distally through the cord of phagocytic cell, and neurilemmal cells begin to form a myelin sheath. The nucleus moves centrally, and Nissl substance begins to reappear.

The changes in the cell body are far less noticeable in small cells and in cells whose Nissl substance is more dispersed, as in unipolar cells.

ide; normal myelin will not stain in this way if similarly pretreated. This reaction forms the basis of the *Marchi method* (Fig. 11–11, p. 241) for staining degenerating myelinated fibers and enables one to trace such fibers in microscopic sections.

In the peripheral nervous system, very shortly after an axon has been severed, the axon tip begins to grow distally, through the cord of proliferating cells, by ameboid extension. There is a marked tendency for each such tip to branch or sprout, but generally one of these branches continues distally for any distance. Such distal growth does not occur unless the cell body survives and begins to reverse the chromatolytic process. The axon regenerates at the rate of a few millimeters a day, at least initially. The rate of growth later becomes considerably less. With regeneration, for those fibers that were myelinated, new myelin is formed by neurilemmal cells. Eventually, the axon establishes contact with whatever structures it previously supplied. The contact may not be normal at first, or the axon may be misdirected during its growth, and functional recovery may be delayed.

Practically speaking, the neurilemmal cords might be regarded as tubes that conduct or direct the growing axon, although the interrelationship is much more complicated.

Regeneration does not occur in the brain and spinal cord, at least to any significant degree. In very young animals, however, neuroblasts may still be present and these may enable some regeneration to occur. Abortive attempts at regeneration (axonal sprouting in the vicinity of the injury) have been observed in the adult, but without evidence of significant regrowth. Apparently the dense glial and collagenous scars that are characteristic of central nervous system injuries are major factors that prevent regeneration. Other, unknown factors are also important, related to differences between warm- and cold-blooded animals. The amazing capacity for regeneration in lower forms of life is familiar to all. Such capacity is retained to a considerable extent in fishes and amphibians, but is less evident in reptiles, and in birds and mammals is practically restricted, so far as the nervous system is concerned, to the peripheral nervous system. If recovery of function in the central nervous system does occur, it is either because the cells are not actually killed or their fibers severed, or because other cells or areas take over their functions.

Widely different agents may produce almost identical changes in nerve cells and fibers. Chromatolysis, which was discussed as a consequence of axonal injury, may follow a direct attack on nerve cells by poisons, bacterial toxins, viruses, and the like, although in such cases recovery is certainly less common. With such direct attacks, chromatolysis is more likely to be followed by cell shrinkage and disappearance. Some diseases and poisons affect only myelinated processes, either their axons or their myelin sheaths, or both, and may produce swelling, demyelination, or disintegration. Any injurious change may be initially irritative and later destructive, so that the functions of involved neurons may be at first enhanced or exaggerated, then later lost.

The degeneration of an axon usually does not involve the succeeding cell with which that axon may be functionally connected. However, if an injury to a group of axons deprives a group of nerve cells of most or all of their afferent input, these cells may die. This reaction of neurons that have not been directly damaged is known as *transneuronal degeneration*.

When a peripheral nerve is cut, hundreds or thousands of fibers are separated from their cell bodies. Function is immediately lost and degenerative changes go on almost simultaneously in each fiber of that nerve. When recovery begins, however, it proceeds at different rates for nonmyelinated (faster rate of regeneration) and myelinated fibers. Recovery is also affected by the manner in which the cut ends of the nerve are united. A close union, without scar formation, favors recovery. Scar tissue prevents proper growth and as a consequence the multiple growing tips often form a swelling or *neuroma* above the scar. Similarly, the loss of a long stretch of nerve prevents recovery unless the gap is bridged in some way.

Growth is not limited to regenerating nerve fibers. For example, when an area of skin is deprived of its nerve supply, branches of the fibers that supply adjacent normal skin may grow into the denervated area and will, of course, reach it before the severed axons can regenerate. Consequently, some return of sensory function may occur long before that calculated on the basis of rate of regeneration.

THE NEURON DOCTRINE

The extraordinary diversity of neurons and the virtual impossibility of demonstrating all of their structural features by any one method or with any one stain accounts for the fact that, decades after the cell theory was propounded, neurons were still not recognized as cellular entities. The concept of the neuron as a distinct cell rather than as a part of continuous reticulum received a major impetus when Deiters, with crude instruments, carried out microdissection of hardened brains which enabled him to isolate single cells of the lateral vestibular nucleus. During succeeding decades, the concept of the neuron received further support from the monumental efforts of Ramón y Cajal, using modifications of Golgi's staining method. It was Waldeyer in 1891 who suggested the name neuron. Subsequently, the development of powerful investigative tools led to an increased understanding of the processes and connections of neurons. Various physiological and pharmacological studies were of major importance; one of the critical advances was provided in 1907 by Harrison who showed that single nerve cells could develop and grow in tissue culture. Nevertheless, the neuron doctrine remained under severe attack. Among the conceptual problems was the inability to explain transmission from one neuron to another if protoplasmic continuity did not exist. The concept of a synapse was put forth by Sherrington; subsequent physiological and pharmacological studies coupled with the advent of more precise instrumentation have finally substantiated the concept of synaptic transmission. It must be emphasized, however, that because the neuron is a morphological unit it is not necessarily a functional unit. The latter may be quite different and may well include non-nervous cells.

SUMMARY

The tissues of the body are composed of cells and intercellular material. Cells consist of protoplasm bounded by a membrane. The protoplasm consists of the cytoplasm and the nucleus. The cytoplasm, which contains organelles such as mitochondria, endoplasmic reticulum, ribosomes, Golgi apparatus, and lysosomes, is the site of most of the biochemical processes of the protoplasm. The nucleus contains the genetic material in the form of nucleic acids.

The adult nervous system consists chiefly of two different classes of cells, neurons, and neuroglia. Neurons possess the same general arrangements and organelles as do other cells, but they are specialized for excitability, conductivity, transmission, and secretion, and they are characterized by processes of variable length. Those processes that conduct toward the cell body are dendrites; those that conduct away from it are axons. Neurons synthesize many compounds, including those necessary for the secretory functions: transmitters, hormones, surface membrane receptors, and enzymes.

Dendrites of multipolar cells are short protoplasmic extensions of the cell body. Dendrites of unipolar and bipolar cells are structurally like axons. An axon is a relatively long process that ends by connecting with another neuron, with an effector, or with a blood vessel. Axons in peripheral nerves are covered by cellular sheaths formed by neurilemmal cells; axons more than 1 or 2 μm in diameter are surrounded by a myelin sheath formed by these cells. Myelin in the central nervous system is formed by oligodendrocytes. Myelin is interrupted by gaps termed nodes of Ranvier.

Axons end in relation to other neurons by means of synapses; or end in relation to effectors (striated muscle, cardiac muscle, smooth muscle, gland cells) by means of neuro-effector junctions; or end in relation to blood vessels for the discharge of neurohormones. Synapses and neuro-effector junctions are specialized for the release of a transmitter from the axon terminal to the succeeding structure, which is then activated or inhibited.

Receptors are specialized structures that detect changes in the environment, that is, changes in energy. All receptors are arrangements of dendrites (or neurons) and non-nervous tissue, so specialized as to be particularly sensitive to one kind of stimulus. A receptor responds to a stimulus by undergoing an electrical change which then initiates nerve impulses.

Neuroglia, ependyma, and neurilemmal cells are non-nervous cells that comprise more than half the bulk of the nervous system. Neuroglia occur in the central nervous system, and consist of macroglia (astrocytes and oligodendrocytes) and microglia. The astrocytes have supporting and other functions, including phagocytosis. Oligodendrocytes are myelin-forming cells. Microglial cells are derived from the monocytes of the blood and serve a phagocytic function. Ependymal cells line the ventricles and central canal. Neurilemmal cells form sheaths for peripheral nerve fibers and are myelin-forming.

New nerve cells cannot be formed in the adult nervous system. If axons are destroyed, their cells of origin undergo chromatolysis. If the axonal injury occurs in the peripheral nervous system, regeneration is possible, seemingly because of the presence of neurilemmal cells which form cords along which the regenerating fibers grow.

NAMES IN NEUROLOGY

OTTO FRIEDRICH KARL DEITERS (1834–1863)

Deiters' great contribution was his demonstration by microdissection of a neuron and its processes. The lateral vestibular nucleus from which he isolated single cells is known as Deiters' nucleus. He died at an early age in Bonn and his outstanding book on the microscopic appearance of nervous tissue was published in 1865 after his death. (Based in part on van der Loos, H.: The History of the Neuron in Hydén, H., editor: The Neuron. Amsterdam, Elsevier, 1967.)

CAMILLO GOLGI (1843–1926)

Golgi was an Italian anatomist who received his medical degree at Pavia and spent all of his active life there as professor of histology. The silver staining method that he devised and first published in 1873 remains a very valuable method for the study of neurons and their relationships. Nevertheless, following the publication in 1883 of his classic paper on the histology of the central nervous system, he became the foremost opponent of the neuron theory by his advocacy of the existence of an axonal net. Golgi was awarded the Nobel Prize in Physiology and Medicine in 1906, which he shared with S. Ramón y Cajal of Madrid. His research was not confined to neuroanatomy. He made important studies in malaria, especially the relation of fever to the development of parasites within the blood.

ROSS GRANVILLE HARRISON (1870–1959)

Harrison is known as the founder of tissue culture and for his demonstration that nerve cells could be grown and maintained in tissue culture. This was a decisive confirmation of the neuron doctrine. He received a Ph.D. from Johns Hopkins University and a medical degree from Bonn. He published his classic paper on the living developing nerve fiber in tissue culture in 1907 while in the anatomy department of Johns Hopkins, and then went to Yale where he spent the rest of his academic life as professor of comparative anatomy. (Harrison, R. G.: Organization and Development of the Embryo. Sally Wilens, editor, New Haven, Yale University Press, 1969.)

VITTORIO MARCHI (1851–1908)

Marchi was an Italian physician who contributed to the establishment of the neuron theory by developing a method for staining degenerating fibers and applying it to experimentally produced lesions.

FRANZ NISSL (1860–1919)

Nissl was a German neuropathologist and psychiatrist who graduated in medicine at Munich and then spent many years at Heidelberg where he developed his method of staining with basic aniline dyes. He discovered what is now termed Nissl substance in nerve cells and also demonstrated the changes that occur in it after axonal injury. Nissl was also active in other fields and reported, for example, on the pathological lesions of the nervous system resulting from syphilis.

SANTIAGO RAMÓN Y CAJAL (1852–1934)

Ramón y Cajal was the greatest of all neuroanatomists. He did so much that is fundamental to present-day knowledge that it is difficult to list his accomplishments. He graduated in medicine from the University of Zaragoza and later worked at Valencia, but it was in Barcelona and Madrid that his major studies of the nervous system were carried out. When he was professor of anatomy at the University of Valencia, he learned of Golgi's method for staining nerve tissue. The method, however, was capricious and undependable. He then conceived the use of embryos in which myelin sheaths are not fully developed and, therefore, less liable to interfere with the impregnation of processes by silver. Using Golgi's method and modifications of it, he was able to demonstrate the morphological independence of neurons. He showed nerve cells in their entirety, their relationships to other neurons, and the presence of synaptic junctions. With this method, and with others which he subsequently developed, he studied almost every portion of the nervous system. He described the fundamental structures of cerebral cortex, cerebellum, retina, spinal cord, and peripheral nerves. His account of degeneration and regeneration is a masterpiece. He demonstrated neuroglial cells in all their detail. In 1906 he shared the Nobel Prize for the Section of Physiology and Medicine with Camillo Golgi.

LOUIS-ANTOINE RANVIER (1835–1922)

Ranvier was a French histologist, best known for his description of the interruptions of myelin sheaths, which now bear his name. He graduated in medicine in Lyon, then became an assistant to Claude Bernard, and in 1875 became professor of histology of the Collège de France in Paris. His first account of nodes appeared in 1871. He also described in detail the perineurium of peripheral nerves.

THEODOR SCHWANN (1810–1882)

Schwann, a German physician, entered the University of Bonn in 1829, then studied at Berlin where he received his M.D. and worked on the physiology of muscle and on the problem of fermentation. In 1839, when he left Berlin for Louvain, he enunciated the cell theory. Later he discussed varicosities of nerve fibers and then described the neurilemmal cells and sheaths which are now named after him. In 1848 he moved to the University of Liège where he chaired Anatomy until his retirement in 1880. (Causey, G.: The Cell of Schwann. Edinburgh, E. and S. Livingstone, Ltd., 1960.)

C. S. SHERRINGTON (1857–1952)

Sherrington, who coined the term synapse, is discussed on p. 125.

HEINRICH WILHELM GOTTFRIED VON WALDEYER (1836–1921)

Waldeyer was a German anatomist who studied at Göttingen and Berlin. In 1891 he published a paper in which he summarized a mass of published data on the morphology of nerve cells and their processes. He concluded that the evidence favored the existence of independent nerve cells to which he applied the term neuron. This fundamental concept then became known as the neuron doctrine. Waldeyer also created the terms "chromosome" and "plasma cell."

AUGUSTUS VOLNEY WALLER (1816–1870)

Waller, an English physician, received his M.D. degree from the University of Paris in 1840. While practicing medicine in London, he traced the degeneration that resulted from the section of various cranial nerves. He established the direction of the degeneration and its limitation to the neuronal processes directly involved. His work formed the basis for important methods of tracing nerve fibers in the nervous system and also helped to establish the neuron theory. Waller later moved to Bonn where he carried out important studies of the autonomic nervous system.

CARL WEIGERT (1845–1904)

Weigert was a German pathologist who contributed immensely to our knowledge of the nervous system by his development of various staining methods. The one applied to myelin sheaths, somewhat modified today, is still one of the most important single stains for nervous tissue. He also stained neuroglia. He was the first to stain bacteria, and he studied the pathological anatomy of smallpox and of Bright's disease.

REFERENCES

The neuroanatomy textbooks cited on p. 159 discuss the microscopic anatomy of the nervous system. The following references contain similar discussions, as well as illustrations of ultrastructure.

Babel, J., Bischoff, A., and Spoendlin, H.: Ultrastructure of the Peripheral Nervous System and Sense Organs. St. Louis, C. V. Mosby, and Stuttgart, Georg Thieme Verlag, 1970.

Bloom, W., and Fawcett, D. W.: A Textbook of Histology. 10th ed. Philadelphia, W. B. Saunders
    Company, 1975.
Burnstock, G.: Structure of smooth muscle and its innervation. Pp. 1–69, in Bülbring, E.,
    Brading, A. F., Jones, A. W., and Tomita, T. (editors): Smooth Muscle. Baltimore, The
    Williams and Wilkins Company, 1970.
Fawcett, D. W.: An Atlas of Fine Structure. The Cell. Philadelphia, W. B. Saunders Company,
    1966.
Ham, A. W.: Histology. 7th ed. Philadelphia, J. B. Lippincott Co., 1974.
Pappas, G. D., and Purpura, D. (editors): Structure and Function of Synapses. New York,
    Raven Press, 1972.
Peters, A., Palay, S. L., and Webster, H. de F.: The Fine Structure of the Nervous System.
    New York, Hoeber, 1970.

The following references deal with neuroglia; see also those cited immediately above.

Bunge, R. P.: Glial cells and the central myelin sheath. Physiol. Rev., *48*:197–251, 1968.
Causy, G.: The Cell of Schwann. Edinburgh, E. & S. Livingston, Ltd., 1960.
Glees, P.: Neuroglia. Oxford, Blackwell, 1955.
Kuffler, S. W., and Nicholls, J. G.: The physiology of neuroglial cells. Ergebn. Physiol. Biol.
    Chem. u. Exper. Pharm., *57*:1–90, 1966.
Watson, W. E.: Physiology of neuroglia. Physiol. Rev., *54*:245–271, 1974.

The following references deal with experimental aspects of degeneration and regeneration.

Guth, L.: Regeneration in the mammalian peripheral nervous system. Physiol. Rev., *36*:441–
    478, 1956.
Guth, L., and Windle, W. F.: The enigma of central nervous regeneration. Exper. Neurol.,
    28:Suppl. 5, 1–43, 1970.
Joseph, B. S.: Somatofugal events in wallerian degeneration: a conceptual overview. Brain
    Research, *59*:1–18, 1973.

The two following references are excellent reviews and discussions of the neuron doctrine. See also Peters *et al.,* cited above.

Shepherd, G. M.: The neuron doctrine: a revision of functional concepts. Yale J. Biol. Med.,
    45:584–599, 1972.
van der Loos, H.: The History of the Neuron, in Hydén, H. (editor): The Neuron. Amsterdam,
    Elsevier, 1967.

CHAPTER 4

EXCITATION, CONDUCTION, AND TRANSMISSION

A fundamental property of cells is excitability, the ability to respond or react to a stimulus, that is, to the application of some kind of energy change. The cellular responses are often quite specific. For example, a gland cell may secrete (or a secreting cell may stop secreting); a muscle cell may contract; a nerve cell may conduct an impulse, or may be prevented from conducting. Most cellular reactions involve oxidative metabolism and are accompanied by the utilization of oxygen and substrates for the provision of energy, the formation of carbon dioxide, and the production of heat.

Many cellular responses to stimuli comprise reactions confined to surface membranes, and often to specialized parts of these membranes. Moreover they are characterized by certain ionic fluxes and electrical charges. These responses are especially prominent in nerve and muscle cells, whose cell membranes are excited (or can be excited) by a variety of stimuli, including artificially applied electrical currents. An additional important feature of membrane reactions is that a response to a locally applied stimulus may spread throughout the entire cell membrane. The nature and manner of the spread and its transmission to other cells make up a part of a field of major biological importance, namely the structure and function of membranes.

The study of cellular activity requires methods and instruments that encompass nearly the entire field of biological research. For example, in studying nerve functions, one may use the end result, such as muscular contraction or glandular secretion. Intrinsic metabolic processes and ion fluxes of nerve and muscle may be analyzed by a variety of physicochemical, biochemical, and pharmacological procedures. Electrical changes may be detected by methods using special electrodes, amplifiers, and recording

instruments (such as a galvanometer, ink writer, cathode-ray os-
cilloscope, or loud speaker). Electrical changes may be initiated
under controlled conditions by using those natural and artificial
stimuli that are easily regulated.

Properties and Functions of Membranes. Membranes are
metabolically active, light, oily layers that are composed of proteins, lipids, and small amounts of carbohydrates. When viewed
under the electron microscope, membranes seem to exhibit regular, almost uniform structural features. On the basis of morphological and other studies, e.g., x-ray diffraction, it has been postulated that membranes consist of a bimolecular lipid layer, with a
layer of protein on its inner and outer aspects. Much of the lipid is
phospholipid (in internal membranes, almost exclusively so). The
phospholipid molecules are polar in structure, each having a head
and two tails. The heads are soluble in water, and the tails relatively insoluble. The arrangement of the lipid molecules reflects
these solubility properties; the heads form the inner and outer
aspects of the membrane where they are adjacent to watery solutions, and the tails meet and form the interior of the membrane.
This lipid bilayer is also the anchorage for the membrane proteins,
some of which lie at or near either surface, whereas others penetrate the membrane and may bridge it completely. These proteins
have various functions. Some provide a structural framework for
the membrane, others act as enzymes, and still others function in
active transport.

It must be emphasized that while membranes may appear
(morphologically) to be stable structures, they are labile and
dynamic, and many of their components have a relatively rapid
turnover. Membranes show specificity as regards structural and
function features according to where they are located, and also
with regard to their protein composition and specific receptor
sites. Finally, ionic fluxes and concentrations and differences in
electrical charges are critically important features. The following
simplified account of excitability characteristics focuses on nerve
cells, but applies also to muscle cells, and in many respects to all
living cells.

The membrane of a "resting" nerve cell is impermeable to the
organic cations (A$^-$) that are produced within the cell and remain
there. It is freely permeable to chloride ions (Cl$^-$), is relatively
permeable to potassium ions (K$^+$), and is much less permeable to
sodium ions (Na$^+$). Hence, a resting nerve cell maintains a high internal concentration of K$^+$ and of A$^-$, and a relatively low internal
concentration of Na$^+$. On the other hand, the extracellular concentrations of Na$^+$ and Cl$^-$ are much higher, and that of K$^+$ is relatively
low. There are also differences in electric charges on either side
of the cell membrane such that the cell is said to be polarized, with
the interior of the cell being negative with respect to the exterior;
the magnitude of this potential difference varies according to the
cell. The interior of nerve cell bodies is about 70 millivolts negative,

that of axons about −80 to −90 mV. This potential difference across cell membranes is termed the *steady* or *resting potential.* It is readily detected in larger neurons or nerve fibers if the tip of an appropriate microelectrode is placed through the membrane into the cytoplasm. This electrode and its partner, which is placed external to the membrane, are connected to an amplifier and thence to a recording instrument (Fig. 4–1).

The differences in ionic concentrations and in electrical charges can be accounted for only in small part by simple diffusion of ions through the cell membrane. One must take into account the balance between the ionic movement from high to low concentration, and the movement due to the attraction between positive and negative charges. K^+, for example, tends to move out of the cell to the extracellular lower concentration, but into the cell toward negative charges (A^-). When the movement of an ion in one direction is equal to the movement in the opposite direction, equilibrium exists. The difference in electric charge across the membrane at equilibrium is termed the *equilibrium potential* of that ion.

The Bernstein membrane theory was a classical hypothesis which treated the resting potential as a *membrane potential* resulting from the equilibrium potentials. One of the assumptions of this early theory was selective ionic permeability, with the membrane being impermeable to sodium. However, several features

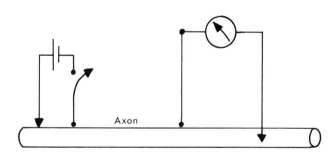

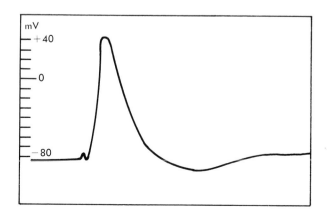

Figure 4–1. Schematic representation of a single nerve fiber and the action potential that can be recorded from it. In the upper figure, the axon is represented as a hollow tube. At the left, two stimulating electrodes connected to a current source are shown touching the fiber. At the right, two recording electrodes are shown (the symbol for the galvanometer represents a direct current amplifier and recording instrument). Where one of the electrodes (a microelectrode with a tip less than 1 μm in diameter) pierces the membrane, a potential difference is recorded, the interior being about −80 mV. When the switch is closed (not shown) and a brief above-threshold pulse of current delivered, the membrane potential is reversed and the exterior becomes about +40 mV, for a total swing of about 120 mV. This is the beginning of the all-or-nothing response. The small deflection immediately preceding the action potential is the "shock artifact" produced by a leakage of stimulating current down the fiber. Note also the positive after-potential.

cannot be explained by the membrane theory as first postulated and which viewed the nerve impulse as a depolarization in which the membrane potential is abolished. Figure 4–1 shows that the nerve impulse actually comprises a reversal of membrane potential, the interior becoming momentarily positive to the exterior (see later discussion). Also, by means of elegant experiments using radioactive tracers and other techniques, it has been shown that sodium does enter the interior of the resting cell to a certain extent but is "pumped out," and that potassium leaks to the outside but is "pumped in." It is noteworthy that sodium is pumped out both against a higher concentration and against a positive (repelling) charge, whereas potassium is pumped in against a higher concentration, but toward an attracting (negative) charge. The Bernstein membrane theory thus has been modified to take into account the various ionic permeabilities. Moreover, it is generally held that there exists what is known as the *sodium-potassium pump* (sometimes as the *sodium pump*), as outlined above. This pump, which helps to maintain the membrane potential and the ionic concentration differences, requires the expenditure of energy derived from the high energy phosphate of adenosine triphosphate (ATP). It also requires the enzyme complex, ATPase, which is located in the membrane.

The precise nature of ionic movement through membranes, whether through pores of various sizes in the membrane, or by coupling with membrane proteins, is still unknown. Moreover, some investigators believe that the membrane potential cannot be explained by the mechanisms outlined above, and that the concentration differences between potassium and sodium can be explained on bases other than the sodium-potassium pump. It is clear that membrane structure and function and active transport are critically important biological problems, many features of which remain to be explained.

EXCITATION

The initiation and conduction of impulses in excitable tissues have been studied mostly in peripheral nerve fibers artificially activated by electrical stimulation (see later discussion). These fibers have characteristic properties that can also be demonstrated by natural stimulation. Among these properties are: electrical excitability, an *all-or-nothing response* to an above-threshold stimulus, non-decremental conduction of impulses; and absolute refractoriness to stimulation during the all-or-nothing response.

The all-or-nothing response (often termed all-or-none) refers to the reversal of membrane potential that is triggered by an appropriate stimulus. It is a potential change that reaches a constant, maximal amplitude that is independent of continued or increased stimulus intensity (just as the powder charge of a bullet determines velocity and force; pulling harder on the trigger after the gun is fired cannot affect a bullet on its way). Unlike the bullet, however, the nerve impulse propagates along the fiber undiminished in magnitude, at a speed which is directly related to fiber diameter (the larger the fiber, the greater the magnitude of change and the faster the speed of conduction). Because this response is all-or-nothing, activity in nerves and tracts is digital in nature. Nerve impulses are either "on" or "off," and vary only in their frequency. Hence, they can be readily measured and counted, and computers are now widely used in such measurements.

It must be emphasized that the all-or-nothing response is a special case of the general property of excitability; it makes possible the conduction of impulses over long distances. The most common reactions of excitable tissues, however, are graded or continuous responses. These vary in intensity or duration with variation in stimulus strength or duration, and the energy output is therefore a function of the energy applied. The graded response spreads decrementally rather than in an all-or-nothing, constant amplitude fashion. It is therefore not digital, and it is more difficult to detect, measure, count, and record.

Graded responses occur especially in the receptive parts of neurons, that is, in nerve cell bodies and dendrites, and in peripheral receptors. They also occur in nerve fibers when stimuli are below the threshold of the all-or-nothing response. Finally, it is graded responses of an excitatory nature that, under normal conditions, "trigger" all-or-nothing responses at transition regions (initial axon segment, nerve fiber terminals in receptors, and synaptic junctions).

CELL BODY AND DENDRITES

When a nerve impulse arrives at an excitatory synaptic junction on the cell body, it initiates a series of events whose electrical changes are shown in Figure 4–2. At the same time the permeability of the membrane to sodium is increased. As the inward flux of sodium increases, the potential difference across the membrane decreases; the membrane is said to undergo a partial or local *depolarization.* This depolarization can be recorded as a potential change termed the *excitatory postsynaptic potential (EPSP)* (an inhibitory synaptic junction can bring about a hyperpolarization known as an *inhibitory postsynaptic potential, IPSP*).

The inward flux of sodium comprises a current flowing through what is termed a *sink* (p. 87). In order to complete the circuit the current must flow outward through adjacent parts of the membrane and return to the sink through extracellular fluid. Where current flows out constitutes a *source*; it also constitutes a stimulus to local depolarization, that is, to a local increase in permeability to sodium. Because the current spreads from the

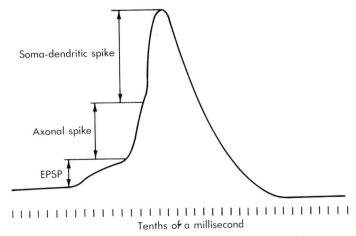

Figure 4–2. Schematic representation of the potential changes recorded when a large nerve cell is activated by an above-threshold excitatory postsynaptic potential resulting from synaptic activity. The rising slope is characterized by three deflections: (1) EPSP, (2) axon spike originating in the initial segment at the axon hillock, and (3) soma-dendritic spike. That the second deflection is an axon spike can be demonstrated by artificially blocking the soma membrane so that it cannot conduct; the axon spike still persists. Moreover, if the conducting part of the axon is stimulated, the impulse traveling centrally (antidromic conduction) invades the initial segment and then the soma and dendrites, producing similar deflections with similar time relationships. Hence, it is generally belived that under normal conditions, the EPSP triggers the axon spike, which is then conducted orthodromically along the axon. (Based on Katz, B.: Nerve, Muscle, and Synapse. New York, McGraw-Hill, Inc., 1966.)

sink in all directions, and the density of flow decreases as the distance from the sink increases, the magnitude of depolarization and, therefore, the amplitude of any recorded change in potential difference decrease with the distance from the sink. The depolarization is said to conduct decrementally, that is, it is a graded response. It should be noted that the responses outlined above can also be obtained if artificial stimuli are used, for example, if a microelectrode is thrust into the interior of the cell and an electric pulse applied (see nerve fiber stimulation, p. 78).

If several adjacent excitatory synapses are simultaneously active, or if several nerve impulses arrive in succession at one synapse, or if the strength of the artificial stimulus is increased, the EPSPs may summate. The inward sodium flux, the depolarization, and the area of outward current flow increase. If the depolarization, no matter how produced, reaches a certain level termed *threshold,* the membrane is so altered that there is a sudden, large increase in permeability to sodium. This regenerative sodium entry is of such a magnitude that the membrane potential is reversed, with the interior becoming positive to the exterior (the total swing is from about −70 mV to about +30 mV, for a total 100 mV change).

The term regenerative is used because the sodium influx now comprises a self-amplifying mechanism; it is independent of the stimulus. The outward flow of current adjacent to the depolarized area is so great that threshold is reached, the membrane potential is reversed, and still more membrane becomes involved in increased current flow. Thus, the membrane reversal spreads throughout the soma as an all-or-nothing response. As it spreads, it reaches the initial axon segment. However, as Figure 4–2 shows, the threshold for the all-or-nothing response of the axon is lower than that for the soma. Hence, if the active synaptic endings are sufficiently close to the axon, the response of the latter will be triggered before the soma is activated. Once the axon is activated, the impulse is conducted distally to the axon terminals. The characteristics of this process are discussed later (p. 77). The all-or-nothing impulse in the soma is conducted outward along the dendrites, although it is uncertain whether the total extent of a dendrite is involved.

When a nerve impulse arrives at an excitatory synapse on a dendrite, the latter is the site of a local change, just as the cell body is. However, the graded responses of dendrites differ in ways that are not yet well understood. Terminally, dendrites are very thin and have a much higher resistance than does the soma. Hence, they are subject to relatively large potential changes (however, they have a high excitatory threshold). There is evidence that the dendritic depolarization may persist for relatively long periods of time, and that the current flow from this maintained dendritic depolarization may serve as a constant stimulus to the cell body and be a factor in repetitive activity in the nervous system. The apical dendrites of cortical neurons have been most extensively studied with regard to these phenomena. It is also of interest that dendrites of some large neurons in some species have been shown to conduct impulses non-decrementally toward the soma under certain conditions. The functional significance of this property is not yet clear.

Unipolar and Bipolar Cells.   The processes of these cells are structurally like axons, but they lack the characteristic initial axon segment. The role of the cell bodies in the conduction of impulses is not well understood, and there is some evidence that the cells may conduct antidromically under certain conditions.

RECEPTORS

Receptors may be regarded as transducers that change energy applied into an electrical response (this definition does not include membrane receptors). This response is a graded one, and receptors are comparable to neuron soma and dendrites in that the graded response is involved in the initiation of all-or-nothing conducted impulses in the nerve fiber that leads away from the receptor.

As indicated previously (p. 53), and as discussed further in Chapters 11 and 12, receptors are classified in a variety of ways, e.g., according to structure, location, nature of exciting stimulus, and connections in the central nervous system. The energy changes that comprise natural stimuli include visible light, changes in temperature, chemical reactions, mechanical distortion, and direct damage. The range is even more remarkable when considered from the comparative standpoint, which reveals receptors specialized in detecting electrical and magnetic fields, and infrared waves.

In spite of the diversity indicated above, receptors share certain response characteristics. When a receptor is stimulated, a local, graded electrical change results that is termed a *receptor potential* or *generator potential.* Just how this is brought about depends upon the nature of the stimulus and the class of receptor. Moreover, its production, i.e., the precise nature of the transducer process, is by no means completely understood. The magnitude of the potential can vary with the strength of the stimulus, and the changes resulting from two or more closely applied stimuli can summate. If the magnitude reaches threshold, the current flow through the nerve terminals of the receptor will be great enough to trigger an all-or-nothing response in the parent nerve fiber, just as occurs at the initial axon segment. Characteristically, the threshold of a given receptor varies randomly with time. Moreover, there is a slight, variable delay between the stimulus application and the initiation of the spike.

For any given receptor, the amplitude of the all-or-nothing response and the rate of its conduction toward the brain or spinal cord are generally the same. The only change that can result from increasing the stimulus strength is an increase in the frequency of impulses. A stimulus just above threshold may initiate only one or but a few impulses. Stronger stimuli give a higher frequency of impulses. Hence, all the information that the brain receives from external receptors consists of "voltage blips" that vary only in frequency and total number.

If a receptor is stimulated repetitively, it may become fatigued, as evidenced by an increase in threshold. If, however, a stimulus is applied to a receptor and maintained at a constant strength, a burst of impulses occurs initially; then the frequency of discharge becomes less and less and either stops or is maintained at a low rate. This phenomenon is known as *adaptation*; it differs according to class of receptor (Figure 4–3). It is not a matter of fatigue, because if the stimulus is even momentarily stopped and then started, impulse discharge usually starts again (exceptions occur, especially in the retina where cells may fire when the stimulus stops). Most people are familiar with adaptation. For example, when one lies in bed with an arm or leg maintained in one position without moving, within a short time one is no longer conscious of the position of that part of the body. Adaptation has occurred and the

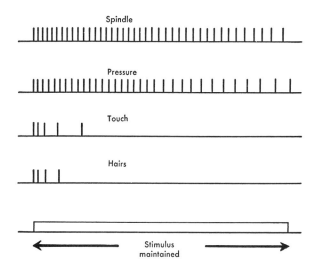

Figure 4–3. Schematic representation of adaptation in sensory endings. Each ending is stimulated for the same length of time, and nerve impulses are shown as if they were being recorded on moving film or paper. When a neuromuscular spindle is stimulated (by maintaining a stretch on its muscle), the spindle fires at a relatively high rate, a rate that decreases only slightly as the stimulus is maintained. A pressure receptor (pacinian corpuscle), on being touched or compressed, likewise continues to fire, but its rate of discharge decreases somewhat more. A touch receptor in skin, and receptors around hair follicles, adapt very rapidly, giving but a few impulses when the stimulus begins.

receptors dealing with the sense of position are not firing. A slight movement, however, interrupts the constant stimulation, nerve impulses are again initiated, and the sense or knowledge of position returns.

Of special interest are the mechanisms whereby the sensitivity of receptors can be changed or controlled by impulses over efferent nerve fibers that end in relation to the receptor. These mechanisms may well be a general property, but they have been studied in some detail only for certain receptors, for example, the neuromuscular spindle (p. 201).

CONDUCTION

The all-or-nothing nerve impulse begins either at the initial axon segment or at the nerve terminal of a receptor. However, the graded responses that comprise the natural triggering mechanisms are often difficult to manage experimentally and our current understanding of nerve impulses has been derived chiefly from studies using controllable artificial stimulation of the conducting parts of axons. Moreover, many of the crucial experiments have been carried out on the single giant axons of squid. These axons range from 0.5 to 1 millimeter in diameter and are therefore large enough to permit the insertion of microelectrodes. In recent years, techniques have been developed that have enabled studies of single large fibers in mammalian nerves to be undertaken.

If the tip of a microelectrode pierces the axolemma of a single fiber, at the moment of entering the cytoplasm it suddenly detects the resting potential, which is about 90 mV negative with respect to the fluid surrounding the axon (Fig. 4–1). If a brief, subthreshold pulse of current is now applied through a pair of stimulating electrodes placed on the immediately adjacent axolemma, certain characteristic changes in the resting potential can be detected and recorded. The outward flow of stimulating current at the cathode so alters the membrane that its conductance to certain ions is increased and the membrane undergoes a partial depolarization. This increase in conductance occurs under the cathode and in the immediately adjacent membrane. The magnitude of this increase depends upon the strength of the stimulus. However, the magnitude decreases as the distance from the cathode increases. Hence, this is a graded or decremental local response.

If the strength of the stimulus is such that the depolarization amounts to 20 to 40 mV, threshold is reached and an *action potential (spike potential)*, i.e., the all-or-nothing response, is triggered. The membrane potential is reversed, the interior becomes 20 to 30 mV positive (Fig. 4–1), and the total change is about 120 mV. Threshold can also be reached if two or more subthreshold stimuli are applied in quick succession; the resulting local responses can summate and thereby reach or exceed threshold.

Graded responses that consist of hyperpolarization instead of depolarization can also be demonstrated. If the polarity of the stimulating electrodes is reversed, so that the anode is nearest the recording electrodes, the current passing inward from the anode decreases the conductance of the membrane. The resulting increase in membrane potential comprises hyperpolarization; it can be recorded as a local, graded response.

The shape and magnitude of a family of curves representing graded responses are shown in Figure 4–4. This figure also shows the origin of an action potential when threshold is reached. When an action potential arises, the current flow longitudinally through the axon and then outward through the membrane (Fig. 4–5) is more than sufficient to reach threshold for a substantially long stretch of membrane. Hence, the action potential is an amplifying mechanism, creating its own propagation, independent of the initiating stimulus. In effect, it is propagated along with what may be regarded as a cable with a high resistance and a leaky surface. A wide "margin of safety" is therefore necessary to insure propagation, and this margin is provided by the density of ionic fluxes that accompany the reversal of membrane potential.

It is to be noted that when an axon is stimulated artificially somewhere along its course, the nerve impulse travels in both directions from the point of stimulation, in contrast to the unidirectional conduction imposed by an origin from a receptor or from the initial axon segment.

The reversal of potential that characterizes the nerve impulse lasts from 0.5 to 2 or more milliseconds, depending upon the diameter and other features of axons. The rising phase of the action potential is steep (hence, the term "spike" potential that is often

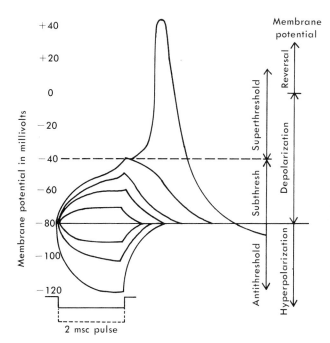

Figure 4-4. A family of curves obtained by stimulating a nerve fiber with a short current pulse of variable strength and polarity. With weak stimulation at the cathode, local membrane depolarization results. As the strength is increased, the local response is greater. Finally, threshold is reached and an action potential results as the membrane potential is reversed. If the polarity of the stimulating electrode is reversed, hyperpolarization results and increases with the magnitude of the stimulus. (Modified from Katz, B.: Nerve, Muscle, and Synapse. New York, McGraw-Hill, Inc., 1966.)

used synonymously for action potential); that of the falling phase is less precipitous (Fig. 4–1). During most of the time occupied by the action potential, the axon cannot be stimulated to fire again, no matter how strong the stimulus. This is the *absolute refractory period.* As the falling phase reflects the return to the resting potential, the axon becomes excitable again, but its threshold is higher. This is the *relative refractory period*; its precise relationship in time with the falling phase varies according to type of axon and the species of animal. In some axons, this may be followed by a short period during which the axon is hyperexcitable; the reasons for this are not fully understood. When the former level of the resting potential is reached, the repolarization usually continues beyond that level, so that for a few milliseconds the membrane is hyperpolarized. This period of hyperpolarization seems to correspond to a *positive after-potential* that can be recorded externally.

A number of elegant experiments using precise physicochemical and electrochemical techniques and radioactive tracers have clarified many of the processes that bring about the potential changes outlined above. The following is a simplified account.

The passage of an artificial electric current outward through the membrane to the cathode brings about a change in the permeability of the membrane (the essential mechanisms of this change are still unknown), characterized by a decreased resistance to ionic fluxes (increase in conductance), and an increase in the

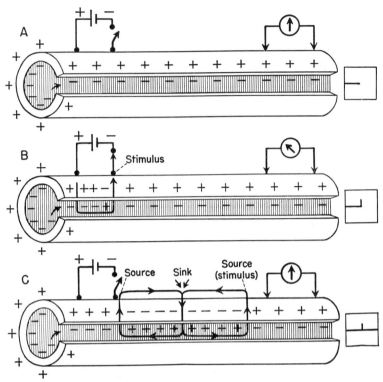

Figure 4–5. Diagram illustrating the initial changes following application of a stimulus to a nerve fiber. A: The fiber is represented as a tube with a strip cut away so as to expose the interior. The stimulating electrodes, indicated by + and −, are at one end and the recording electrodes at the other. The electrical charges internal and external to the membrane are also indicated. B: When the switch is closed, a battery current flows from the positive electrode into the fiber and out through the membrane back to the negative electrode (cathode), bringing about the change in membrane conductance. Some of the stimulating current leaks down the nerve, instantaneously for all practical purposes, and is recorded as a small deflection (inset at right). This is the shock artifact and indicates the moment of stimulation. C: The effect of current flow out through the membrane is to initiate the conduction of a nerve impulse. The impulse is represented as two dipoles, each consisting of current flow (not the stimulating current from the battery) within a region indicated by the reversal of electrical charges. The current flow out through the membrane in the leading dipole acts as a stimulus, just as did the artificial current from the battery. According to conventional methods, the recording instrument will not show a deflection until the region of negativity passes under the first electrode (see Figures 4–11 and 4–12).

movement of sodium into the axon (Fig. 4–6). The resulting graded responses for both axon and cell body have been outlined previously. Threshold is reached when the entry of sodium is high enough to balance the simultaneous inward movement of chloride and the outward movement of potassium. At threshold, any slight increase in stimulus strength is sufficient to trigger the nerve impulse. Its onset is signaled by a further but massive lowering of membrane resistance (increase in conductance), coupled with a massive sodium entry. Thus, unlike the resting potential, which is potassium-dependent, the action potential is sodium-dependent, and cannot be brought about if sodium is absent from its external fluid (local anesthetics act by blocking sodium entry and thereby preventing conduction). The ionic current flow that results from sodium entry spreads longitudinally through the axon and out through its membrane to return through extracellular fluid to the entry zone (sink). The outward ionic current acts as the stimulus for further membrane depolarization and increased sodium entry, and is of a magnitude so great as to more than insure that threshold is reached and the impulse propagated. The massive sodium entry, therefore, comprises a regenerative or amplifying process which is independent of stimulus strength.

The longitudinal extent of membrane occupied by an action potential at a given instant ranges from a few millimeters to several centimeters, and in the largest, most rapidly conducting fibers may reach 5 or 6 centimeters. In such fibers, the current flow may spread beyond a length of fiber that is blocked by cold or by a local anesthetic, and may be sufficient to enable the nerve impulse to jump the block. Whatever the length of the nerve fiber occupied by a nerve impulse, the rapid increase in sodium conductance is a transient phenomenon. As it brings about the ionic current flow that stimulates at a distance, the entry at a given point is quickly inactivated and is converted into a greatly increased potassium conductance (Fig. 4-6). This leads to an accelerated movement of potassium out of the axoplasm to the exterior, and thereby to a rapid fall (return) of the inside potential to the resting level (and beyond, as potassium efflux leads to the hyperpolarization mentioned previously). The potassium efflux then rapidly shuts itself off and the sodium-potassium pump becomes operative again.

The various changes outlined above involve oxidative metabolism and are accompanied by the uptake of oxygen, the formation of carbon dioxide, and the production of heat.

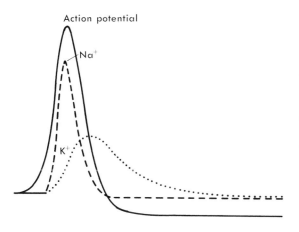

Action potential

Na^+

K^+

Figure 4-6. Simplified representation of increase in conductance of Na^+ (for inward movement) and of K^+ (for outward movement) in relation to the action potential. Note the differing time relationships. (From Hodgkin, A. L., and Huxley, A. F., in J. Physiol., *117*:500–544, 1952.)

FIBER SIZE, EXCITABILITY, AND CONDUCTION

Fibers of large diameter are more excitable, that is, have lower thresholds, than do smaller fibers. Moreover, their action potentials are larger, shorter, and faster. In cats and many other animals, the largest fibers are about 20 μm in diameter. In fibers of this size, the average duration of an action potential is about 0.5 millisecond, and it conducts at about 120 meters per second. In human beings, however, fibers of similar size conduct more slowly, at 60 or 70 meters per second or less. Fibers of similar size in cold-blooded animals conduct still more slowly (dropping the temperature of warm-blooded animals results in a decrease in speed of nerve conduction and amplitude of action potential).

Nonmyelinated fibers (in vertebrates these are nearly always 1 or 2 μm or less in diameter) have much higher thresholds, their spike potentials last longer (2 milliseconds or more), and they conduct impulses more slowly (one meter per second or less).

Strength-Duration Curves. As is evident from preceding accounts, stimulation of a cell or an axon takes place during the rate of change of a stimulus or of the applied energy. When artificially stimulated by an electric current that is turned on and left on, so that a constant current is said to flow, stimulation occurs when the current is turned on (at the *make*) and when it is turned off (at the *break*). However, the current has to flow for a certain finite time in order to be effective (the time varies according to fiber diameter and certain other characteristics). If brief electric pulses are used (that is, currents that are turned on and off rapidly), it is found that as the pulses become shorter and shorter, they have to be made stronger and stronger in order to stimulate. Finally, the duration of a pulse becomes so brief that it will not stimulate, no matter how strong it is made. This accounts for the fact that high frequency currents may not stimulate, no matter how great the voltage (however, other electrical effects may occur). It is of interest that the ordinary sinusoidal house current of 50 to 60 cycles and 110 to 220 volts is one of the most effective stimulators, and therefore one of the most dangerous of currents.

The curve illustrated in Figure 4–7 is a *strength-duration curve* showing the relationship of the strength of the stimulus to the time during which it acts. That strength of current which, when acting over an infinite time, is just sufficient to stimulate is known as the *rheobase*. If a current of twice the rheobase is chosen, and the shortest time during which this can flow and still stimulate is determined, then this time is known as the *chronaxie* or *excitation time.* Chronaxie is an arbitrary but useful measure of excitability which has rather characteristic values for different tissues. More useful, however, are strength-duration curves (Figs. 4–8 and 4–9).

If electrodes are applied to a normal muscle and electric shocks are given, the contractions that follow are actually the result of stimulating the motor nerve of the muscle. If the times taken

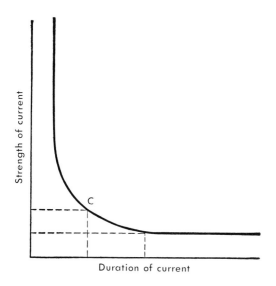

Figure 4-7. Graph illustrating relationship of current strength and duration. The horizontal portion of the curve indicates the rheobase, the least strength of current which, if flowing an infinite time, is just sufficient to stimulate. A current of less strength will never stimulate, no matter how long it flows. A current of twice rheobase strength reaches threshold after a time interval known as chronaxie, *C*. The vertical portion of the curve indicates that the stronger a current, the shorter its excitation time. Currents of high frequency act over such short times that they may never stimulate, no matter what their intensity.

for varying strengths of current to stimulate are determined, a strength-duration curve is obtained which is characteristic for nerve (Fig. 4–8). The chronaxie, which is one point of the curve, is less than 1 millisecond. But if electrodes are applied to a muscle deprived of its nerve supply, the contractions following electric shocks are the result of direct stimulation of muscle fibers. The time during which current must flow is considerably longer. Hence, the curve has a different shape and the chronaxie is much greater. Therefore, in a muscle which is partially denervated, some muscle fibers (the denervated ones) will respond to direct stimulation and others (the normal ones) will respond to nerve impulses.

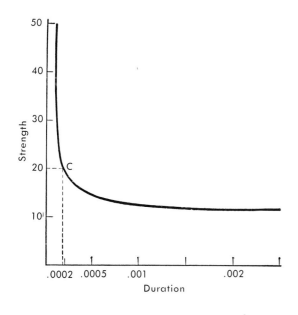

Figure 4-8. Strength-duration curve of a tibialis anterior muscle. The nerve supply is intact, so the curve is actually that of nerve. The chronaxie, C, is less than 0.2 millisecond. (Modified from Adrian, E. D., in Brain, *39*:1–33, 1916.)

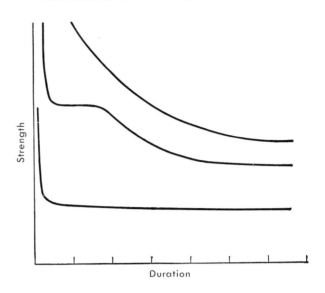

Figure 4–9. Composite graph which allows comparison of the shapes of the various strength-duration curves. *Top curve:* Denervated muscle, the curve being that for the muscle. Although it cannot be shown in a composite graph, the chronaxie may be more than 50 times greater than that of normal muscle. *Middle curve:* Partially denervated muscle, there being a mixture of two curves, one for normal muscle and nerve and another for denervated muscle. *Bottom curve:* Normal muscle and nerve, the curve being similar to that of Figure 4–8. (Modified from Adrian, E. D., Brain, *39*:1–33, 1916.)

As Figure 4–9 shows, the curve is complex in shape, indicating that it is composed of the two simpler ones with different time relationships.

The strength-duration curve of Figure 4–7 shows the level below which a current, no matter how long it flows, will not stimulate. Nevertheless, as was pointed out previously, subthreshold stimuli produce local, graded responses. Hence, when a constant current of subthreshold strength is applied, the nerve under the cathode becomes more excitable as the local depolarization occurs. However, the sodium entry decreases, as does potassium efflux, even though the current is still flowing. The converse occurs at the anode. This decline from maximum excitability during the period of constant current flow is known as *accommodation*, and the various changes are shown in Figure 4–10.

Saltatory Conduction. Complex nervous systems need information that reaches them rapidly. The "amount" of information that can be transmitted over a single nerve fiber is limited because each single conducted nerve impulse is "on" or "off," and can vary only in the frequency, that is, the number of impulses per unit time. Hence, the "amount" of information received by the brain depends upon the number of nerve fibers carrying impulses to it, and the frequency of impulses carried by these fibers. Rapid conduction and higher frequency can be provided by large fibers, because resistance to ionic flow decreases with increasing fiber diameter, just as the resistance of a large copper wire or cable is less than that of a small one. However, an increase in nerve fiber size beyond a certain diameter is not compatible with the requirement of a great number of signal channels; the peripheral nerves and the central tracts would be disproportionately large. Moreover, leakage is greater in larger fibers. In vertebrates, increased speed of conduction and decrease in cable losses are provided by myelinated fibers. The myelin sheath comprises an insulating segmented sheath of low capacity with very little leakage as the action potential propagates. The outward flow of ionic current is concentrated where the axolemma is exposed, namely, at the nodes of Ranvier. Hence, successive stimulation occurs only at successive nodes, rather than as a continuous process such as is characteristic of nonmyelinated fibers. In effect, it is as if the impulse skips from node to node, thereby greatly increasing the speed of conduction. This is known as *saltatory conduction.*

Recording From Groups of Fibers. Action potentials may be recorded from the external aspect of a single fiber by suspending the fiber on two recording electrodes in a chamber with a moist atmosphere. As the action potential reaches the first recording electrode, a potential change is recorded as shown in Figure 4–11. Because both electrodes are external to the membrane the first electrode records an action potential that is negative with respect to the interior of the fiber, and also with respect to the fluid around the second recording electrode. The direction of polarity is reversed as the action potential passes by the second electrode. Thus, a *diphasic* record is obtained. If that part of the fiber between

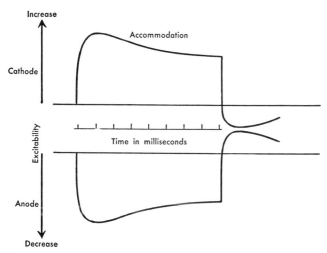

Figure 4–10. Diagram of excitability changes in nerve during the passage of a current for a short period of time. Note that the nerve under the negative electrode (cathode) increases in excitability very quickly, but this excitability slowly decreases (accommodation) as the current continues to flow, and drops very abruptly when the current is turned off. In fact, the nerve momentarily becomes less sensitive than it was before the current was applied. Converse changes occur in that part of the nerve under the positive electrode (anode). (Based on Erlanger, J., and Blair, E. A., in Am. J. Physiol., *99*:108–128, 1931; and Ruch, T. C., and Patton, H. D., editors: Physiology and Biophysics. 20th ed. Philadelphia, W. B. Saunders Company, 1973.)

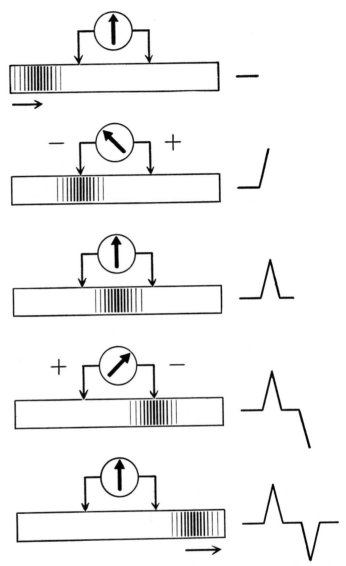

Figure 4–11. Conventional schematic representation of recording conducted activity. The long rectangle is a nerve on the surface of which are two electrodes (arrows) connected to a galvanometer in which the direction of conduction is indicated by an arrow. As an excitatory or negative change (vertical lines) comes under the first electrode, current flows from positive to negative, as indicated. When the impulse is between the electrodes, no current flows and the record returns to the base line. When it reaches the second electrode, current again flows from positive to negative, but in a direction opposite to that recorded first. When the impulse is past the electrode, no current flows. Thus a diphasic record is obtained.

the two electrodes is killed by crushing, or is inactivated by a local anesthetic, the nerve impulse will not reach the second electrode (unless the two are closer together than the length of axon normally occupied by the potential reversal). With the axon thus damaged, a *monophasic* record is obtained, that is, a record of the change under the first electrode only.

Monophasic and diphasic records are distortions of the true form of the recorded response, which is *triphasic* at each electrode. The triphasic form is not readily demonstrable when recording from an axon isolated in an artificial chamber, because the fluid surrounding the nerve fiber is much reduced in amount, and the external, longitudinal flow of current is altered or impeded. A single axon in its normal situation within a nerve in the body is surrounded by extracellular fluid and other conducting tissue, and the current flow associated with nerve impulses spreads in all directions. The interpretation of recorded potential changes involves geometry in three dimensions, and their conduction is often termed *volume conduction*. One can consider this conduction as if two whirlpools were moving along a fiber (Fig. 4–12). Each whirlpool or *dipole* consists of lines of current flow inside a fiber, out through the membrane at the source, back through extracellular fluid, and into the fiber through the membrane. The convergence of the entering lines of both dipoles is the sink. The leading dipole is associated with propagation, since its current, on flowing outward, acts as a stimulus. The trailing dipole is associated with recovery processes. Thus, the first change to be detected by the recording electrode is a positive one, brought about by the outward flow of current of the leading dipole. Next is what is usually termed the action potential, namely, the change at the sink (surface negative to the electrode, positive in the interior). Finally, the third part of the triphasic potential represents positivity as current in the trailing dipole flows outward.

Some kind of volume conduction recording is generally involved in the usual electrical records obtained from intact animals, and from human beings during a variety of diagnostic tests. For example, nerve impulses can be initiated in and recorded from peripheral nerves by electrodes placed on the overlying skin. The *electrocardiogram*, which is the record of the spread of excitation through the heart, can be detected by electrodes placed on the skin. Likewise, electrodes on the scalp can detect the complex, spontaneous electrical activity of the brain, the record of which comprises the *electroencephalogram*.

If a whole peripheral nerve is being studied, whether removed and placed in a moist chamber or whether it is in its normal place in the body, the recorded response is much more complicated than that of a single fiber. The nerve has fibers of many different sizes, excitability characteristics, and conduction rates. Hence, as Fig. 4–13 shows, if all the fibers in a nerve are stimulated simultaneously and if the recording electrodes are sufficiently far away,

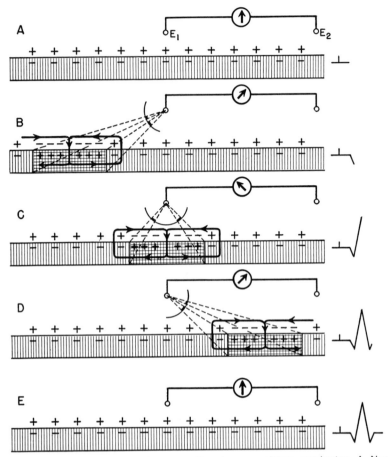

Figure 4–12. Diagram indicating recording from a volume conductor. *A,* Nerve fiber with electrical charges. At some distance from the nerve, separated by body fluid and tissue, are two electrodes, E_1 and E_2, connected to a recording instrument. E_2 is considered to be far enough away so that it can be neglected in this discussion. At some distance away a stimulus has been applied (not shown), and the shock artifact is shown at the right. *B,* The nerve impulse is conducting toward E_1, and the leading dipole is indicated completely. In order to determine the sign of any recorded potential, lines are drawn from E_1 to each end of the planes separating depolarized from polarized regions. With E_1 as a center, part of a circle is drawn. The length of arc included between each pair of lines is an indication of sign, in the following manner: The pair of lines to the right occupies a longer arc than does the other pair, and the surface of the fiber included by these two lines is positive, whereas that included between the other two is negative. Therefore, E_1 is "looking at more positivity than negativity," and a small positive deflection will be recorded. *C,* Both dipoles are under E_1, and the surfaces included by the lines are both negative; therefore a large negative deflection is recorded. *D,* Both dipoles are past E_1, which is again "looking" at positivity, and a small positive change is again recorded. *E,* The dipoles are relatively far away, and the triphasic change is completed. If E_2 were now represented as being affected, another triphasic change would be recorded, but with opposite signs.

the form of the recorded response is determined by the fact that the larger fibers have greater action potentials, conduct faster, and will reach the recording electrodes first. The action potentials of a group of fibers of varying sizes therefore become more and more out of phase as they travel along the nerve. These differences have led to a classification of nerve fibers into A, B, and C types, according to conduction rates and other features. The A fibers are myelinated and are subdivided into *alpha, beta, gamma,* and *delta* types. The *alpha* fibers are the largest and fastest conducting (the terminology is confusing because some of the *alpha* fibers are sensory, yet the term is generally restricted to the motor fibers that supply the extrafusal fibers of skeletal muscle; Fig. 10–3, p. 202). The *beta* and *delta* fibers are sensory, and the *gamma* fibers are motor to the intrafusal fibers of skeletal muscle (p. 201). The B fibers are preganglionic autonomic fibers, which are usually myelinated (not present in the saphenous nerve of Figure 4–13), and the C fibers are nonmyelinated. Unfortunately, other classifications are also in use. For example, afferent fibers from muscle are often classified as Group I, II or III, depending upon size and other characteristics (p. 205).

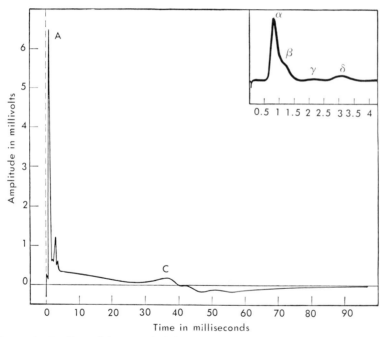

Figure 4-13. Potentials recorded from mammalian saphenous nerve several centimeters from the point of stimulation. Rapidly traveling nerve impulses reach the electrodes first and are recorded as the *A* elevation. Following the *A* elevation by a considerable interval is the *C* elevation, representing nonmyelinated fibers. The inset shows the *A* elevation recorded from the cat saphenous nerve 6 cm from the point of stimulation. Since the recording rate is faster, the *A* components, *alpha, beta, gamma,* and *delta,* are dispersed to a greater degree and represent the algebraic summation of potentials recorded from fibers varying from 2 to 16 μm in diameter. An intermediate or *B* elevation is recorded only from nerves containing preganglionic autonomic fibers, which are myelinated, but differ considerably from *A* fibers in duration of spike potential and type of after-potential. (From Gasser, H. S., in Ohio J. Sci., *41*:145–159, 1941; and Gasser, H. S., in Proc. A. Res. Nerv. & Ment. Dis., *23*:44–62, 1943.)

Finally, in considering whole nerves, it is worth pointing out that as the ionic current produced by an active fiber flows through extracellular fluid, it also flows through adjacent inactive fibers and can change their excitability. This action on adjacent fibers, when the fibers are damaged or cut, may play a role in certain painful conditions that sometimes follow peripheral nerve injuries (p. 239).

TRANSMISSION

The term transmission refers to the events that follow the arrival of nerve impulses at synaptic junctions or at neuromuscular or neuroglandular junctions. In the brain and spinal cord of vertebrates, transmission usually involves the release of chemical mediators at synaptic junctions, although in some instances, current flow across an electrical synapse or a gap junction comprises the activating mechanism. Chemical mediators are also released at neuromuscular and neuroglandular junctions.

Our current knowledge of chemical transmission and synaptic mechanisms has come chiefly from many years of investigation of the various neuromuscular junctions. Major advances in recent years have come from pharmacological studies of receptors in cells, from pharmacological and electrophysiological studies of single motor neurons in the spinal cord of the cat (and, more recently, other large neurons in the brain), from the electron microscope in morphological studies, and because of the reemergence of the Golgi stain as an important analytical method. Of outstanding importance have been carefully designed experiments involving the development of microelectrodes for intracellular and extracellular recording, and of a variety of experimental, biochemical, and pharmacological procedures. Examples are the use of radioactive tracers, microchemical analyses, iontophoresis (the application of compounds by micropipettes to the surface or the interior of single cells), electrophoretic analyses, and the alteration of structure and function by pharmacological means.

There are certain criteria to be met in order that a chemical can be classified as a chemical mediator or transmitter. Nerves should have the enzymes needed to synthesize the transmitter. The transmitter should be released when the nerves are stimulated, and it should then react with a specific receptor in the membrane of the postjunctional cell so as to produce a biological response. Mechanisms should exist for rapidly terminating the actions of the transmitter. On the basis of these criteria, acetylcholine and norepinephrine are now established as neurotransmitters. Other putative transmitters include various catecholamines (dopamine and epinephrine), other monoamines (serotonin), inhibitory amino acids (*gamma* aminobutyric acid and glycine), excitatory amino acids (glutamic acid and aspartic acid), and possibly other compounds such as adenosine derivatives and various polypeptides. Some transmitters are either excitatory or inhibitory, depending upon their site of action and the receptor mechanism involved.

The following account deals chiefly with the sequence of events and the electrical changes involved in transmission. The biochemistry and pharmacology of transmitters are discussed in Chapter 5.

SYNAPTIC TRANSMISSION

Synaptic transmission can be either electrical or chemical. Electrical synapses occur in association with certain giant nerve fibers in fishes, they are present in certain parasympathetic ganglia, such as the ciliary ganglia of young birds, and they are common in the developing nervous system. The synaptic endings of electrical synapses are large, and the cleft is a gap junction. Apparently, the current flow from the nerve impulse in the axon terminal is sufficient to depolarize the membrane of the succeeding nerve cell and cause it to discharge.

Chemical transmission, which was first studied in smooth muscle, involves a sequence of reactions comprised of a number of discrete steps, many of which are not yet fully understood. A specific transmitter is synthesized in the axon terminals by enzymes that are synthesized in the cell body and transported to the axon terminals. Both synthesis and storage occur in the synaptic vesicles, although some may occur in the cytoplasm, depending on the transmitter. When a nerve impulse arrives at and depolarizes the synaptic ending, the transmitter is liberated in multimolecular packets or quanta. The released transmitter then diffuses across the synaptic cleft and combines with a receptor in the membrane of the succeeding nerve cell or of the effector. The term receptor refers to sites of membrane specialization where the combination of transmitters or other compounds with specific membrane proteins is followed by certain cellular changes or reactions. In the case of nerve cells, the transmitter-receptor union brings about changes in ionic permeability of the membrane, perhaps by increasing or decreasing pore size. This in turn results in changes in ionic flow through the membrane. Such changes may be excitatory, that is, they may produce a local depolarization of the membrane. This local graded response, either by itself or in combination with other, nearby local changes, may be of sufficient magnitude and involve enough area of the membrane, so that the depolarization spreads and becomes self-propagating. On the other hand, the transmitter may be inhibitory, that is, it may hyperpolarize the membrane and thereby prevent discharge or stop ongoing activity. Whether excitatory or inhibitory, action is soon stopped, either by enzymatic "destruction" or by uptake of transmitter into the axon terminals.

The time for the total sequence of events, from the arrival of the nerve impulse at the synaptic ending until the biological response of the postjunctional cell, may be as short as 0.5 millisecond. This time is spoken of as *synaptic delay.*

Any one neuron synthesizes only one transmitter. Hence, for neurons supplying skeletal muscle, the transmitter, acetylcholine, is the same at the terminals of the collateral branch of the initial segment as it is at the motor ending.

Excitatory Synapses.   One example is the synaptic endings formed by preganglionic autonomic fibers in peripheral autonomic ganglia. The transmitter is acetylcholine. Normally there is a random, spontaneous discharge of a few quanta out of the nerve terminals, into and across the synaptic cleft. The combination of acetylcholine and the receptor protein leads to a very small local depolarization which comprises a miniature graded response. Also present in the receptor is a specific enzyme, acetylcholinesterase, which hydrolyzes the acetylcholine into choline and acetic acid. The choline then becomes available again for the synthesis of acetylcholine.

Just how acetylcholine (or any other transmitter) is released is still not clear. It may be that the synaptic vesicles are discharged by a process termed *exocytosis,* in which the vesicles fuse with the presynaptic membrane and are then released into the synaptic cleft. It is also possible that the vesicles open up and allow the transmitter to diffuse or be carried through the presynaptic membrane, after which the vesicles close. Such an opening and closing mechanism would likely require the presence of a contractile protein in the vesicle membrane.

When a nerve impulse arrives at a nerve ending, the depolarization of the membrane causes an increase in the rate of discharge of transmitter. Calcium ions are necessary for this increase in the release of the transmitter. It is postulated that when the depolarization occurs, the permeability of the presynaptic membrane to calcium increases. The flux of calcium from extracellular fluid through the membrane is followed by the release of transmitter, and the development of a graded response or local depolarization greater in magnitude than the miniature, random changes mentioned above. This larger local change is the excitatory postsynaptic potential (EPSP) mentioned earlier. The EPSP may be large enough to trigger off an action potential at the initial axon segment, and it may also be large enough to trigger an action potential in the cell body (Fig. 4–2). Moreover, two or more EPSPs, either adjacent and simultaneous, or one closely following the other in the same area, may summate and reach threshold (*spatial* and *temporal summation*).

Other putative excitatory transmitters in the autonomic and central nervous system are discussed in Chapter 5.

Inhibitory Synapses.   Transmitters that bring about inhibition of neurons are less well understood. Whatever the transmitter(s) may be (at the terminals of certain spinal cord interneurons it is very likely the amino acid glycine), its release at axosomatic and axodendritic synapses brings about an increase in membrane resistance, as well as a local hyperpolarization so that the membrane becomes less excitable. The local potential change is known as the inhibitory postsynaptic potential (IPSP). This kind of inhibitory synapse is sensitive to strychnine, that is, the local application of strychnine blocks the inhibitory mechanism and may be followed by spontaneous discharges of the postsynaptic neuron.

Another amino acid, *gamma* aminobutyric acid (GABA), is known to be a powerful inhibitor of certain crustacean muscles. It now seems likely that in mammalian nervous system, GABA is the transmitter that is responsible for presynaptic inhibition. In the axo-axonal synapses in which this kind of inhibition occurs, it may be that GABA acts by depolarizing the second axon terminal to such a degree that the loss of excitatory transmitter renders ineffective the further depolarization produced by the arrival of a nerve impulse. This kind of inhibitory mechanism is sensitive to picrotoxin, in contrast to the strychnine sensitivity of the other type of inhibitory synapse.

NEUROMUSCULAR TRANSMISSION

Skeletal (Striated) Muscle. The neuromuscular junction in skeletal muscle is a synapse that has been studied in great detail. The information and understanding derived from these studies paved the way for many investigations of ganglionic and central synapses. It was in the neuromuscular junction or end plate that the random, small, local spots of depolarization now termed *miniature end plate potentials* were found. It was determined that these local fluctuations were due to the random release of multimolecular packets or quanta of the transmitter acetylcholine, which then combined with the receptor. It was subsequently found that similar changes occurred in neurons, as described above.

When the nerve impulse arrives, and calcium is present, an amount of acetylcholine is released sufficient to produce, as it combines with receptor molecules, a large local depolarization, the *end plate potential* (Fig. 4–14). This local change, which often reaches or exceeds 50 mV, quickly exceeds the threshold of the muscle fiber. The muscle fiber then "fires off." The propagated wave of membrane depolarization then initiates the contractile mechanism of the fiber. How this is brought about is not yet clear, although calcium is known to be essential for the activation of the contractile proteins in muscle.

In normal muscle, the acetylcholine receptors are concentrated at the end plate. In developing muscle, acetylcholine receptors are scattered over the surface of the muscle, and when a

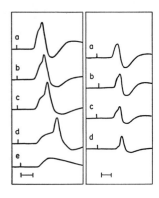

Figure 4–14. Records of end plate potentials of a single muscle fiber. In the left-hand column, the initial short deflections signal the stimulation of the motor nerve to the muscle fiber. In *a*, there is a compound deflection that, in *b-d*, breaks up into end plate potential and muscle action potential upon the application of curare at increasing strengths. In *e*, the preparation is deeply curarized, and only the end plate potential is left. In the right-hand column, the initial, short deflection signals the stimulation of the motor nerve to a single muscle fiber. In *a*, one electrode is on the end plate. In *b*, one electrode is on the nerve-muscle junction. In *c* and *d*, the electrode is placed at increasing distances from the end plate. Note that the end plate potential decreases in amplitude, indicating that it is not a conducted potential, but rather a local change. (Data from Kuffler, S.: J. Neurophysiol., 5:18–26, 1942.)

muscle is denervated, acetylcholine receptors again appear in great numbers on the surfaces of the muscle cells.

Cardiac (Striated) Muscle. As outlined previously, the heart contains specialized muscle cells that form the conducting system. Propagated impulses over these cells electrically activate the regular cardiac muscle cells, and the activation then spreads throughout the heart across the end-to-end gap junctions between the cardiac muscle cells. The cells of the sinu-atrial node are pacemakers and exhibit rhythmic depolarization and repolarization. Their rhythmic discharge is responsible for the regular contraction and relaxation of the heart. The rate of firing of the nodes is regulated by nerve impulses that reach them. Some of the nerve fibers release norepinephrine; the general action of norepinephrine on the nodal cells is an excitatory one, that is, it increases the rate of nodal firing. Other nerve fibers release acetylcholine, which is inhibitory to the intrinsic activity of the nodes. Further details of the nerve supply of the heart are given with the autonomic nervous system (p. 337).

Smooth Muscle. As indicated previously, some smooth muscle bundles are heavily innervated by postganglionic autonomic fibers. In these instances, nearly every smooth muscle cell has large numbers of close contacts with the varicosities of the nerve fibers; some of these contacts are synaptic junctions. The transmitter at these junctions may be either acetylcholine or norepinephrine, depending upon the organ. If the excitatory nerve fibers to one of the densely innervated bundles are stimulated, there occurs a transient, local depolarization in each smooth muscle cell. This depolarization is termed an *excitatory junction potential.* If this potential reaches threshold, a conducted spike potential is triggered, and is followed by contraction. Repetitive subthreshold stimulation leads to the summation of junction potentials.

Miniature excitatory junction potentials have also been observed, and are probably due to the random quantal release of transmitter.

In most smooth muscle bundles, the innervation is less dense and may even be sparse. In such instances the transmitter diffuses through extracellular space, and its action is further mediated by the spread of excitation from one muscle cell to another across gap junctions.

Many smooth muscle cells, especially those in hollow organs, possess intrinsic activity, that is, act as pacemakers. In such instances, the nerves supplying these cells act chiefly to regulate the spontaneous activity. Also, in the digestive system there are intrinsic neurons that are to a large degree independent of the external nerve supply, and whose transmitters may be acetylcholine and norepinephrine, or others as yet undetermined.

The precise nature of a smooth muscle response depends upon the nature of the receptors, which selectively recognize and combine with the neurotransmitter. Among the known receptors are those for acetylcholine, *alpha* and *beta* receptors for norepinephrine, and a receptor for dopamine. (These are discussed further in Chapter 5.)

NEUROGLANDULAR TRANSMISSION

Many gland cells are activated by neurotransmitters across junctions that in nearly every aspect resemble synapses (p. 53). The transmitters are acetylcholine or norepinephrine. The suprarenal medullae and the salivary and sweat glands have been most widely studied in this regard. The cells of the salivary glands, which are inexcitable except by nerve stimulation, exhibit resting potentials and, upon activation by a transmitter, a *secretory potential*. This depolarization is probably largely dependent upon an increased permeability to potassium. It is a part of a complex series of events that include this change in membrane potential, followed by the secretion of fluid, electrolytes, and protein, and an increase in metabolic rate. It is interesting that when acetylcholine is the transmitter, the saliva is relatively low in volume but viscous, whereas when norepinephrine activates the cells, the saliva is much higher in volume and more watery.

SUMMARY

All membranes consist of a bimolecular lipid layer, with a layer of protein on its inner and outer aspects. The ionic permeabilities of the membrane of a resting nerve cell, together with the electric charges on either side, are such that the interior of the nerve cell and its processes is 70 to 90 mV negative with respect to the adjacent extracellular fluid. A sodium-potassium pump is involved in maintaining the membrane potential and the ionic concentration differences.

A conducted nerve impulse comprises a reversal of membrane potential, the interior becoming momentarily positive to the exterior. It is an all-or-nothing response. The more common responses to stimulation, however, are graded responses. These occur chiefly in the receptive parts of neurons. When synaptic endings are activated, the membrane undergoes a local partial depolarization known as an excitatory postsynaptic potential (EPSP). If the synapse is inhibitory, the membrane undergoes a local partial hyperpolarization known as an inhibitory postsynaptic potential (IPSP). The EPSP is accompanied by an inward flux of sodium. If the flux and the depolarization are great enough so that threshold is reached, the sodium entry suddenly increases, becomes independent of stimulus strength, and initiates a sequence of events resulting in stimulation of the initial axon segment and a conducted nerve impulse. Basically similar events follow stimulation of receptors and result in a conducted nerve impulse in the nerve fiber terminal.

The self-propagating, all-or-nothing nerve impulse makes possible conduction over long distances and is characterized by constant magnitude and rate of conduction, both of which depend upon fiber diameter. Myelinated fibers have larger, more rapidly conducting impulses characterized by saltatory conduction, in which the impulse "jumps" from one node of Ranvier to the next. During and after the passage of an impulse, there are absolute and relative refractory periods, as well as negative and positive action potentials.

Nerve impulses can be recorded in the intact body. Owing to the fact that the current flow is through extracellular fluid as well as active nerve, the conduction is often termed volume conduction. Other examples are the electrocardiogram and the electroencephalogram.

Transmission comprises the events that follow the arrival of nerve impulses at synapses and neuromuscular and neuroglandular junctions. Synaptic transmission may be electrical, but is commonly chemical. A specific chemical transmitter is synthesized by the nerve cell. It is released by the arrival of a nerve impulse and crosses the synaptic cleft and combines with a receptor in the postsynaptic membrane, thereby initiating a biological response. It is then enzymatically inactivated or taken up by the presynaptic nerve fiber. The events at neuromuscular and neuroglandular junctions are similar.

Acetylcholine and norepinephrine are established transmitters. Other putative transmitters include various catecholamines (dopamine and epinephrine), other monoamines (serotonin), inhibitory amino acids (*gamma* aminobutyric acid and glycine), excitatory amino acids (glutamic acid and aspartic acid), and possibly adenosine derivatives and various polypeptides. Some of the transmitters may be either excitatory or inhibitory.

NAMES IN NEUROLOGY

JULIUS BERNSTEIN (1839–1917)

Bernstein was a German physiologist who studied in Berlin and was an assistant to Helmholtz in Heidelberg, but who spent most of his active career in Halle. In carrying out his electrophysiological studies over many decades, he used the capillary electrometer to measure nerve currents, and invented the rheotome by which he analyzed and timed the nerve impulse. In 1902 he published his concept (already expressed to some extent in earlier papers) that membrane potentials in nerve and muscle are generated because of special membrane permeability to potassium, and impermeability to anions inside and cations outside. This hypothesis is now known as the Bernstein membrane theory.

REFERENCES

The following are accounts of a generally advanced nature, dealing with broad aspects of cellular excitability and conduction.

Bennett, M. R.: Autonomic Neuromuscular Transmission. Cambridge, at the University Press, 1972.
Brazier, Mary A. B.: The Electrical Activity of the Nervous System. 3rd ed. Baltimore, The Williams and Wilkins Company, 1968.
Davies, M.: Functions of Biological Membranes. London, Chapman and Hall, and New York, Halsted Press, 1973.
Eccles, J. C.: The Physiology of Synapses. New York, Academic Press, 1964.
Hodgkin, A. L.: The Conduction of the Nervous Impulse. Liverpool, Liverpool University Press, 1964.
Hubbard, J. I., Llinás, R., and Quastel, D. M. J.: Electrophysiological Analysis of Synaptic Transmission. Baltimore, The Williams and Wilkins Company, 1969.
Katz, B.: Nerve, Muscle, and Synapse. New York, McGraw-Hill, Inc., 1966.
Katz, B.: The Release of Neural Transmitter Substances. Liverpool, Liverpool University Press, and Springfield, Ill., Charles C Thomas, 1969.
Ruch, T. C., and Patton, H. D. (editors): Physiology and Biophysics. 20th ed., Philadelphia, W. B. Saunders Company, 1973.

The following papers are valuable for their reviews of important aspects of nerve conduction and transmission.

Bishop, G. H.: Natural history of the nerve impulse. Physiol. Rev., 36:376–399, 1956.
Catton, W. T.: Mechanoreceptor function. Physiol. Rev., 50:297–318, 1970.
Douglas, W. W., and Ritchie, J. M.: Mammalian nonmyelinated nerve fibers. Physiol. Rev., 42:297–334, 1962.
Schneyer, L. H., Young, J. A., and Schneyer, C. A.: Salivary secretion of electrolytes. Physiol. Rev., 52:720–777, 1972.

Chapter 5

BIOCHEMISTRY AND PHARMACOLOGY OF THE NERVOUS SYSTEM

Chemical studies of the nervous system were pioneered primarily by Thudichum. However, after his death in 1901, research in this field lagged behind anatomical and physiological studies. It was not until appropriate research methods and instrumentation became available some decades later, and when the significance and application of research findings began to be appreciated, that neurochemistry became an established subject. Today it involves nearly every aspect of neural function, from membranes and receptor sites to the behavioral mechanisms of organisms.

Neuropharmacology probably received its major impetus with the experimental studies of smooth muscle and the heart near the beginning of this century. Today it is a subject of immense importance, closely linked with neurochemistry, and dealing especially with the mechanisms of action and the rational use of therapeutic agents.

An understanding of these two fields is essential to an understanding of the normal functions of the nervous system. It is equally essential to an understanding of the actions of drugs and of the mechanisms and treatment of many neurological disorders. Moreover, it is now recognized that many metabolic disorders can be correlated with specific cellular functions, and that many are inherited and can be detected before birth. For example, when hereditary disorders cause specific lysosomal (hydrolytic) enzymes to be missing or defective in action, certain macromolecular carbohydrates or lipids cannot be metabolized, and they therefore accumulate in nerve cells. A number of such "storage" diseases are known and nearly all are associated with mental retardation. An example is infantile amaurotic familial idiocy, a genetic defect produced by a defective lysosomal enzyme, hexosaminidase A, which normally splits the sugar from a ganglioside (lipid-polysaccharide complex). Because of the enzyme defect, there is a massive accumulation of the ganglioside in nerve cells, many of which are destroyed. The disease begins before birth and can be detected before birth by tests of the amniotic fluid for the enzyme. The infants become deaf, blind, and paralyzed from progressive brain deterioration and die within two or three years after birth. It should be emphasized that more than 60 genetic diseases can now be diagnosed before birth, and many of these are lysosomal enzyme defects.

GENERAL METABOLISM

The metabolism of the nervous system in general is high. Although the rate of oxygen consumption in resting peripheral nerve is about the same as it is in resting muscle, that in the central nervous system is about thirty times as great. The needs of the nervous system for high energy and rapid turnover are related to transmitter synthesis, release, and uptake, to rapid conduction and ion pumping, to intracellular transport, and to complex synthetic mechanisms in both neurons and glial cells.

Central Nervous System. Respiratory quotients, calculated from cerebral arterial and venous differences and from a variety of flow and uptake measurements, clearly show that glucose and oxygen are the prime sources of metabolic energy for the brain. The substances, carbon dioxide, lactic acid, and pyruvic acid, account for the glucose used by the human brain under normal conditions. However, during long-term decrease in available glucose (for example, during starvation or with severe liver damage), other metabolites are used. The most likely ones appear to be butyrate and certain amino acids. In a person at rest, about 20 per cent of inspired oxygen is removed from the blood by the brain (a significant part of the general circulation supplies the brain). Sleep does not decrease overall cerebral metabolism, but surgical anesthesia, diabetic coma, uremia, and hepatic coma are accompanied by decreased cerebral oxygen consumption.

Glucose is not only the main source of energy, but it is also the major carbon source for a wide variety of simple and complex molecules. For example, much of this carbon appears in amino acids and their derivatives.

Glucose reserves in the nervous system are low, and the brain is therefore highly dependent upon its blood supply. Glycogen in the brain serves as a carbohydrate reserve; much of it is stored in cytoplasmic granules.

Peripheral Nervous System. Information about the metabolism of the peripheral nervous system has been obtained chiefly by studying isolated peripheral nerves. Such studies show that peripheral nerves differ from the central nervous system in that their respiratory quotient is 0.8 instead of 1, indicating that they utilize noncarbohydrate as well as carbohydrate. For example, if a peripheral nerve is removed and placed in a warm, moist chamber, oxygen consumption may continue at the usual rate, and the ability to conduct may persist for hours, even after the utilization of carbohydrate has stopped. An active peripheral nerve is not metabolically restricted to glucose, but may derive energy from some as yet unknown metabolite.

Exogenous glucose likewise seems to be the main substrate for resting metabolism in sympathetic ganglion cells. However, although glucose utilization is accelerated during activity, the substrate for metabolism during activity is not glucose. The significance of increased glucose utilization during activity is uncertain.

REGULATORY MECHANISMS

Carbohydrates. All of the enzymatic components of the classic glycolytic pathway (glucose to pyruvate and lactate) have been found in brain tissue and appear to be in the cytoplasm outside of mitochondria. Elegant microchemical studies on the dynamics of the substrates of this pathway have clearly shown the roles of phosphocreatine and glycogen as energy stores maintaining adenosine triphosphate (ATP) homeostasis (Fig. 5–1). The final common pathway of oxidation of carbohydrate, fat, and protein, that is, the citric acid cycle, through which acetyl–CoA is completely oxidized to carbon dioxide and ultimately to water, takes place in the mitochondria. The energy derived from this oxidative metabolism is channeled into the energy-rich phosphorous bonds of creatine phosphate and ATP. Microchemical studies have shown that these oxidative processes are more prominent wherever mitochondria are more numerous. Moreover, the beginning of these processes in the fetal brain can be correlated with the appearance of mitochondria.

The hexose monophosphate shunt pathway also makes a contribution to cerebral carbohydrate metabolism, but the extent of this contribution is uncertain.

The brain is especially sensitive to oxygen lack and glucose deficiencies. A few minutes' deprivation of oxygen is usually sufficient to kill many neurons. Metabolic disorders that interfere with glucose metabolism (e.g., diabetes, liver damage, starvation) may have profound effects on brain functions. Also of major importance are congenital disorders in intermediary metabolism, especially those involving lysosomal enzymes, as mentioned previously.

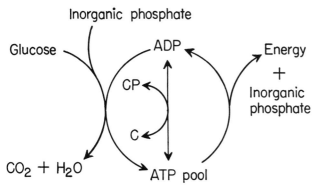

Figure 5–1. A schematic representation of the transfer of energy from glucose metabolism. Energy latent in the glucose molecule is evolved in the form of a high energy phosphate group. The hydrolysis of most common organic phosphate esters evolves 2000 to 4000 calories per mole, while certain of the organic phosphates produced in glucose metabolism yield 10,000 to 16,000 calories per mole. These high energy phosphate groups are used by the cell in the form of the nucleotide, adenosine triphosphate (ATP), which is synthesized by the cell from adenosine diphosphate (ADP), inorganic phosphate and energy. Although a pool or reserve supply of ATP is available, the cell calls upon a secondary energy carrier, creatine phosphate (CP), during sudden bursts of activity. In the resting state some ATP is used to synthesize CP, which is then reconverted to ATP at the appropriate time.

Lipids.   Lipids, which are critically important constituents of membranes, comprise almost half of the dry weight of the brain. They serve both as structural components and as functional participants in brain activity. Three major categories comprise most of the lipids of the normal nervous system: *cholesterol, sphingolipids,* and *glycerophospholipids* (there is not yet complete agreement on lipid terminology, and some variation in terms is encountered). Fatty acids are important parts of all complex lipids, but free fatty acids and triglycerides are present in the brain only in very small amounts. The lipids of gray and white matter differ in total concentration and in their individual distribution, especially with respect to membrane structures.

Interference with the biosynthesis and degradation of the various lipids leads to many neurological disorders, such as demyelinating diseases, as well as the hereditary storage diseases due to lysosomal enzyme deficiencies.

Proteins and Amino Acids.   Proteins form nearly 40 per cent of the dry weight of the brain. Although relatively few of them have been completely characterized, they function as enzymes, hormones, and structural elements; they probably function in transport systems as well. The importance of their synthesis and turnover in the nervous system is indicated by the prominence of the endoplasmic reticulum, Golgi apparatus, and ribosomes in neurons, and by the mechanisms of axonal transport and synaptic transmission. Proteins consist of long chains of *alpha*-amino acids linked by peptide bonds. The general scheme of their synthesis has been well defined. The genetic material, DNA, directs the synthesis of the three types of RNA, which are: transfer RNAs, each of which combines with a single amino acid and transports it to ribosomes; messenger RNAs, which direct the insertion of amino acids into the polypeptide chain; and ribosomal proteins, which help to form the ribosomes of the protein-synthesizing complex (a group of ribosomes linked by a strand of mRNA). The polypeptide then takes on its ultimate three-dimensional form. Most proteins become linked with carbohydrates to form *glycoproteins.*

The 20 different amino acids from which proteins are formed reach the brain from the blood stream mostly by active transport across the blood-brain barrier. A number of these amino acids are synthesized from intermediates arising from the aerobic breakdown of glucose during the citric acid cycle. The essential amino acids (those that cannot be synthesized) are obtained from the diet. The predominant amino acids in the nervous system are glutamate, glutamine, aspartate, *N*-acetylaspartate, and *gamma*-aminobutyrate, and usually comprise more than two-thirds of the free *alpha*-amino acids in the central nervous system. Glutamate, for example, is present in higher concentration in the brain than in any other organ of the body.

The active metabolic and direct role of amino acids in other than protein synthesis is indicated by the number of important amino acid derivatives (epinephrine, norepinephrine, dopamine, serotonin, melatonin, and peptide hormones), and by the fact that some amino acids (glycine, glutamic acid, aspartic acid, and *gamma*-aminobutyric acid) are putative transmitters.

Disorders of protein and amino acid metabolism are important causes of many neurological and behavioral problems, and interference with their functions forms the basis of many drug actions. For example, some psychic energizers and depressants act by displacing active molecules from receptors or by inhibiting their breakdown (e.g., monoamine oxidase inhibitors). Hereditary disorders of amino acid metabolism secondary to enzyme deficiency are often accompanied by neurological symptoms and mental retardation. Phenylketonuria (a hereditary phenylalanine hydroxylase deficiency in which phenylalanine is not transformed into tyrosine) is the most publicized of this class of disorders, but many others have been described. All are frequently associated with mental retardation, emphasizing the importance of proteins in the development of the brain.

Nucleoproteins. Nucleoproteins are conjugated proteins associated with the nucleic acids, ribonucleic acid (RNA) and deoxyribonucleic acid (DNA). Nerve cells have the highest content of ribonucleic acid (RNA) of any somatic cell of the body and a correspondingly high rate of protein turnover. This has spurred some elegant experimental work on the synthesis and characterization of RNA in single cells during the learning process and considerable speculation about the role of proteins or RNA as memory molecules. It has been shown that puromycin, an inhibitor of protein synthesis, inhibits the development of long term (but not short term) memory in some species.

Ribonucleic acid (RNA) is present in the nucleolus, small quantities are found in chromosomes, and it is present in large amounts in the Nissl substance (rough or granular endoplasmic reticulum). Deoxyribonucleic acid (DNA) is present only in the nucleus. Nucleic acids in general are large polymers of subunits or nucleotides, which in turn are composed of a pentose unit, a purine or pyrimidine base, and phosphoric acid. Nucleoproteins are depleted during intense activity of the nerve cell, are depleted or altered during chromatolysis, and are involved in some way in regenerative processes.

Vitamins.   Vitamins (or derivatives formed from them in the body) usually function as cofactors for enzymes. Accordingly, vitamin deficiencies may interfere with neural functions and cause neurological disorders. Deficiencies of the vitamin B group are especially likely to cause diseases that include severe neurological signs and symptoms. For example, thiamin is a cofactor in the oxidative decarboxylation of pyruvic *alpha*-ketoglutaric acids and its deficiency may result in brain stem involvement, neuritis, or beriberi. Nicotinic acid (niacin) is involved in the transfer of hydrogen or electrons and its deficiency is responsible for pellagra, in which the pathological signs include chromatolysis and degeneration of large neurons. The cobalamins (vitamins B_{12}), are closely related metabolically to folic acid; their deficiencies are involved in the production of megaloblastic anemia which is often accompanied by demyelinating disorders.

Hormones.   Hormones are important constituents of certain nerve cells, especially in the hypothalamus (p. 349) where neurosecretory cells form vasopressin and oxytocin. These are carried by axonal transport to the neurohypophysis where they are discharged into the blood stream. Other hypothalamic neurons form releasing factors that activate the release of adenohypophysial hormones.

INORGANIC CONSTITUENTS

In general, cerebral tissue has a fairly constant water content; water forms 85 per cent of the gray matter and 70 per cent of the white matter. Potassium and sodium are among the most important cations and are discussed elsewhere (p. 70). Other minerals are present, but their functions are largely unknown. Iron is present in nerve cells, and there are regional differences in its concentration. Copper is also present, and there are indications that it has an important function. In hepatolenticular degeneration, there is an abnormal excretion of amino acids, and copper is present in especially high concentrations in the degenerating liver and basal ganglia. There is also evidence that an abnormality of copper metabolism may be concerned in certain demyelinating diseases affecting sheep. Copper is usually associated with a particular protein in the blood, ceruloplasmin, the level of which is markedly decreased in hepatolenticular degeneration.

TRANSMITTERS AND RECEPTORS

In recent years the study of enzymes associated with the synthesis and metabolism of transmitters has proved extremely valuable in evaluating synaptic mechanisms. Some of the results are discussed below, and are outlined in Table 5–1, which lists the putative transmitters, the enzymes that synthesize them, and the suggested neuronal pathways in which these transmitters function.

Acetylcholine. Acetylcholine is synthesized in the cytoplasm of axon terminals from acetyl-CoA, which is of mitochondrial origin, and choline, which enters from extracellular fluid (Figs. 5–2, 5–3). The reaction is catalyzed by the cytoplasmic enzyme *choline acetylase (choline-O-acetyltransferase),* which is strongly localized in the synaptic endings. Once synthesized, acetylcholine is loaded into synaptic vesicles (the vesicles are synthesized in the cell body and reach the synaptic endings by axonal transport). Acetylcholine is released when the ending is depolarized by the arrival of a nerve impulse and calcium enters the terminal. The released acetylcholine may diffuse away, it may be hydrolyzed, or it may combine with specific macromolecules in the receptor mechanism of the postsynaptic membrane (Fig. 5–3). A number of nonspecific cholinesterases can hydrolyze acetylcholine, but the specific enzyme in the receptor is *acetylcholinesterase,* which rapidly hydrolyzes the acetylcholine to acetic acid and choline; the choline can then re-enter the process of acetylcholine synthesis. The enzymatic hydrolysis of acetylcholine can be blocked by the drugs *eserine (physostigmine)* or *neostigmine,* which thereby indirectly accentuate the actions of acetylcholine. Evidence relating to these effects is offered by the treatment of the disease *myasthenia gravis.* In this disease, when muscles are used they become weak and many of them seem, to all intents, paralyzed. But after a variable period of rest, activity can be resumed only to have the weakness set in again. In many cases, the use of neostigmine offers striking relief for a few hours or days. This compound, by destroying cholinesterase, makes possible a more efficient acetylcholine function. It is presumed that in myasthenia gravis, acetylcholine is deficient or is abnormally inactivated at neuromuscular junctions.

Table 5–1.   Putative Neurotransmitters, Their Synthetic Enzymes, and Some Proposed Neuronal Pathways.

Putative Transmitter	Synthetic Enzymes	Suggested Neuronal Pathways
Dopamine	Tyrosine hydroxylase Aromatic-L-amino decarboxylase	Nigro-striatal Meso-limbic Tubero-infundibular Superior cervical ganglion inter- neurons Retinal interneurons
Noradrenaline (Norepinephrine)	Tyrosine hydroxylase Aromatic-L-amino acid decarboxylase Dopamine-β-hydroxylase	Post-ganglionic sympathetic Ventral brain stem–limbo-cortical pathway Locus coeruleus–limbo-cortical pathway Brain stem-spinal cord Locus coeruleus–cerebellum
Adrenaline (Epinephrine)	Tyrosine hydroxylase Aromatic-L-amino acid decarboxylase Dopamine-β-hydroxylase Phenylethanolamine-N-methyl transferase	Adrenal medulla parenchymal cells Brain and peripheral sympathetic of the frog
Serotonin	Tryptophan hydroxylase Aromatic-L-amino acid decarboxylase	Brain stem–spinal cord Brain stem–diencephalon- telencephalon
Acetylcholine	Choline acetylase	Skeletal motor system Post-ganglionic parasympathetic Septal-hippocampal Striatal interneurons
GABA	Glutamic acid decarboxylase	Purkinje cell-interpositus and Deiters' nuclei Globus pallidus-substantia nigra Retinal interneurons Hippocampal interneurons
Glycine	(Synthetic route not proven)	Spinal cord interneurons

(From McGeer, P. L., and McGeer, E. G., Prog. Neurobiol., 2:69–117, 1973. By permission of the authors and publisher.)

The receptor mechanism with which acetylcholine combines is a complicated structure in which the combining macromolecule is probably a lipoprotein. However, the precise nature of the receptor differs according to which of the four types of cholinergic

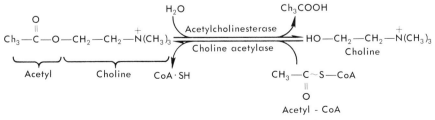

Figure 5-2. Formation and breakdown of acetylcholine.

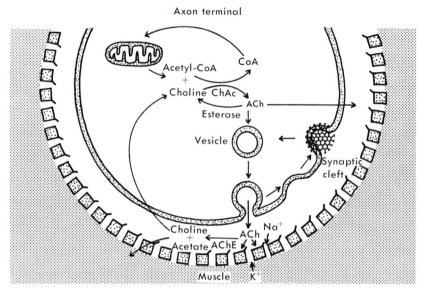

Figure 5–3. Neuromuscular transmission at the subcellular level. The stippled portion of the diagram represents muscle. Note the synthesis in the cytoplasm of acetylcholine (ACh) from acetyl-CoA (of mitochondrial origin) and choline (from extracellular fluid); the reaction is catalyzed by choline acetylase (ChAc). ACh is incorporated into vesicles. These fuse with the membrane and quanta of ACh are discharged into the synaptic cleft; the vesicles are then recovered and refilled with ACh. In the synaptic cleft, ACh either combines with receptors on the muscle surface (squares), thus activating ionic gates; or it diffuses away from the cleft; or it is broken down by acetylcholinesterase (AChE). Following the hydrolysis, some of the choline is taken up by the nerve terminal. (From Hubbard, J. I., and Quastel, D. M. J. cited: Micropharmacology of vertebrate neuromuscular transmission. Ann. Rev. Pharmacol., *13*:199–216, 1973. By permission of the authors and publisher.)

synapses or junctions are involved. These are (1) the neuromuscular junction in skeletal muscle, (2) the neuromuscular junction in smooth muscle and cardiac muscle and in the neuroglandular junction, (3) the synapses in autonomic ganglia, and (4) certain central nervous system synapses. For example, in autonomic ganglion cells and in motor end plates, there are receptors that are termed *nicotinic.* When the drug *nicotine* is applied in low concentrations to ganglion cells and motor end plates, it stimulates, whereas in high concentrations it depresses and blocks synaptic transmission. Acetylcholine does likewise, and its actions on ganglion cells and motor end plates are termed its *nicotinic effect.* However, where acetylcholine is released to act on smooth muscle cells (instance number 2 above), its effects are termed its *muscarine action* (the drug *muscarine* acts on smooth muscle much as acetylcholine does). The muscarine action is blocked by the drug *atropine.* A slow muscarine effect also occurs in ganglion cells. Nicotinic and muscarinic receptors (mostly the latter) occur in central synapses, and their various physiological roles are discussed elsewhere (p. 111).

A very large number of drugs have actions that can mimic, impede, or block specific steps in synaptic transmission, both by acetylcholine and by other transmitters. These drugs are often used in the investigation of normal function; many have therapeutic value, and many have profound ill effects on neural function. It is a matter of great importance that some of the narcotic drugs may compete for and take over certain receptor sites. Opiate receptors, for example, have been described on the membranes of nerve cells in the central nervous system. The classical paralyzing effect of *curare* was traced to its effect on the motor end plate. Subsequently, *d-tubocurarine,* one of the many alkaloids of crude curare, was shown to block acetylcholine transmission by competing for the receptor site.

Biogenic Amines.   These include the catecholamines (especially *dopamine, norepinephrine,* and *epinephrine*) and the indole amine, *serotonin (5-hydroxytryptamine, 5-HT).* The synthesis, uptake, storage, release, and metabolism of these compounds are now known in considerable detail. The four prerequisite enzymes (Fig. 5–4) are synthesized in the cell body and are transported to the axon terminals.

The precursor for catecholamine synthesis is the amino acid *tyrosine* (Fig. 5–4). Tyrosine, which is also derived from *phenylalanine* by hydroxylation, is transported into the nerve cell and is then converted to *dopa.* The enzyme *tyrosine hydroxylase* which catalyzes this reaction is highly specific, to such an extent that it is the rate-limiting step in the synthesis of norepinephrine. Inhibition of this enzyme virtually prevents the synthesis of norepinephrine. The next step is the formation of dopamine by the decarboxylation of dopa (see p. 386 for a discussion of the use of l-dopa in the treatment of neurological disorders in which certain nerve cells are deficient in dopamine). The conversion of dopa is catalyzed by *dopa-decarboxylase,* a relatively non-specific cytoplasmic enzyme which can decarboxylate other aromatic amino acids, such as 5-hydroxytryptophan and histidine.

Dopamine enters synaptic vesicles and in some neurons is released as a transmitter. Many of these dopamine neurons also contain melanin in their cytoplasm (substantia nigra, p. 139). Melanin, which is also the pigment of skin and hair, is derived from dopa. In other neurons, dopamine is hydroxylated to form norepinephrine (noradrenaline), a step which is catalyzed by *dopamine-B-hydroxylase,* an enzymatic reaction that requires ascorbic acid and oxygen.

In the medulla of the adrenal glands of mammals norepinephrine is converted to epinephrine (adrenaline), which, when released, enters the blood stream as a circulating hormone. This final step in the synthesis of catecholamines is catalyzed by *phenylethanolamine-N-methyltransferase,* an enzyme that is selectively localized in the adrenal medulla. Corticosteroids from the adrenal cortex control the synthesis of this enzyme, and these

COMPOUND	STRUCTURAL FORMULA	ENZYMATIC PROCESS	ENZYME

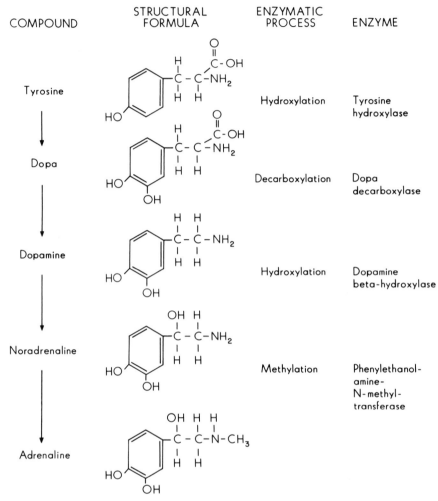

Figure 5-4. The sequential synthesis of the catecholamines.

corticosteroids in turn are controlled by the hypophysial hormone, adrenocorticotropic hormone (ACTH). It is also of interest that dopamine, norepinephrine, and epinephrine may have regulatory roles in ganglionic transmission (p. 342).

The various steps in the release and metabolism of catecholamines are shown in Figure 5–5. Probably most of the released transmitters are taken up by the axon terminals. In addition, two main metabolic pathways are involved. One is deamination by *monoamine oxidase (MOA)*, a relatively nonspecific enzyme that is localized in mitochondria. The other is *catechol-O-methyltransferase (COMT)*, which is located mainly outside the synaptic ending, probably closely associated with the adrenergic receptor. Any norepinephrine that enters the circulation (Fig. 5–5) is metabolized chiefly in the liver, as is epinephrine.

The receptors of the postsynaptic membrane are of special interest. Two types have been described, *alpha* and *beta*. These two types "recognize" norepinephrine and, in certain instances, circulating epinephrine (there is also a dopamine receptor). The *alpha* receptor probably serves a regulatory function; a high level of norepinephrine in the synaptic cleft activates the receptor, which then shuts off further transmitter release. The *beta* receptor initiates the biological response. It activates adenylate cyclase, which then converts the cellular energy carrier ATP to cyclic AMP. The latter then brings about the response of the postjunctional cell, whether that response be contraction or secretion. For exam-

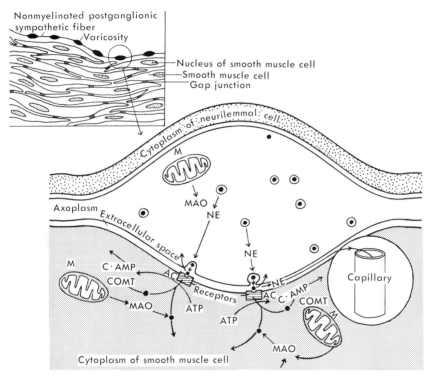

Figure 5–5. Upper left figure: Schematic diagram of a nonmyelinated post-ganglionic sympathetic fiber coursing along a bundle of smooth muscle fibers (the associated neurilemmal sheath is omitted). The axon shows varicosities (see Figure 3–27, p. 52), one of which is shown in the lower figure (but not in solid black). The smooth muscle cells are characterized by gap junctions. The distances between the cells and between the cells and the nerve fiber are exaggerated. *Lower figure*: One of the varicosities is shown forming a synaptic junction with a smooth muscle cell. Norepinephrine (NE) is synthesized in the vesicles by dopamine beta hydroxylase and is then released during exocytosis. The NE then combines with the receptor, and adenylate cyclase (AC) is activated and converts the cellular energy carrier adenosine triphosphate (ATP) to cyclic AMP (C.AMP). The latter then stimulates the biological response. The effects of NE can be prevented by monoamine oxidase (MAO), of mitochondrial origin, or terminated by diffusion to the blood, or by uptake into the varicosity, or, postjunctionally, by being metabolized by MAO or by catechol-O-methyltransferase (COMT). (Modified from Devine, C. E., and Simpson, F. O., in New Z. Med. J., *67*:326–333, 1968. By permission of the authors and publishers.)

ple, in the pineal body, cyclic AMP stimulates the synthesis of the enzyme that catalyzes the conversion of serotonin in the first of a series of steps in the synthesis of melatonin (a hormone that inhibits the activity of the sex glands).

Many drugs are powerful agents in the study of neurotransmitters. For example, it is known that there is a fairly consistent relationship between the biogenic amines and affective or behavioral states in that drugs that depress or inactivate epinephrine synthesis centrally cause sedation or depression, whereas the converse is generally associated with stimulation or excitement. The drug *reserpine* seems to act by releasing norepinephrine from vesicles (it is then deaminated within the terminals) so that endogenous stores of norepinephrine are reduced. This is the basis for the use of reserpine as a depressant or tranquilizer. Antidepressant drugs such as *imipramine* and *chlorpromazine* appear to slow the spontaneous release of norepinephrine, which then accumulates. A build-up of norepinephrine may also occur if monoamine oxidase is inhibited. *Amphetamine,* which is used as a psychic stimulant, has such an action. Table 5–2 indicates some of the drugs that interfere with the various steps in biosynthesis, and whether or not they mimic sympathetic or parasympathetic actions (see also Chapter 15 on the Autonomic Nervous System).

The catecholamine transmitters act peripherally in smooth muscle and cardiac endings and in certain autonomic ganglion cells. In the central nervous system, catecholamine-synthesizing cells comprise an important group in the core of the brain stem, with widespread axonal distribution to the cerebellum, cerebral cortex, and limbic system (p. 390). Within this group, dopamine cells are located in the substantia nigra. Norepinephrine cells are located in the pons and medulla oblongata.

Serotonin (5-HT) is a biogenic amine that stimulates a variety of smooth muscle cells and which, in addition, probably has important functions in a variety of central mechanisms, such as the regulation of sleep and of body temperature (p. 323), and which may be involved in certain behavioral disorders and pathological conditions. Serotonin is known to be synthesized by specific groups of cells in the brain stem (p. 319) and it is probably the transmitter for these cells.

Serotinin is synthesized from the amino acid *tryptophan.* This is hydroxylated to 5-hydroxytryptophan, and this is then decarboxylated to 5-HT.

Amino Acids.   It is likely that acetylcholine and the catecholamines comprise only a small fraction of the transmitters in the central nervous system. It appears more and more certain that various amino acids act as transmitters, and these may be classified as inhibitory and excitatory. The putative inhibitory amino acids are *gamma*-aminobutyric acid (GABA) and glycine. GABA is present in considerable concentration in all regions of the central nervous system. All neurons are sensitive to it, especially

Table 5–2. Actions of Drugs on Synaptic and Neuroeffector Transmission.

Mechanism of Action	System	Drugs	Effect
1. Interference with synthesis of transmitter	Cholinergic	Hemicholinium	Depletion of ACh
	Adrenergic	α-Methyl-p-tyrosine	Depletion of norepinephrine
2. Metabolic transformation by same pathway as precursor of transmitter	Adrenergic	α-Methyldopa (Aldomet)	Displacement of norepinephrine by false transmitter (α-methylnorepinephrine)
3. Blockade of transport system of axonal membrane	Adrenergic	Imipramine, amitriptyline	Accumulation of norepinephrine at extracellular sites
4. Blockade of transport system of storage granule membrane	Adrenergic	Reserpine	Destruction of norepinephrine by mitochondrial MAO, and depletion from adrenergic terminals
5. Displacement of transmitter from axonal terminal	Cholinergic	Carbachol	Cholinomimetic
	Adrenergic (rapid, brief)	Ephedrine, tyramine	Sympathomimetic
	Adrenergic (slow, prolonged)	Guanethidine	Depletion of norepinephrine from adrenergic terminal
6. Prevention of release of transmitter	Cholinergic	Botulinus toxin	Anticholinergic
	Adrenergic	Bretylium	Antiadrenergic
7. Mimicry of transmitter at postsynaptic receptor	Cholinergic Muscarinic Nicotinic	Methacholine Nicotine	Cholinomimetic Cholinomimetic
	Adrenergic Alpha Beta	Phenylephrine Isoproterenol	Sympathomimetic Sympathomimetic
8. Blockade of endogenous transmitter at postsynaptic receptor	Cholinergic Muscarinic Nicotinic	Atropine d-Tubocurarine, hexamethonium	Cholinergic blockade Cholinergic blockade
	Adrenergic Alpha Beta	Phenoxybenzamine Propranolol	α-Adrenergic blockade β-Adrenergic blockade
9. Inhibition of enzymatic breakdown of transmitter	Cholinergic	Anticholinesterase agents (physostigmine, diisopropyl-phosphorofluoridate [DFP])	Cholinomimetic
	Adrenergic	MAO inhibitors (pargyline, nialamide, tranylcypromine)	Accumulation of norepinephrine at certain sites; potentiation of tyramine

(From Koelle, G. B., Anesthesiology, 29:643–653, 1968. By permission of the author and publisher.)

those in the cerebral cortex as well as some in the brain stem. GABA brings about a marked increase in membrane permeability to chloride, it may well act presynaptically, and it is blocked by picrotoxin. GABA is derived from another amino acid, glutamic acid, by decarboxylation. Glycine is probably similar to GABA in increasing chloride permeability, but it probably acts on the postsynaptic membrane.

The putative excitatory amino acids are l-glutamic acid and

l-aspartic acid, both of which have similar excitatory actions that are especially pronounced in the cerebral cortex. The main source of l-glutamic acid is glucose, by way of the citric acid cycle. It is the more powerful of the two transmitters, and there is more of it in the central nervous system than any other amino acid, and more of it there than anywhere else in the body.

Histamine.   Histamine is present in parts of the central nervous system and is derived from the amino acid *histidine.* It has been postulated to be a transmitter, but this has not been proved.

Cyclic AMP and Prostaglandins.   The complexity of synaptic transmission is indicated by the fact that adenylate cyclase and cyclic adenosine monophosphate (cyclic AMP) are important components of the biological responses triggered by synaptic mechanisms, as described above and illustrated in Figure 5–5. Prostaglandins may also play a role. These are a group of closely related substances, all derivatives of the parent compound prostanoic acid. The prostaglandins have widespread and diverse actions. One of the earliest effects observed was stimulation of uterine smooth muscle. A role in synaptic transmission has been postulated, possibly by interaction with the adenyl cyclase-cyclic AMP system. For example, the spontaneous firing of Purkinje cells in the cerebellum may be inhibited by the iontophoretic application of norepinephrine (or cyclic AMP). The simultaneous application of the appropriate prostaglandin inhibits the norepinephrine stimulation of cyclic AMP formation.

SUMMARY

Oxygen consumption in the central nervous system is about 30 times as great as that in resting peripheral nerve or muscle. Glucose and oxygen are the prime sources of energy under normal conditions. All of the enzymatic components of the glycolytic pathway are present in the brain, and the final common pathway is the citric acid cycle. The brain is especially sensitive to oxygen lack and glucose deficiencies.

Lipids are critically important membrane constituents and comprise almost half of the dry weight of the brain. Most of the lipids are cholesterol, sphingolipids, and glycerophospholipids. Interference with the biosynthesis and degradation of the various lipids leads to many neurological disorders, such as demyelinating disorders and hereditary lysosomal storage diseases.

Proteins form nearly 40 per cent of the dry weight of the brain. They function as enzymes, hormones, structural elements, and in transport systems. Of the 20 different amino acids from which proteins are synthesized, a number are putative transmitters, and other putative transmitters are derived from amino acids. Disorders of protein and amino acid metabolism are important causes of many neurological and behavioral disorders, and interference with their functions forms the basis of many drug actions.

Nucleoproteins are conjugated proteins associated with the nucleic acids RNA and DNA, which direct and carry out the metabolic activity of cells.

Vitamins or their derivatives usually function as cofactors for enzymes, and vitamin deficiencies may interfere with neural functions and cause neurological disorders.

The various neurotransmitters are synthesized by enzymes that are synthesized chiefly in cell bodies. The various steps in the total synthetic sequence for a given transmitter begin in the cytoplasm of the cell body and end in the axon terminals, with axoplasmic flow being an essential transport mechanism. The putative transmitters include acetylcholine, the biogenic amines (dopamine, norepinephrine, epinephrine, serotonin), the excitatory amino acids (l-glutamic acid and l-aspartic acid), and the inhibitory amino acids (gamma-aminobutyric acid and glycine). Cyclic AMP and possibly the prostaglandins also seem to have important roles in synaptic transmission.

NAMES IN NEUROLOGY

JOHANN LUDWIG WILHELM THUDICHUM (1829–1901)

Generally called the father of the chemistry of the brain, Thudichum, a London physician of German birth, first practiced medicine and then, in 1864, began the study of what are now called lipochromes or carotinoids. He and his assistants then carried out the first systematic attempts to isolate and characterize the chemical composition of the brain. The results of their work were published in 1884 as *A Treatise on the Chemical Constitution of the Brain Based Throughout Upon Original Researches,* London, Baillière, Tindall & Co. Revised edition, Tübingen, Pietsker, 1901. Thudichum clearly recognized the importance of his contributions, but decades were to elapse before extensive study in the field began again. Thudichum actively practiced medicine (otolaryngology) and later in life he wrote two books, one on cookery and one on wines.

REFERENCES

The following are major texts in neurochemistry and pharmacology.

Albers, R. W., Siegel, G. J., Katzman, R., and Agranoff, B.: Basic Neurochemistry. Boston, Little Brown and Company, 1972. A first-rate presentation, dealing with basic concepts.
Goodman, L. S., and Gilman, A. (Editors): The Pharmacological Basis of Therapeutics. 4th ed. New York, The Macmillan Company, 1970. The definitive work in this field, a superb book.
Hers, H. G. and Van Hoof, F. (Editors): Lysosomes and Storage Disease. New York, Academic Press, 1973. A well-organized, comprehensive account.
McIlwain, H., and Bachelard, H. S.: Biochemistry and the Central Nervous System. 4th ed. Baltimore, The Williams and Wilkins Company, 1971. Edinburgh, Churchill, Livingstone. A detailed treatise on neurochemistry.
Phillis, J. W.: The Pharmacology of Synapses. Oxford, Pergamon Press, 1970. An excellent, relatively short book, clearly written.

Stanbury, J. B., Wyngaarden, J. B., and Frederickson, D. S.: The Metabolic Basis of Inherited Disease. 2nd ed. New York, McGraw-Hill Book Company, 1966. An excellent volume on an important aspect of neurological disorders.
Turner, R., and Richens, A.: Clinical Pharmacology. Baltimore, The Williams and Wilkins Company, 1973. Edinburgh, Churchill, Livingstone. A short, well-written account.

The following are papers and reviews on specific aspects of neurochemistry and neuropharmacology.

Axelrod, J.: Noradrenaline: fate and control of its biosynthesis. Science, *173*:598–606, 1971. The lecture given by Dr. Axelrod in 1970 when he received the Nobel Prize for his work on catecholamine biosynthesis.
Axelrod, J.: Neurotransmitters. Sci. Amer., *230*:58–71, 1974. A fine example of a short scientific review written for the general scientific public by one of the world's leading investigators.
British Medical Bulletin: Catecholamines. vol. *29*, 1973. A collection of excellent, relatively short accounts of various aspects of catecholamine properties and biosynthesis.
Hubbard, J. I., and Quastel, D. M. J.: Micropharmacology of vertebrate neuromuscular transmission. Ann. Rev. Pharmacol., *13*:199–216, 1973.
Krnjević, K.: Chemical nature of synaptic transmission in vertebrates. Physiol. Rev., *54*:418–540, 1974.
McGeer, P. L., and McGeer, E. G.: Neurotransmitter synthetic enzymes. Prog. Neurobiol., 2:69–117, 1973.
Schildkraut, J. J. and Kety, S. S.: Biogenic amines and emotion. Science, *156*:21–30, 1967.

Chapter **6**

SIMPLE NEURONAL CONNECTIONS AND REFLEX ARCS

This chapter is an introduction to the functional organization of neurons, preliminary to more detailed discussions in later chapters. Its purpose is to illustrate the organization of reflex connections in the spinal cord and to emphasize the importance of coordinated excitation and inhibition in reflex activity.

A simple, unconditioned reflex act may be defined as a relatively fixed pattern of response or behavior that is similar for any given stimulus. The pupil of the eye constricts when a light is flashed in the eye. A hand inadvertently set on a hot object is immediately jerked away; the withdrawal is partially completed before pain is felt. A few drops of a weak acid may be placed on the skin of a frog that has had its brain destroyed. The animal attempts to get rid of the irritating agent by making active, coordinated limb movements. These movements do not take place if the spinal cord is destroyed or if the nerves between the cord and the leg have been cut. The pathway consists of afferent nerves by which impulses initiated when receptors are stimulated reach the gray matter of the spinal cord; after synaptic transmission within the cord, impulses leave by way of efferent nerves which transmit them to the appropriate muscles. The total pathway is termed a *reflex path* or *reflex arc* and can function independently of higher centers. This independence, however, is rarely characteristic of normal activity.

TYPES OF REFLEXES

Reflexes are often classified according to the least number of neurons by which their pathways can be represented. Such paths

115

are useful abstractions; however, they rarely, if ever, operate in such isolated form.

Three-Neuron Reflex Arcs. There are a variety of such reflexes, perhaps best exemplified by the reflex withdrawal of a limb in response to a painful stimulus. The impulses travel centrally and are widely distributed within the spinal cord so that, after synapsing with *interneurons (intercalated* or *internuncial neurons),* they activate many motor cells. Thus, reflex flexion at several joints may follow a painful stimulus to a relatively small area of skin. Figure 6–1 illustrates the simplest abstraction of such an excitatory mechanism, specifically, one involving at least three neurons. Three-neuron reflexes may also be initiated by stimulation of receptors in deep tissues (in reflex components of walking) and are the most common type of reflex involving skeletal muscle.

Two-Neuron Reflex Arcs. Certain reflexes may be represented by a pathway of two neurons (Fig. 6–2). Nearly everyone is familiar with the knee jerk, which is elicited by tapping the tendon of the quadriceps femoris muscle just below the patella (knee cap). This stretches the muscle, and the receptors stimulated include *neuromuscular spindles* (described on p. 201). The resulting nerve impulses reach the spinal cord over fibers that synapse with motor neurons in the ventral gray matter. The axons of these cells transmit impulses to the muscle originally lengthened, which then contracts and regains its former length.

This *phasic* type of *stretch* or *myotatic reflex* is a rather restricted or local type of response. In its simplest form, it involves two neurons and, therefore, one area of synaptic junctions. The nerve fibers concerned are large and conduct rapidly. Since there is also a minimum of synaptic delay, the resulting reflexes are among the fastest known. Myotatic reflexes are further characterized by the fact that the motor discharge is mainly restricted to the muscle that was stretched. The knee jerk is called a phasic type of

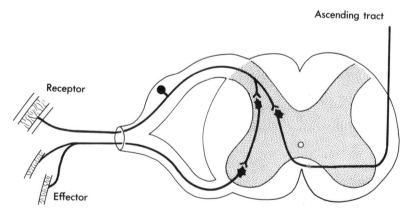

Figure 6–1. Diagram illustrating how impulses from a cutaneous receptor reach an effector (skeletal muscle), by a three-neuron arc involving an interneuron in the gray matter at the level of entrance into the spinal cord. Impulses may also reach the brain by way of an ascending tract.

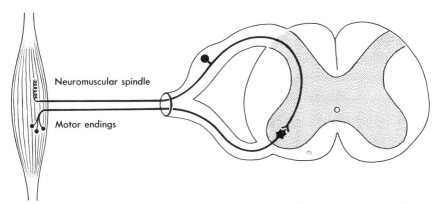

Figure 6–2. Diagram of a two-neuron reflex, from a spindle in a muscle to motor neurons that supply the same muscle.

stretch reflex because the muscle is stretched quickly, and the spindles within it are stimulated at the same time. Consequently, the resulting nerve impulses travel centrally as a synchronous volley, much like a volley from a rifle squad when the rifles are fired simultaneously. The reflex discharges from the spinal cord are likewise in phase, so that muscle fibers are activated at the same time. The result is a quick, reflex muscular contraction, lasting but a short time; hence the term "jerk."

There are also *static* types of stretch reflexes. If a muscle is slowly stretched, varying numbers of spindles are stimulated, some at first and some later as the stretch increases or is maintained. The result is an irregular, or asynchronous, discharge from these endings, much as if the members of a rifle squad were firing in sequence or at random. The reflex motor discharge is likewise asynchronous, and muscle fibers are activated at different times. The result is a more sustained contraction, but one in which at any one time only a relatively few muscle fibers may be in action.

Muscles are stretched when their antagonists contract, and also when joints are flexed as a result of the effect of gravity upon a limb. It is ordinarily held that antigravity muscles are so sensitive to the latter situation that they always exhibit static stretch reflexes, to the extent that they have what is called *postural contraction* or *tone.* It is also held that neurologically controlled tone may be present in muscles which are not strictly postural. However, the presence of such tone under all postural conditions is debatable. A muscle can be so relaxed that no electrical or mechanical activity can be detected. What tone it then possesses is a result of its inherent elasticity and not of neurological mechanisms. Furthermore, in human beings in an upright, comfortable position, with feet fairly well apart, there is little if any electrical or mechanical activity in the antigravity muscles until there is a fairly considerable deviation or flexion (p. 200). In other words, the structure and arrangement of human joints are such that in an upright static position they provide maximum stability. Little if any muscular effort is needed. Reflex mechanisms are of course easily demonstrated upon deviation from the mechanically stable situation. It should be emphasized that most experimental work on stretch reflexes has been carried out on animals such as cats, in which conditions are only partially comparable.

COORDINATION OF REFLEX ARCS

Reflexes are generally much more complicated than the simple abstractions just presented. They occur over the brain stem as well as the spinal cord, often involve smooth muscle and glands as well as striated muscle, and in many instances may be conditioned (p. 427). In intact organisms, the initiating impulses may also traverse fibers that reach the cerebral cortex, where they may be interpreted as sensations. But reflexes are not dependent upon this. A painful stimulus may be followed by a reflex response before the subject experiences pain (or even may occur without the knowledge of pain). Responses may occur after the spinal cord has been severed above the level over which the reflex takes place. Although a subject under general anesthesia feels no pain, reflexes can be elicited by appropriate stimuli, provided that the anesthesia is not too deep.

To the casual observer, a reflex is an apparently simple and relatively isolated mechanism of which the knee jerk is a splendid example. The response is an extension of the leg. But is it so simple? In order for this to happen, the opposing muscles (flexors of the leg) must give way to a degree corresponding to the extension. The flexor muscles relax, the relaxation being brought about by inhibitory mechanisms taking place in the gray matter of the spinal cord. Indeed, nearly every reflex involves coordinated excitatory and inhibitory mechanisms (the various transmitters and synapses involved are discussed on p. 92). The inhibitory mechanism just mentioned is known as *reciprocal inhibition* or *Sherrington's inhibition,* and can be brought about by a variety of central actions. The fibers carrying impulses from muscle receptors enter the spinal cord and, in traversing gray matter toward their synapses with motor neurons, give branches to inhibitory neurons (Fig. 6–3), whose axons synapse with and inhibit the motor neurons supplying flexor muscles. Another way of providing inhibition is through the Renshaw cells, which are activated by the collaterals of motor neurons (Fig. 6–3). The axons of Renshaw cells inhibit adjacent motor neurons. The functional role of Renshaw-cell inhibition is still not clear. Moreover, the Renshaw cell may be inhibited by other interneurons, the net result being excitatory. There are a variety of interneurons, some inhibitory, some excitatory, with varying intraspinal connections. These are discussed in somewhat more detail on pp. 227 and 290.

Let us return to the protective reflex, cited on p. 115, brought

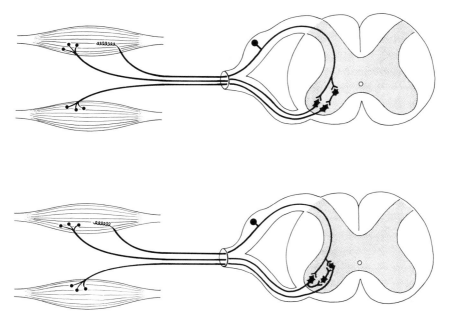

Figure 6-3. *Top:* Schematic representation of a two-neuron reflex with a collateral given to an interneuron which is inhibitory to the motor neuron supplying the antagonistic muscle. *Bottom:* Schematic representation of another mechanism of inhibition, namely the Renshaw cell (p. 125), which is activated by collaterals of motor cells and which in turn is inhibitory to adjacent motor cells. More complicated interneural connections may end in axo-axonal synapses (not shown), where pre-synaptic inhibition may occur. It is also postulated that Renshaw cells may inhibit interneurons; the motor neurons are thereby released from inhibition and appear to be facilitated. (Modified from Wilson, V. J., in Sci. Amer., *214*:102–110, 1966.)

about in a frog by placing a few drops of a weak acid on the skin of its leg. The reflex is complex because a number of muscles are involved in the withdrawal movement. These are supplied by motor fibers from more than one segment of the cord. Therefore, the cells with which the entering dorsal root fibers synapse in turn synapse with motor neurons at the same level and also send axons up and down the cord to motor neurons at other levels (Fig. 6–4). These ipsilateral connections provide for widespread reciprocal responses.

These responses are further complicated by the necessity, in many cases, of contralateral responses. Suppose that a painful stimulus is applied to the bottom of the foot. The entire lower limb may be withdrawn or jerked away. The weight of the body must then be supported by the opposite lower limb whose muscles, therefore, contract strongly. There is an anatomical basis for such a response. In addition to the connections of interneurons cited earlier, axons cross the midline of the spinal cord and reach motor neurons at many levels (Fig. 6–5). Motor impulses thus reach muscles in the opposite limb; this again is accompanied by the necessary reciprocal inhibition.

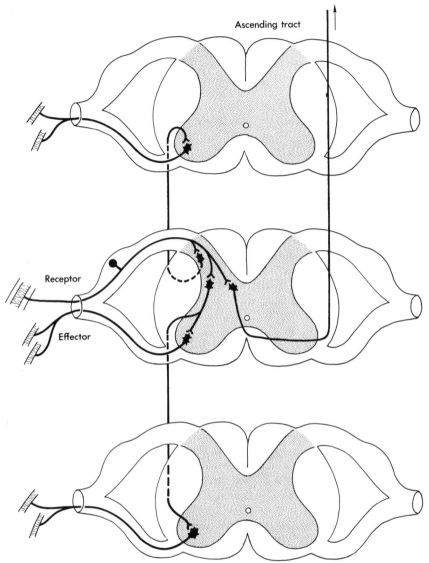

Figure 6–4. Diagram of the connections by which impulses from a receptor reach motor neurons at different cord levels. This accounts for multisegmental, ipsilateral responses.

These examples illustrate the remarkable degree of coordination of two equally significant interacting mechanisms, namely, excitation and inhibition. When one group of muscles contracts, certain other muscles must either contract or relax to a like degree. This may be a local reflex activity or it may be a part of "voluntary" muscular activity (p. 197).

Reflexes are not as invariable as the definition of a reflex would indicate. For instance, receptors (or their parent fibers) may be stimulated so that a muscle reflexly contracts. But when the stimulation stops and impulses can no longer be recorded from the sensory nerve fibers, the muscle may continue to contract for many milliseconds during which time impulses can be recorded from the motor nerve fibers. This is an *after-discharge.* The branching of entering fibers is such that impulses can traverse paths containing varying numbers of interneurons and thus reach motor neurons at different times, thereby providing for a succession of discharges from them. Furthermore, it has been postulated that some of the interneurons in the gray matter form closed circuits that can continue to excite a motor neuron after impulses have ceased entering the cord (Fig. 6–6). The

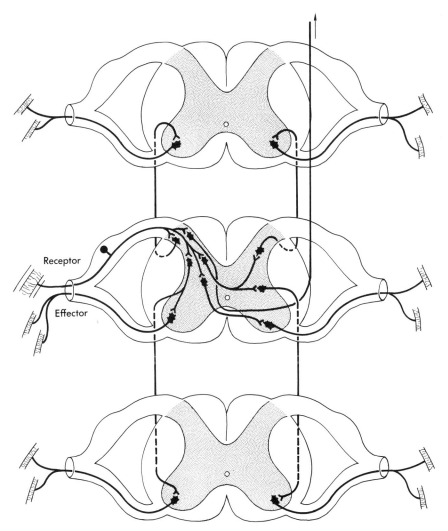

Figure 6–5. Diagram of the connections by which impulses from a receptor reach motor neurons at various levels on both sides of the spinal cord. This accounts for multisegmental, ipsilateral, and contralateral responses.

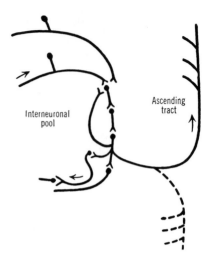

Figure 6–6. Diagram of an interneuronal pool. Connections are such that an ascending tract may convey impulses derived from several afferent fibers, each of which impinges on the closed circuit. Arrows indicate direction of conduction.

multiple and closed circuits just outlined may be characteristic of gray matter throughout the central nervous system. The degree to which afferent fibers overlap in making synapses with interneurons and motor neurons provides another basis for variability. Figure 6–7 illustrates how reflexes elicited by stimulation of different afferent fibers may either summate or become occluded.

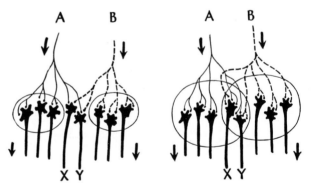

Figure 6–7. Diagram illustrating facilitation (*left*) and occlusion (*right*). It is arbitrarily assumed that impulses at two synaptic junctions are necessary to stimulate a motor neuron. *Left:* Afferent fiber *A* forms two junctions with each motor neuron in the encircled field, but only one each with motor neurons *X* and *Y*. An impulse over *A* therefore causes three neurons to discharge. The same situation obtains for *B*. But if impulses arrive over *A* and *B* simultaneously, not only will the six encircled neurons discharge, but also *X* and *Y*, since these will have two active junctions each. The reflex response will be greater than could be postulated from the result of stimulating *A* and *B* separately. *Right:* Afferent fiber *A* forms two junctions with each of five motor neurons, as does *B*. But *X* and *Y* are common to both, so that impulses over *A* and *B* simultaneously cause 8, and not 10, neurons to discharge. The reflex response is less than could be postulated from the result of stimulating *A* or *B* separately.

Finally, it should be emphasized that the interneurons and their various patterns of connections are influenced by impulses arriving over descending pathways as well as by those entering over sensory fibers. These descending impulses, which can vary the level of excitability, are discussed in the chapters on motor and sensory pathways (pp. 197 and 220), and also those on the spinal cord and brain stem (pp. 287 and 300).

REFLEXES AND BEHAVIOR

It might seem justified to consider the reflex arc a basic unit of the nervous system. The isolation and study of clear-cut reflexes would support the concept that the nervous system is composed of a series of such arcs, integrated and controlled by higher centers. Indeed, such a concept is commonly encountered. But can we really conceive of the nervous system as a mass of stereotyped patterns? The answer is no. The reflex should be regarded as a local, highly-differentiated mechanism, the study of which affords little insight into higher-level functions.

The concept that the reflex arc is the basic unit of the nervous system arose in part because of the supposition that reflexes are the first recognizable patterns to appear in the embryo. There are, however, no anatomical or physiological data that adequately support this hypothesis. Rather, it seems more likely that the basic organization of the nervous system develops according to a genetically programmed pattern, and that the first activity to occur in the embryo may result from spontaneous discharges of motor neurons, before or independent of the appearance of reflex connections. These matters are discussed further in Chapter 9, on the development of the human nervous system.

CLINICAL VALUE OF REFLEXES

Reflexes are important in clinical practice, because an examination of them may yield information about the nature and location of neurological disorders. In relation to clinical testing, reflexes are often classified as superficial, deep, special, and abnormal.

Superficial reflexes are those elicited by cutaneous stimulation. If the skin of the abdominal wall is scratched, the abdominal muscles contract. The toes flex if the sole of the foot is scratched. These responses are of the three-neuron or flexor type.

Deep reflexes are elicited by tapping a tendon and are of the stretch or myotatic type. Those commonly tested are the *ankle jerk,* by tapping the tendo calcaneus (Achilles tendon, p. 124), with resulting plantar flexion of the foot; the *knee jerk,* by tapping the quadriceps femoris tendon just below the patella, the leg extending; the *biceps jerk,* by tapping the biceps brachii tendon and obtaining a flexion of the forearm; and the *triceps jerk,* by tapping the tendon of the triceps brachii muscle, the forearm extending.

Special reflexes involve structures other than skeletal muscles. When a light is flashed upon the eye, the diameter of the pupil lessens, thus restricting the amount of light which can enter the organ. Some of the more important special reflexes are discussed in Chapters 14 and 15.

Abnormal or *pathological reflexes* are those not present normally or are exaggerations of normal ones. Disorders of the spinal cord or higher centers are the common causes, and the reasons for them are discussed in Chapter 10.

SUMMARY

In reflex mechanisms, nerve impulses from the periphery reach the central nervous system and are then relayed back to the periphery, where a response occurs. Receptors, central connections, neuroeffector junctions, and effectors are parts of reflex arcs.

The simplest of these are two-neuron arcs for stretch or myotatic reflexes, and three-neuron arcs for flexor or superficial reflexes.

Reflex responses involve not only contractions, but also relaxations, of opposing muscles. A number of muscles may be involved in or be subsidiary to a reflex. Ipsilateral and contralateral connections within the cord provide for these.

Reflexes are local, highly differentiated mechanisms that are unconditional, and which are not to be regarded as the basic developmental units of the nervous system.

The clinical examination of reflexes may enable one to determine the nature and location of neurological disorders.

NAMES IN NEUROLOGY

ACHILLES, SON OF PELEUS AND THETIS

Legend has it that Thetis dipped the child Achilles in the waters of the River Styx, and that he became invulnerable except in that part of the heel by which she held him. From this arises the proverbial term, "heel of Achilles." It was here that he later received a mortal wound during the siege of Troy. The tendo calcaneus, by which the calf muscles attach to the calcaneus or heel bone, is termed the *tendo Achillis* (this synonym was first used in 1693, according to J. H. Couch, Canad. Med. Assoc. J., *34*:688, 1938), and the reflex elicited by tapping this tendon is the Achilles reflex.

BIRDSEY RENSHAW (1911–1948)

In a classic paper published in 1948, Renshaw described the electrophysiological properties of interneurons in the spinal cord that are excited by antidromic activation of motor axons. (Forbes, A.: Birdsey Renshaw, J. Neurophysiol., *12*:81, 1948).

SIR CHARLES SCOTT SHERRINGTON (1857–1952)

There is scarcely a phase of neurophysiology in which this noted English physiologist was not a pioneer or a leading investigator. A few of his most important contributions are studies of muscular rigidity, reciprocal innervation, physiology of synapses, many types of reflexes, the activity of the cerebral cortex, and functions of the inner ear. In his famous book *The Integrative Action of the Nervous System* (New Haven, 1906), he introduced new and far-reaching concepts of nervous function, in the course of which he discussed in detail the synapse and transmission across it. It is difficult to do justice to the extent of his contributions to our understanding of the nervous system. So much that is known today can be traced to an original work by Sir Charles that one can do no more than state that this is the situation. He was as pre-eminent in neurophysiology as Jackson was in clinical neurology and Ramón y Cajal in neuroanatomy.

REFERENCES

For discussions of structure and function of reflex arcs see those references cited on pp. 159 and 219.

Riss, W. (editor): Do Renshaw Cells Exist? Brain, Behav., Evol., *4*:1–96, 1971. This issue consists of two excellent and important papers, one by W. D. Willis and the other by M. E. and A. B. Scheibel, which present differing views of the Renshaw cell.

Chapter 7

THE HUMAN BRAIN
AND SPINAL CORD

During the course of development in the embryo, the central nervous system becomes a tubular structure, and this tubular arrangement is present in the adult, although in a considerably modified form (Chapters 2 and 9).

The brain and spinal cord are protected by the *skull,* the *vertebrae,* and their ligamentous connections. The brain occupies the cranial cavity in the interior of the skull. This cavity is commonly of 1200 to 1500 ml capacity. There are numerous openings or *foramina* in the base of the skull for blood vessels and nerves. Through an especially large one, the *foramen magnum,* the medulla oblongata of the brain is continuous with the spinal cord (Fig. 7–1).

The vertebrae are irregularly shaped bones joined so as to form a long column. Each vertebra has a heavy body from which an arch extends backward, enclosing a large opening, the *vertebral foramen.* The vertebrae are arranged so that the foramina form a continuous channel, the *vertebral canal.* The spinal cord occupies the vertebral canal and extends from the foramen magnum to about the level of the first or second lumbar vertebra. There are lateral openings between the vertebrae, the *intervertebral foramina,* through which nerves and blood vessels run.

Seven *cervical* vertebrae are present in the neck; twelve *thoracic* vertebrae in the chest or thorax; five *lumbar* vertebrae in the abdomen, a *sacrum* and a *coccyx* in the pelvis (the sacrum develops before birth as five sacral vertebrae that later fuse into a single bone, and the coccyx is a small bone that represents several vertebral segments).

The brain and spinal cord are surrounded and protected by three layers of non-nervous tissue collectively called *meninges.* From without inward, these are the *dura mater (pachymeninx),* the

126

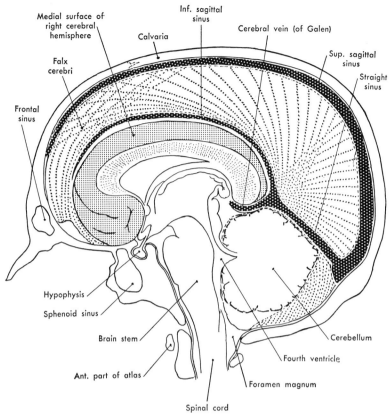

Figure 7-1. Diagram of a median section of skull and brain showing relationship of various parts of brain to skull and dura mater. The falx cerebri and its contained sinuses are also shown in Figure 7-2. Veins in the cerebral hemispheres empty into the sinuses. Blood flows posteriorly and, from the junction of straight sinus and superior sagittal sinus, is carried by other sinuses (not shown) to the internal jugular veins.

arachnoid, and the *pia mater.* The last two are known as the *leptomeninges.* The dura mater (Figs. 7-1 and 7-2) is a tough fibrous membrane that is lined on its inner aspect by flat cells. When bone is removed preparatory to entering the cranial cavity, the dura mater is the first meningeal layer to be encountered. The dura mater serves as the periosteum for the inner aspect of the cranial bones. In certain regions the dura mater contains venous channels or *sinuses* that carry venous blood from the brain to veins in the neck and thence to the heart. In the vertebral canal, the dura mater is separated from bone by an interval, the *epidural space,* which contains fat and many small veins. A comparable space is not found in the cranial cavity except when artificially produced, for example, by bleeding between skull and dura mater after trauma (p. 147).

The arachnoid, which lies just internal to the dura mater, is a thin membrane of reticular fibers; its outer and inner aspects are

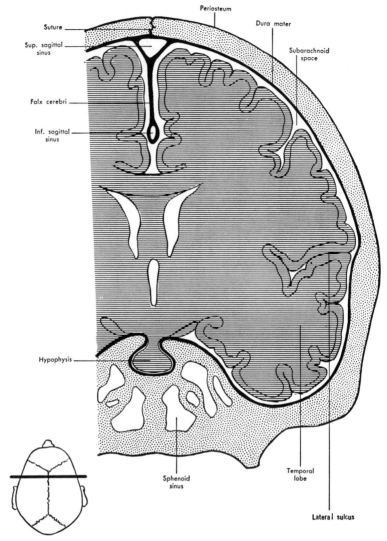

Figure 7–2. Diagram of a coronal section of skull and brain, showing certain features of the dura mater (the arachnoid and pia mater are not shown). The small figure shows the plane of section. Note that the dura mater forms a fold (falx cerebri) between the cerebral hemispheres, and contains two venous sinuses. This plane is at right angles to that of Figure 7–1. Note also that the dura mater is continuous through the suture with periosteum on the outer surface of the skull.

lined by flat and oval cells. The potential space between the arachnoid and the dura mater is termed the *subdural space.* Immediately around the brain and spinal cord is the pia mater, which is connected to the arachnoid by a fine network of connective tissue trabeculae. The pia mater is a delicate membrane of reticular and elastic fibers that is closely applied to the brain and spinal cord. The outer part of the pia mater is more loosely arranged and contains the blood vessels that supply the brain and spinal cord. The space between the arachnoid and the pia mater, the *subarachnoid space,* contains the extraventricular cerebrospinal fluid. The subarachnoid space is shallow over the convexity of the brain, but at the base of the brain and in the lateral sulci is arranged into capacious spaces termed *cisterns.*

THE BRAIN

The brain, which is also known as the *cerebrum* or *encephalon,* consists of the forebrain, midbrain, and hindbrain. As described in Chapters 2 and 9, the forebrain is subdivided into the telencephalon and the diencephalon. Most of the telencephalon forms the two *cerebral hemispheres* that in turn form the bulk of the brain. The midbrain is also known as the mesencephalon. The hindbrain is subdivided into the pons, medulla oblongata, and cerebellum. The term brain stem refers to the midbrain, pons, and medulla oblongata, and often includes the diencephalon as well. These regions collectively form a stem or stalk between the expanded cerebral hemispheres and the spinal cord.

The cavity of the embryonic neural tube persists in the adult brain and spinal cord as the ventricles and the central canal.

Cerebral Hemispheres. The huge size of the hemispheres relative to the rest of the brain is due, in humans as in most other primates, to the massive development of neocortex and of cortical and subcortical regions concerned with motor, sensory, and higher mental functions.

A prominent longitudinal fissure partially separates the two hemispheres. This fissure is occupied by a downward projection or fold of dura mater, the *falx cerebri.* When the arachnoid and pia mater are removed, it is seen that the hemispheres are folded or convoluted. The convolutions are called *gyri;* the depressions or intervals between gyri, *sulci.* Most gyri and sulci are named, and the more constant of these are shown in Figures 7–3 to 7–8.

Thus, between the *central sulcus* and *precentral sulcus* is the precentral gyrus, a region concerned in motor activities. There is considerable individual variation in size, shape, and position of gyri and sulci, and none can be identified with certainty unless arachnoid and pia mater are removed.

Some sulci divide the hemispheres into separate parts called *lobes.* Each lobe supposedly has specific functions. To a certain extent this is true; the occipital lobe, for example, is concerned with vision. However, the assignment of clear-cut functional properties to lobes may be quite arbitrary. The lobes are shown in Figure 7–4. The *frontal lobe* is in front of the central sulcus, the *parietal lobe* behind it and above the lateral sulcus. The *temporal lobe* is below the lateral sulcus. The *occipital lobe* is posterior to temporal and parietal lobes, but there is usually no definite sulcus

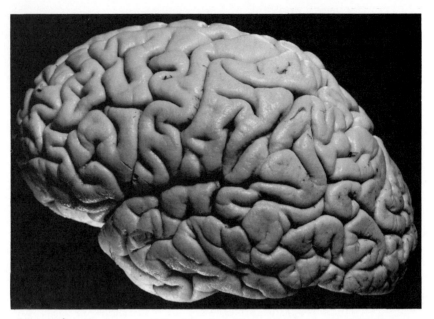

Figure 7-3. Photograph of the lateral surface of human cerebral hemisphere. The cerebellum and hindbrain have been removed by a section through the midbrain, and the arachnoid and pia mater have been stripped from the surface of the hemisphere.

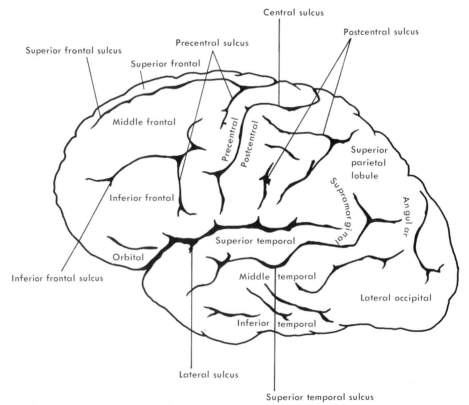

Figure 7-4. Outline sketch of the lateral surface of the cerebral hemisphere shown in Figure 7-3. The gyri are directly labeled (except the superior frontal) and the sulci are indicated by leaders.

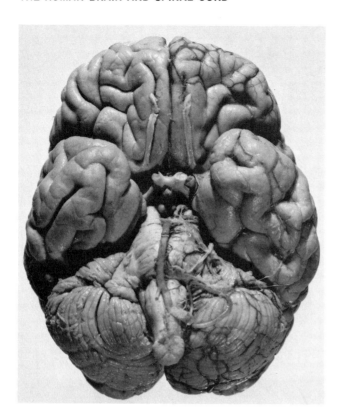

Figure 7-5. Photograph of the inferior aspect of the brain. The arachnoid and pia mater have been removed from the right half. (From Gardner, E., Gray, D. J., and O'Rahilly, R.: Anatomy. 4th ed. Philadelphia, W. B. Saunders Company, 1975.)

separating them on the lateral surface of the hemisphere. Figures 7–9 and 7–10 show the medial aspect of the hemisphere and the major sulci and gyri.

The two hemispheres are united by several bands (commis-

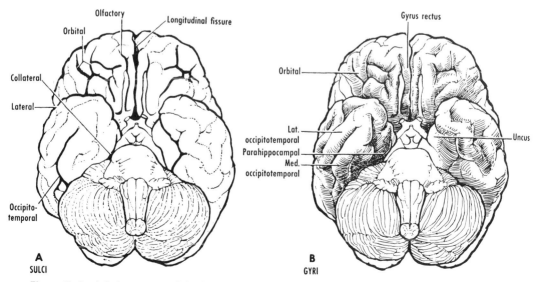

Figure 7-6. Inferior aspect of the brain shown in Figure 7–5. A shows the sulci; B shows the gyri. (From Gardner, E., Gray, D. J., and O'Rahilly, R.: Anatomy. 4th ed. Philadelphia, W. B. Saunders Company, 1975.)

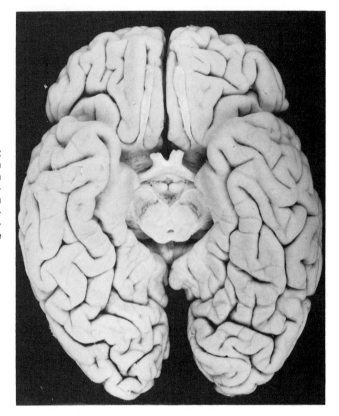

Figure 7–7. The inferior aspect of the brain with the brain stem removed by a section through the midbrain. (Photograph number 3 from Bossy, J.: Atlas du Système Nerveux. Paris, Editions Offidoc., 1971. Reproduced by permission of the author and the publisher.)

sures) of nerve fibers that cross the median plane. The most prominent of these is the *corpus callosum* (Fig. 7–14).

The diencephalon is formed by the thalamus, and just below it, the hypothalamus (Figs. 7–9, 7–10, 7–14, and 7–15).

Base of Brain. The nerves connected to the brain, and the arteries supplying it, enter or leave from below, that is, from the inferior or ventral aspect. Hence the brain must be removed and its base studied. Figures 7–5 to 7–8 show the base of the brain, including the brain stem and parts of the frontal, temporal, and occipital lobes.

All of the cranial nerves are attached to the base of the brain, from the base of each of the frontal lobes to the medulla oblongata. These nerves are discussed in Chapter 8.

Also at the base of the brain is the *circulus arteriosus (circle of Willis),* formed by communications between branches of the internal carotid and basilar arteries, and from which branches are distributed to the brain.

Midbrain. The front of the midbrain is formed by the two *cerebral peduncles,* which contain nerve tracts connecting the cerebrum with brain stem and spinal cord (Fig. 7–11). On the posterior surface of the midbrain are four rounded eminences. The upper two are the *superior colliculi,* the lower two the *inferior* *colliculi.* The posterior limit of the diencephalon, at the junction of the diencephalon and midbrain, is marked by a small, oval body, the *pineal body* or *epiphysis,* which is attached to the brain stem in the median plane, just above the superior colliculi. The pineal body often becomes calcified with advancing age, and hence more radio-opaque. It thereby becomes visible in radiograms and thus serves as a useful landmark or reference point in interpreting radiograms of the brain and skull.

Pons and Medulla Oblongata. The midbrain continues below into a massive, rounded structure, the pons, which serves in part as a bridge or connection between the two cerebellar hemispheres. The pons continues below into the medulla oblongata, which in turn continues into the spinal cord, the junction being at the level of the foramen magnum. The front of the medulla oblongata is marked by the longitudinally directed *anterior median fissure,* on each side of which is an elevation, the *pyramid.* Lateral to the upper part of each pyramid, and separated from it by the *anterior lateral sulcus,* is an ovoid elevation, the *olive.*

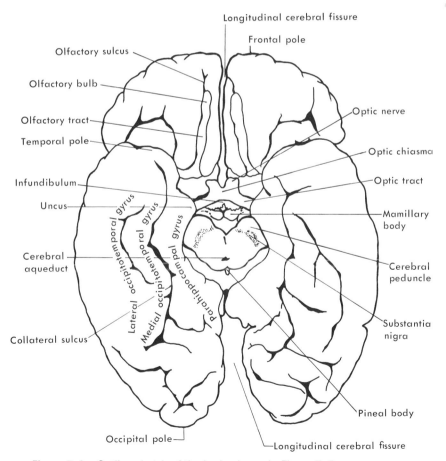

Figure 7-8. Outline sketch of the brain shown in Figure 7-7.

Two vertebral arteries enter the cranial cavity through the foramen magnum, ascend in front of the medulla oblongata, and unite to form the basilar artery. This in turn ascends in front of pons and midbrain and ends by dividing into the two posterior cerebral arteries, which enter the circulus arteriosus (Fig. 7–21).

Cerebellum. The cerebellum is a deeply fissured structure behind the brain stem, formed of two hemispheres connected by a median portion, the *vermis.* The cerebellum is connected to the brain stem by paired peduncles, whose position and direction are shown in Figure 7–11. The *superior cerebellar peduncles* connect the cerebellum and the midbrain, the *middle cerebellar peduncles* connect the cerebellum and the pons, and the *inferior cerebellar peduncles* connect the cerebellum and the medulla oblongata.

The Ventricular System. Figures 7–9, 7–10, and 7–14 to 7–18 show some of the parts of the ventricular system. Figure 7–12 shows a cast of the ventricles, and Figure 7–13 two pneumo-encephalograms (p. 157). There is a *lateral ventricle* in the interior of each cerebral hemisphere. Each lateral ventricle joins the front end of the *third ventricle* by an *interventricular foramen.* The third ventricle is a narrow space within the diencephalon. Posteriorly it is continuous with the *cerebral aqueduct* (*aqueduct of Sylvius*). The aqueduct is a narrow channel within the midbrain, continuous below with the *fourth ventricle,* between

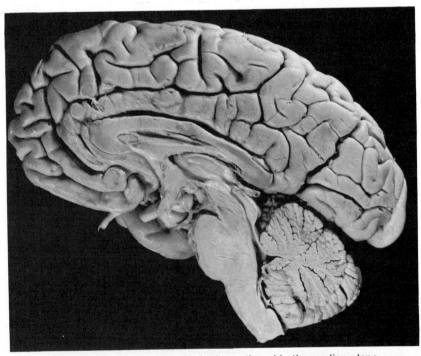

Figure 7-9. Photograph of a brain sectioned in the median plane.

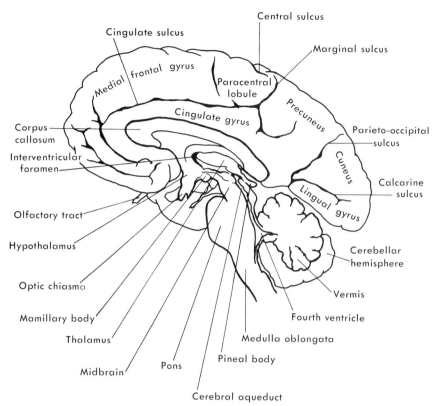

Figure 7–10. Outline sketch of the brain shown in Figure 7–9. The gyri are labeled directly and the sulci and other structures are indicated by leaders.

the cerebellum behind, and pons and medulla oblongata in front. The fourth ventricle continues below into a narrow channel, the *central canal,* which is present in the lower part of the medulla oblongata and throughout the length of the spinal cord.

Below the cerebellum, the fourth ventricle is roofed by a thin membrane in which there is an opening, the *median aperture,* by means of which the ventricle communicates with the subarachnoid space. A *lateral aperture* on each side also provides a communication between the fourth ventricle and the subarachnoid space. The ventricles and central canal are lined by *ependyma,* a single layer of cells that are often ciliated. In the lateral, third, and fourth ventricles there are complex tufts of small blood vessels and ependymal cells which form the *choroid plexuses.* These plexuses are concerned with the formation of cerebrospinal fluid. This fluid circulates through the ventricles, enters the subarachnoid space, and is eventually absorbed into the venous system (p. 152).

The floor of the fourth ventricle is formed by the pons and medulla oblongata (Fig. 8–3). There is, in the median plane, a *median sulcus,* lateral to which are various elevations. Below

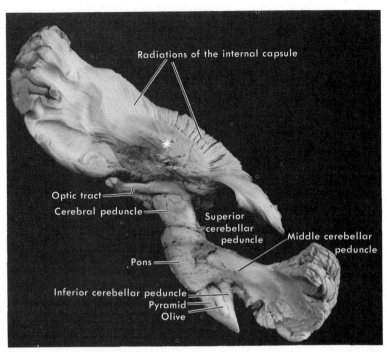

Figure 7-11. Photograph of the left lateral aspect of the human brain stem dissected so as to show the internal capsule and the cerebellar peduncles. Only a small part of the superior cerebellar peduncle is visible because it lies on the dorsal aspect of the brain stem. ✳ indicates the mass formed by the putamen and globus pallidus lateral to the internal capsule.

the lower end of the fourth ventricle are two elevations on each side of the median plane, the *fasciculus gracilis* and *fasciculus cuneatus,* marking nerve tracts ascending from the spinal cord.

Gray and White Matter of the Brain.   If a cerebral hemisphere is cut into slices (Figs. 7–14 and 7–15), certain structural features are evident. The cortex, in fresh brains, is grayish in appearance, and is accordingly termed gray matter, in contrast to white matter. Gray matter is composed largely of glial cells and bodies of nerve cells, whereas white matter is formed largely by processes or fibers of nerve cells (p. 44). Figures 7–14 and 7–15 also show that the interior of the hemispheres is composed partly of white matter, and partly of well demarcated areas of gray matter known collectively as *basal nuclei* or *basal ganglia.* In each hemisphere, these masses of gray matter form a medial and a lateral group, which are separated by a band of white matter known as the *internal capsule.* Each internal capsule emerges from the base of the brain as a cerebral peduncle; it contains nerve fibers which connect the medial and lateral groups of basal ganglia. These interconnecting fibers give the region a striated appearance, and the connected structures are collectively termed the *corpus striatum.*

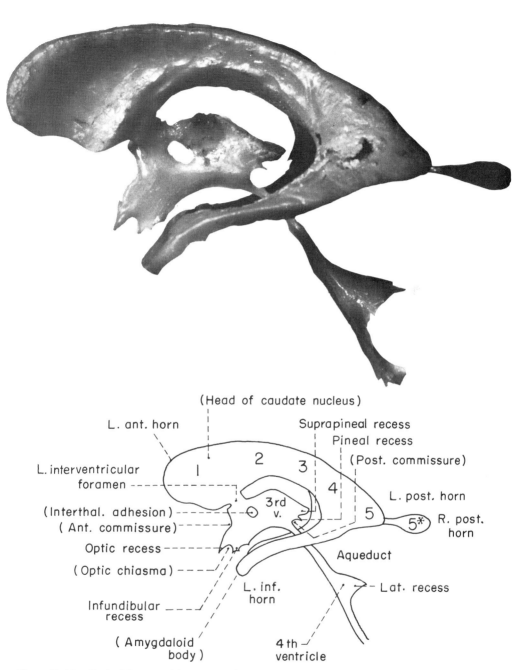

Figure 7–12. Cast of the ventricles of the brain, left lateral aspect. The key diagram below shows the various parts of the ventricular system; related, solid structures are indicated in parentheses. In this brain, the right posterior horn is considerably longer than the left. The numbers indicated for the lateral ventricle refer to parts of the lateral ventricle, each of which has different relationships. (From Gardner, E., Gray, D. J., and O'Rahilly, R.: Anatomy. 4th ed. Philadelphia, W. B. Saunders Company, 1975. Courtesy of Dr. David Tompsett, Royal College of Surgeons of England, London.)

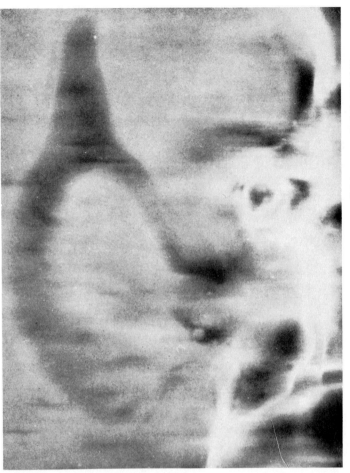

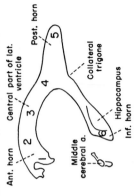

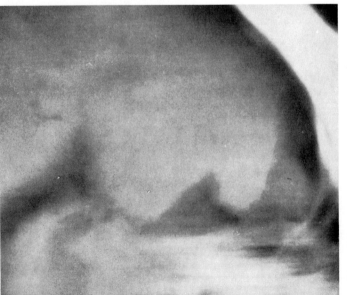

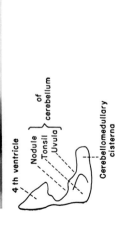

Figure 7-13.   See opposite page for legend.

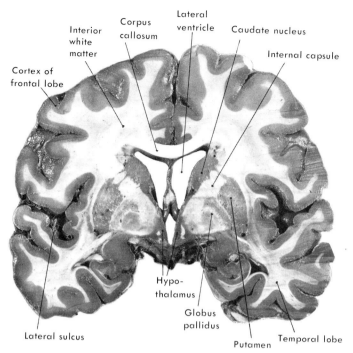

Figure 7–14. Photograph of a coronal slice of brain, stained by a Berlin blue reaction that accentuates the gray matter and leaves white matter relatively unstained.

Figure 7–16 illustrates a slice through the midbrain. There are two masses of gray matter in an intermediate position. In the fresh condition, they are pinkish and are accordingly named the *red nuclei.* Just in front of each nucleus, in the cerebral peduncle, is an area, the *substantia nigra,* in which the nerve cells contain the pigment melanin.

Figures 7–17 and 7–18 are slices of pons and medulla oblongata. These show that white matter is found anteriorly; mixtures of white and gray matter, the *reticular formation,* are intermediate; and gray matter is next to cerebral aqueduct, fourth ventricle, and central canal.

The slices shown in Figures 7–17 and 7–18 include parts of the cerebellum. As is true of the cerebral cortex, the cortex of the

Figure 7–13. Pneumo-encephalographic tomograms. *Left:* Pneumoencephalographic tomogram showing the fourth ventricle. A key diagram is situated below the photograph. *Right:* Tomogram showing the lateral ventricle of one side. The anterior horn is only partially filled. A key diagram is located below the photograph. (From Gardner, E., Gray, D. J., and O'Rahilly, R.: Anatomy, 4th ed. Philadelphia, W. B. Saunders Company, 1975. Courtesy of G. DiChiro, M.D.: An Atlas of Detailed Normal Pneumoencephalographic Anatomy, 1961, and Charles C Thomas, Publisher, Springfield, Illinois.)

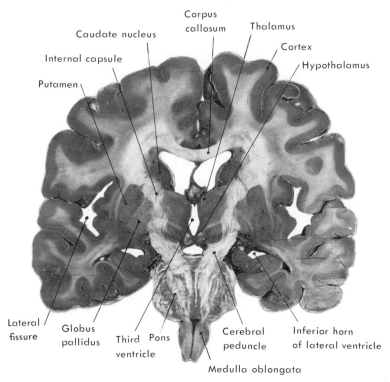

Corpus callosum
Thalamus
Caudate nucleus
Cortex
Internal capsule
Hypothalamus
Putamen
Lateral fissure
Globus pallidus
Third ventricle
Pons
Cerebral peduncle
Inferior horn of lateral ventricle
Medulla oblongata

Figure 7–15. Photograph of a coronal slice of brain, posterior to that of Figure 7–14, and stained by the same method. This is in approximately the same plane and same region as the microscopic sections of Figures 17–6 and 17–7 (pp. 383 and 384).

cerebellum is composed of gray matter. The cerebellar peduncles and the interior of the cerebellum are composed of white matter. But within the interior of the cerebellum, in and near the roof of the fourth ventricle, are paired masses of gray matter, among which are the *dentate nuclei* (Fig. 7–18) and several others known collectively as *roof nuclei.*

Figure 7–16. Transverse slice of midbrain. Staining as for Figure 7–14.

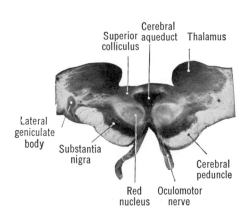

Cerebral aqueduct
Superior colliculus
Thalamus
Lateral geniculate body
Substantia nigra
Red nucleus
Oculomotor nerve
Cerebral peduncle

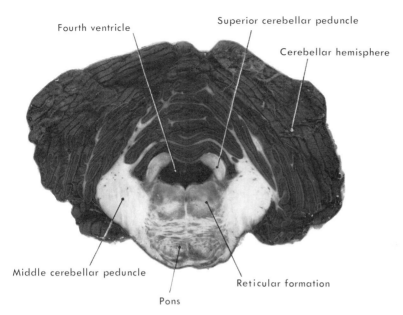

Figure 7–17. Transverse slice of pons and cerebellum. Staining method as for Figure 7–14.

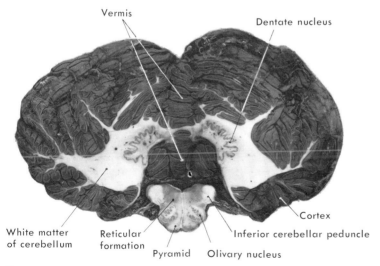

Figure 7–18. Transverse slice of medulla oblongata and cerebellum. Staining method as for Figure 7–14.

THE SPINAL CORD

Figure 7–19 shows the brain and spinal cord, with attached spinal nerves. It illustrates the general shape and length of the spinal cord, which does not occupy the whole length of the verte-

Figure 7–19. The brain and spinal cord with attached roots and ganglia, based on a dissection by Dr. M. C. E. Hutchinson, Department of Anatomy, Guy's Hospital Medical School. Note the relative sizes of the cerebral and cerebellar hemispheres. The longitudinal cerebral fissure, which separates the two cerebral hemispheres, contains the falx cerebri. The horizontal cleft between the occipital lobes and the cerebellum is occupied by the tentorium cerebelli. Note the changing obliquity of the spinal roots in their craniocaudal progression. Their attachment to the spinal cord partially obscures the cervical and lumbar enlargements, the extents of which are approximately indicated on the left side. The cauda equina is undisturbed on the right side and has been fanned out on the left to facilitate identification of its individual components. The labels on the right indicate the first cervical, first thoracic, first lumbar, and first sacral nerves. (From Warwick, R., and Williams, P. L., editors: Gray's Anatomy. 35th British edition. Philadelphia, W. B. Saunders Company, 1973.)

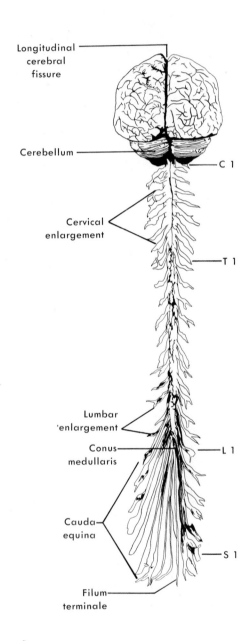

bral canal, but rather ends at the level of the lower part of the first lumbar vertebra or the upper part of the second. Below this level the vertebral canal is occupied by meninges, including subarachnoid space, and nerve roots. A thin, fibrous strand, the *filum terminale,* continues downward from the spinal cord as a prolongation of the pia mater. Below, it is fused with the dura and continues to the back of the coccyx.

In the median plane the spinal cord shows posteriorly, a slight longitudinal groove, the *posterior median sulcus.* A continuous series of nerves, the *dorsal roots,* enters the *posterior lateral sulcus* of the spinal cord at regular intervals (Fig. 7–20). A *posterior intermediate sulcus* is commonly present between the lateral and median sulci, in the upper half of the spinal cord. A variable number of small arteries and veins is present on the posterior surface of the cord. In the cervical region the arteries are usually present as a *posterior spinal artery* on each side.

Anteriorly, in the median plane, the spinal cord has an anterior median fissure, occupied by the *anterior spinal artery,* and one or two small veins. *Ventral roots* leave at regular intervals from the anterolateral region of the spinal cord.

The spinal cord has *cervical* and *lumbar enlargements,* corresponding to the attachments of dorsal and ventral roots supplying the limbs. The collection of roots in the spinal canal below the spinal cord resembles the tail of a horse, hence the name *cauda equina* given to this collection.

A slice through any level of the spinal cord reveals a characteristic structure (Fig. 7–20). In contrast to the cerebral hemispheres, gray matter is found in the interior, surrounded by white

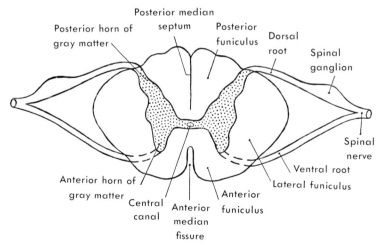

Figure 7–20. Transverse section of spinal cord, showing spinal roots and arrangement of white and gray matter. Note that a septum continues inward from the posterior median sulcus to divide the white matter into two posterior funiculi. Compare with Figure 13–2 (p. 289).

matter. The gray matter is arranged somewhat like the letter H, with
anterior and *posterior horns,* and a connecting bar of gray matter.
A *lateral horn* is also present in the thoracic part of the spinal
cord. The central canal lies in the connecting bar. Not uncommon-
ly, in the adult, the canal is obliterated at various levels.

The spinal cord is generally referred to as *segmental* in organization (see p. 10), and the longitudinal extent of spinal cord
to which a pair of right and left spinal roots is attached constitutes
a segment of the spinal cord.

Nerve fibers leaving the anterior horns enter ventral roots.
Nerve fibers of dorsal roots, entering the spinal cord at the posterior lateral sulcus, reach the posterior horns.

The white matter of the spinal cord is arranged into *funiculi.*
A septum extending inward from the posterior median sulcus
divides the white matter into two *posterior funiculi.* In the upper
half of the spinal cord, and especially in the cervical region, a
thin septum extending inward from each posterior intermediate
sulcus divides each posterior funiculus into a laterally placed
fasciculus cuneatus and a medially placed *fasciculus gracilis.*
These are continuous with the corresponding fasciculi of the
medulla oblongata.

Each *lateral funiculus* is the white matter between dorsal and
ventral root fibers. Each *anterior funiculus* is the white matter
between the ventral root fibers of that side and the anterior median
fissure.

The white matter of the spinal cord contains nerve tracts
connecting dorsal and ventral root fibers with various parts of
the spinal cord, and with the brain. The gray matter contains
cells concerned with sensory impulses, with the activity of muscles, and with the functions of various viscera, glands, and blood
vessels.

BLOOD SUPPLY

ANATOMICAL DISTRIBUTION

The blood vascular system is designed to bring blood to or
away from the *capillaries,* which are usually 10 μm or less in
diameter and which are tubes composed of endothelial cells.
All exchanges between blood and cells take place through the
endothelial cells of these tiny vessels. The *arteries,* which proceed from the heart, distribute blood to various large regions of
the body. The smallest of the arteries (*arterioles*) are highly contractile and are thus able to regulate the amount of blood entering
a given region or organ. The capillaries themselves may also open
or close and thus affect the amount of blood circulating in an area.
From the capillaries, blood enters small vessels, the *venules.*
These in turn form larger vessels, the *veins,* by which the blood is
ultimately returned to the heart. The number of capillaries in the

body is so great that, if all were open at once, there would not be enough blood to fill them. In any given structure, such as a muscle, most capillaries are closed except during marked activity. In certain parts of the body, notably skin and intestine, direct anastomoses between arterioles and venules are common. These *arteriovenous anastomoses* bypass the capillary circulation. If open, they shunt blood past a given capillary network and thereby prevent exchange from occurring or, in the case of skin, prevent cooling of the blood.

The blood vessels supplying the nervous system form an extensive capillary bed, especially in gray matter such as the cerebral cortex. The blood supply of the brain and spinal cord, however, presents a number of special features. Anastomoses between major arterial branches on the surface of and within the brain are limited, and arteriovenous anastomoses are absent. The arteries that enter the brain acquire a special relationship to glial cells, and the capillaries possess endothelial cells of a special nature, which limits or blocks the passage of large molecules (see blood-brain barrier, p. 149). Finally, the cerebral circulation is characterized by autoregulation — that is, blood flow is relatively independent of changes in blood pressure (p. 149).

Blood Supply of the Brain. The blood supply of the contents of the cranial cavity is derived from two pairs of arteries in the neck. These are the *common carotid* and the *vertebral arteries.*

The common carotid arteries ascend in the neck; below the base of the skull, each divides into an *external* and an *internal carotid artery,* certain branches of which supply cranial structures. Each internal carotid artery enters the cranial cavity through a canal in the base of the skull, emerges alongside the optic chiasma, and divides into an *anterior* and a *middle cerebral artery.* The two anterior cerebral arteries are united by a small communicating branch.

The vertebral arteries ascend in foramina in the transverse processes of the cervical vertebrae and enter the cranial cavity through the foramen magnum. On the ventral surface of the brain stem they join to form a single arterial stem, the *basilar artery.* This artery ascends in front of the brain stem and ends by dividing into two *posterior cerebral arteries.* Each of these is joined to the corresponding internal carotid artery by a communicating branch. The various branches at the base of the brain thus form the circulus arteriosus. The arrangement of this circle and the branches issuing from it are illustrated in Figure 7–21. The circulus arteriosus may serve as an anastomotic channel if one of its component or contributing arteries is occluded.

Figure 7–22 shows the distribution of the cerebral arteries to the lateral aspect of the brain; the medial aspect is supplied by the anterior and posterior cerebral arteries. The branches to the brain comprise two sets. One, the leptomeningeal, courses in the subarachnoid space on the lateral and medial aspects of the

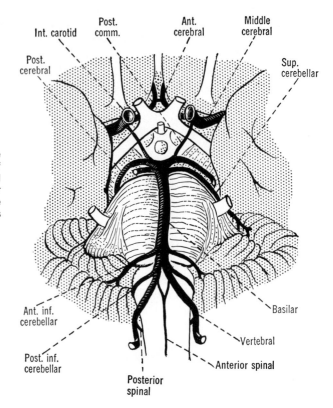

Figure 7-21. Drawing of the circulus arteriosus at the base of the brain. All small branches and ramifications of various larger branches have been omitted. The anterior communicating artery is not labeled.

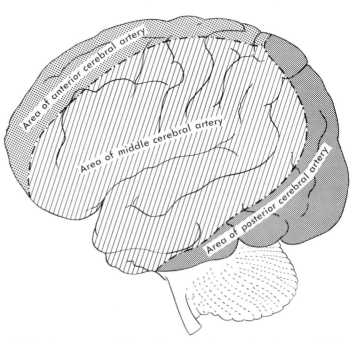

Figure 7-22. The approximate portions of the lateral surface of the hemisphere supplied by the cerebral arteries.

brain, giving branches that penetrate and supply the cortex and white matter. The other set, the striate and perforating branches, arrive from the major arteries at the base of the brain, quickly traverse the subarachnoid space, and enter the brain to supply the basal ganglia, white matter, and hypothalamus. In addition, the posterior cerebral artery gives choroidal branches to the choroid plexuses, as does the internal carotid or middle cerebral artery.

The brain is drained by two sets of veins. One is the deep or great cerebral venous system which eventually empties into dural venous sinuses, and thereby reaches the internal jugular veins. Another set drains the superficial part of the brain and also empties into dural venous sinuses.

The brain stem is supplied by surface branches and short penetrating branches of the basilar artery and its superior cerebellar branch, and also by branches of the vertebral arteries. The cerebellum is supplied by major branches of the vertebral and basilar arteries. The veins that drain the brain stem and cerebellum empty into the dural sinuses.

Venous blood has potential routes of exit from the cranial cavity other than by the internal jugular veins, for example, by emissary veins through the skull and by veins that traverse various foramina to empty into extracranial veins.

Blood Supply of the Meninges (Dura Mater). The main blood supply of the dura mater is by the middle meningeal branches of the external carotid arteries. Each ascends through a foramen in the base of the skull and then lies between the dura mater and the skull. Their special importance is that they may be torn or otherwise damaged in skull injuries. In such cases there is severe bleeding which, because it occurs between the dura mater and the skull, is known as extradural or epidural hemorrhage, and which may cause severe symptoms because of pressure on the brain.

Blood Supply of the Spinal Cord, Spinal Roots, and Spinal Nerves. An anterior spinal artery arises from each vertebral artery (Fig. 7–21). The two arteries join and form a single artery that descends in the anterior median fissure of the spinal cord. It is reinforced by medullary branches, which join it at irregular intervals, and it gives branches to the anterior part of the spinal cord (Fig. 7–22).

A posterior spinal artery arises from each vertebral artery (Fig. 7–21). Each descends along the posterior aspect of the spinal cord, and each usually breaks up into plexiform channels in the lower part of the spinal cord.

The various arteries also give rise to small branches that form a plexus on the surface of the spinal cord.

The spinal branches (Fig. 7–23) that traverse the intervertebral foramina and give rise to radicular and medullary branches are derived from the vertebral and other arteries in the neck,

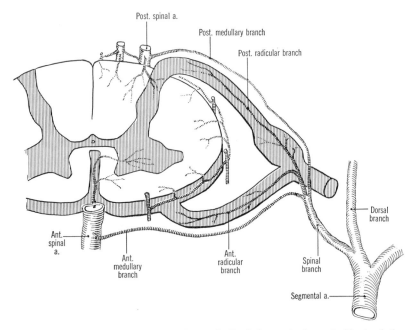

Figure 7-23. The arterial supply of one half of the spinal cord. Most of the extensive branching within the substance of the cord has been omitted. Note that two posterior spinal arteries are present (only one is labeled).

from the posterior intercostal arteries in the thorax, and from the lumbar and lateral sacral arteries in the abdomen and pelvis.

The veins that drain the spinal cord are segmentally arranged. Together with veins in the epidural space they exit through intervertebral foramina as intervertebral veins; blood eventually drains into major veins that empty into the right atrium of the heart.

ANGIOGRAPHY

The nervous system is frequently affected by disorders of its blood supply. These disorders may result, for example, in occlusion of a vessel by a thrombus (a clot) or by an embolus (a mass of material such as a clot or groups of cells or bacteria that originate elsewhere and travel in the blood until they stop and block a vessel). In such instances the area of the nervous system deprived of its blood supply softens and degenerates. The results may be severe and even fatal. Diseased blood vessels may also give way; the resulting hemorrhage is usually fatal. These various vascular disorders affecting the brain are familiar under the lay terms "stroke" or "apoplexy."

Among the procedures used to diagnose vascular disorders, and also other neurological involvements such as tumors, is *angiography.* A radio-opaque material is injected into an artery in the neck, arm, or thigh, and the head and neck x-rayed as the material circulates through the cranial vessels; the vessels of the spinal cord can also be demonstrated by angiography. This diagnostic procedure has proved to be a valuable method for determining the normal pattern of the blood supply of the central nervous system in living individuals (Figs. 7–24 and 7–25).

CEREBRAL BLOOD FLOW

Blood flow through the brain is high, being about 15 to 20 per cent of the cardiac output at rest (about 750 ml per minute). The flow increases with increased activity of the brain, especially in the gray matter. The high utilization of oxygen and glucose and the lack of energy stores make it critical that blood flow, and therefore the delivery of oxygen and glucose, be as constant as possible in the face of factors that tend to change blood flow.

A variety of techniques have been developed to measure blood flow. Among these is the use of an inert, diffusible gas, such as nitrous oxide, which is breathed and the difference between arterial and venous concentrations thus determined. Radioactive tracers may be injected into the cerebral circulation. It is now evident that the circulation and its control are enormously complicated, that major differences in flow exist between gray and white matter, and that autoregulation exists, that is, the maintenance of constant flow in the face of wide changes in perfusion pressure (the difference between mean arterial pressure and venous pressure). Autoregulation is accomplished by a dilation of small cerebral arteries when blood pressure is reduced, and by a constriction of these vessels when blood pressure is increased. However, the mechanisms that provide for autoregulation are still not known with certainty. The nerves supplying the cerebral blood vessels may be involved. Carbon dioxide undoubtedly plays a role in that an increase in carbon dioxide tension leads to an increase in cerebral blood flow. Oxygen tension, pH, and circulating metabolites probably also are involved. This field of investigation continues to be heavily dependent upon the development of techniques that allow measurements to be made in living individuals.

BLOOD-BRAIN BARRIER

The arteries that supply the central nervous system lie first in the subarachnoid space, as do the veins (Fig. 7–26). They then penetrate the surface glial membrane, and are accompanied for a short distance by leptomeningeal sheaths (arachnoid and pia mater) with their contained subarachnoid space. However, these

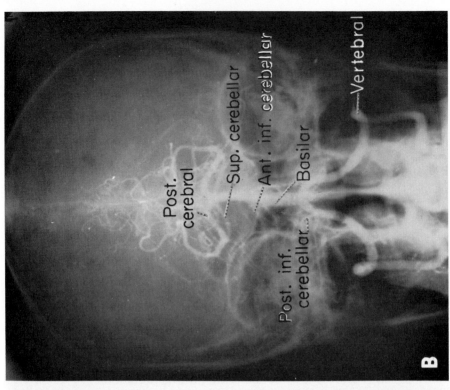

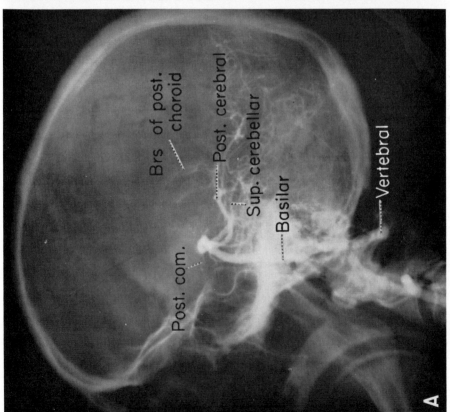

Figure 7–24. Vertebral arteriograms *in vivo.* A: Lateral view; B: Posterior-anterior view. (From Gardner, E., Gray, D. J., and O'Rahilly, R.: Anatomy. 4th ed. Philadelphia. W. B. Saunders Company, 1975. Courtesy of E. S. Gurdjian, M.D., and J. E. Webster, M.D., Department of Neurosurgery, Wayne State University School of Medicine, Detroit, Mich.)

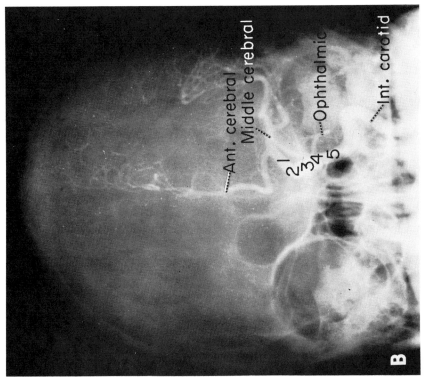

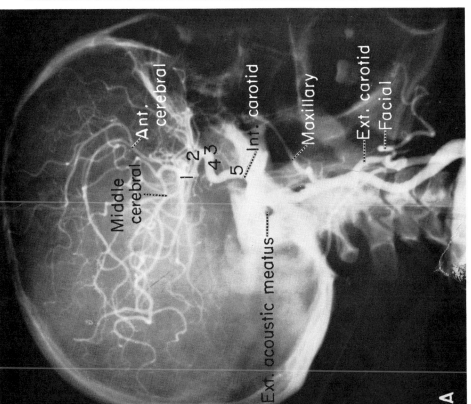

Figure 7–25. Internal carotid arteriograms *in vivo.* A: Lateral view; B: Postero-anterior view. The numerals from 1 to 5 refer to portions of the internal carotid artery as it ascends through the base of the skull. (From Gardner, E., Gray, D. J., and O'Rahilly, R.: Anatomy. 4th ed. Philadelphia. W. B. Saunders Company. 1975. Courtesy of E. S. Gurdjian, M.D. and J. E Webster, M.D., Department of Neurosurgery, Wayne State University School of Medicine, Detroit, Mich.)

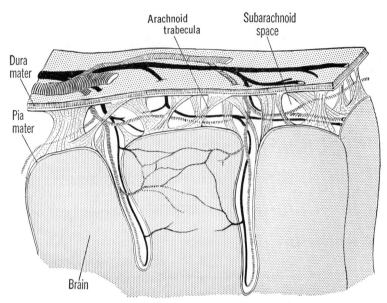

Figure 7-26. Schematic representation of meninges, blood vessels, and nervous tissue. Arteries (black) and veins are shown as they pierce the dura mater and run in the subarachnoid space, which is filled with cerebrospinal fluid. Blood vessels that enter the brain are ensheathed by a prolongation of the pia mater. The subarachnoid space is prolonged for a short distance along the larger vessels.

sheaths are soon replaced by glial investments that become more pronounced as capillaries are approached. The capillary network of the central nervous system is extensive, especially in the gray matter. What is of unique importance, however, is that these capillaries have permeability characteristics that are fundamentally different from those of capillaries elsewhere in the body. The endothelial cells form a continuous rather than a fenestrated layer (Fig. 7–27). These endothelial cells, with their tight junctions and externally applied basement membrane (glial end feet are external to the basement membrane), form the *blood-brain barrier.* This barrier is a major obstacle to the free movement of substances from the blood to the brain. In fact, the diffusion of most substances is definitely limited, except for lipid-soluble compounds and water. This barrier may prevent potentially therapeutic drugs from reaching the brain.

CEREBROSPINAL FLUID

Cerebrospinal fluid is a clear, colorless fluid, only slightly heavier than water, which fills the ventricles and subarachnoid space. In recent years, particularly with the aid of radioactive tracers, studies of ions and nonelectrolytes have shown that cerebrospinal fluid is not a simple filtrate of blood plasma. The fluid has higher concentrations of sodium, chloride, and magnesium ions than does plasma, whereas the concentrations of potassium, calcium, urea, and glucose are lower. Moreover, the cerebrospinal fluid contains few if any cells (usually 0 to 5 lymphocytes per cubic mm), and very little protein (45 mg/ 100 ml or less). The formation of cerebrospinal fluid is considered to be a secretory process, requiring energy.

The choroid plexuses are the major sites of formation of the cerebrospinal fluid, although it is possible that some fluid in the extracellular spaces of the brain diffuses through the gap junctions between ependymal cells and enters the cerebrospinal fluid. In the choroid plexuses, however, tight junctions are present just as they are between the endothelial cells of intracerebral capillaries (Fig. 7–27). When a substance such as glucose is injected into the blood, it escapes rapidly into the surrounding tissues, including those of the brain. However, it takes much longer

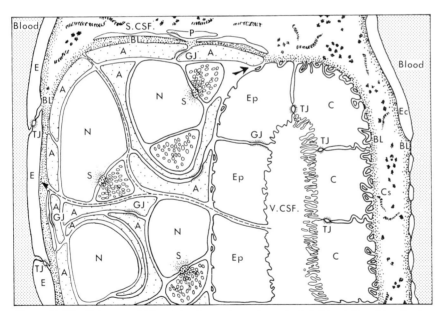

Figure 7–27. Schema of blood, brain, and cerebrospinal fluid relationships in the mouse. A: Astrocytic process. BL: Basal lamina. C: Choroid plexus epithelium. Cs: Choroid plexus stroma. E: Endothelium of parenchymal vessel. Ec: Endothelium of choroid plexus vessel. Ep: Ependyma. GJ: Gap junction. N: Neuron. P: Pia. S: Synapse. S.CSF.: Cerebrospinal fluid of subarachnoid space. TJ: Tight junction. V.CSF: Cerebrospinal fluid of ventricles. The dashed line follows two typical open pathways connecting ventricular cerebrospinal fluid with the basement membrane of parenchymal blood vessels and with the basement membrane of the surface of the brain. The thick arrow (top) indicates a "functional leak" whereby substances crossing the fenestrated endothelium of the choroid plexus can pass along the choroidal stroma to enter the parenchyma of the brain at the root of the choroid plexus. A "leak" in the opposite direction could also occur, as indicated by the arrow point. (From Brightman, M. W., and Reese, T. S., in J. Cell. Bio., *40:*648–677, 1969. Courtesy of the authors and the publisher.)

for it to appear in the cerebrospinal fluid, and equilibration may take hours. Hence it seems that there is a barrier (the *blood–cerebrospinal fluid barrier*) between the blood and the cerebrospinal fluid. This barrier is undoubtedly in the choroid plexuses, and is due chiefly to the barrier to diffusion presented by the tight junctions. However, many substances that are injected into the cerebrospinal fluid diffuse readily into the brain, even though they may not cross the blood-brain barrier. The diffusion in such instances is between ependymal cells (other than those of the choroid plexuses) and their gap junctions.

Cerebrospinal fluid circulates through the ventricles, from lateral to third to fourth. It enters the subarachnoid space through the median and lateral apertures of the fourth ventricle. It then circulates around the brain and spinal cord and is absorbed into the venous blood. This occurs chiefly through small tufts or villi of arachnoid tissue which project into the dural venous sinuses (Fig. 7–28). Villi are also found with the veins just external to the spinal dura mater and absorption may occur here. It is also possible that some fluid may seep along cranial and spinal nerves to be absorbed by tissue lymphatics.

The circulation of cerebrospinal fluid results from the net formation at the choroid plexuses and the bulk absorption into the venous sinuses. It has been shown, especially by the use of radioactive isotopes injected into a ventricle or into the lumbar subarachnoid space, that the cerebrospinal fluid after leaving the fourth ventricle and entering the adjacent cistern flows chiefly upward in front of the brain stem. It then moves over the lateral aspect of the hemisphere (Fig. 7–29) and can be detected at the superior longitudinal sinus within 12 to 24 hours after injection.

The volume of cerebrospinal fluid within the ventricles and subarachnoid space is normally about 120 to 140 ml. It is estimated that an average of 0.37 ml is formed each minute. This means that the turnover of cerebrospinal fluid takes, on the average, about six hours.

The normal pressure of the cerebrospinal fluid is about 100 to 200 mm of water (see below). The rate of formation of cerebrospinal fluid is relatively independent of its pressure, but the latter is affected by many conditions. The effect of blood hydrodynamics may be shown by a maneuver carried out while measuring its pressure during a *lumbar puncture.* If both internal jugular veins are compressed manually in the neck, there is shortly a prompt rise in the pressure of cerebrospinal fluid, because the venous occlusion prevents blood from leaving the cranial cavity. Venous pressure promptly rises, and the gradient of pressure between the arterial side in the choroid plexuses and the venous side in the dural sinuses decreases. Since arterial blood continues to enter the cranial cavity, the only result can be a general increase in cerebrospinal fluid pressure.

In carrying out a lumbar puncture by thrusting a puncture

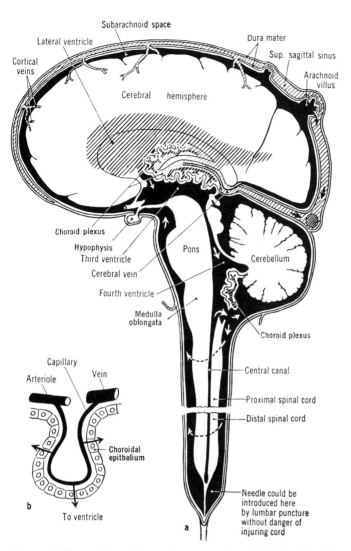

Figure 7-28. *a,* Circulation of cerebrospinal fluid (in black); arrows indicate the direction of circulation. The drawing represents a median section of the nervous system and therefore shows third ventricle, cerebral aqueduct, fourth ventricle, and central canal, with the approximate size and location of one of the lateral ventricles indicated by oblique lines. Note the aperture in the fourth ventricle by which fluid reaches the subarachnoid space. Note also one of the arachnoid villi through which fluid enters venous blood in a dural sinus. *b,* Fundamental plan of choroid plexuses. Cerebrospinal fluid is formed from blood plasma and passes through choroidal epithelium into the ventricular space. (Modified from Rasmussin, A. T.: The Principal Nervous Pathways, 3rd ed. Macmillan Company, 1945.)

needle between the third and fourth lumbar vertebrae into the subarachnoid space, the pressure of the cerebrospinal fluid can be measured by an attached manometer. Figure 7–28 shows that, since the spinal cord ends above this level, there is no danger of injuring it by such a puncture. In the horizontal or

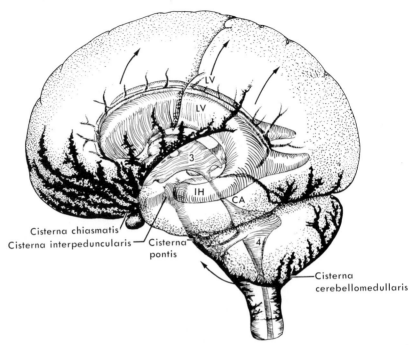

Figure 7-29. The general arrangement of the ventricles within the brain and the major cisterns of the subarachnoid space. The arrows indicate the circulation of the cerebrospinal fluid upward in front of the pons, and then upward and over the convexity of the hemisphere toward the superior sagittal sinus (the sinus is not shown). The amount of fluid in the cisterna cerebellomedullaris is de-emphasized so as not to obscure the central canal. LV, lateral ventricle. IH, inferior horn of lateral ventricle. CA, cerebral aqueduct. 3, third ventricle. 4, fourth ventricle, continuous below with the central canal. (From Dandy, W., in Bull. Johns Hopkins Hosp., *32*:67–75, 1921.)

recumbent position, cerebrospinal fluid pressure ordinarily amounts to 10 to 20 mm of mercury (approximately 100 to 200 mm of water) at the level of the lumbar puncture. The lumbar pressure is higher in the erect position. Abnormal conditions, such as the growth of a tumor, by obstructing circulation, may cause the total intracranial pressure to rise to 400 or more mm of water. Cerebrospinal fluid may also be withdrawn through the needle and examined for bacteria, cells, or chemical compounds not normally present. The fluid may be tested for various serological reactions, such as tests for syphilis. Fluid that is withdrawn may be replaced by air, or by an opaque oil. Since the air or oil may be detected by radiography, the position of a mass, such as a tumor, which may interfere with normal cerebrospinal fluid dynamics, may be determined. Anesthetics, such as procaine, may also be introduced for spinal anesthesia.

Air may also be introduced into ventricles by means of a needle thrust through the brain into the ventricles after a small hole is drilled in the skull cap. A *ventriculogram* is a radiogram of ventricles filled with air. The subarachnoid space of the cranial cavity may be visualized by air introduced at lumbar puncture (*pneumoencephalography*).

The composition and hydrodynamics of cerebrospinal fluid are important from a clinical standpoint. Infections and metabolic disorders, for example, may cause significant changes in content and composition. As mentioned above, abnormal masses such as tumors may interfere with the circulation of the fluid. If, for example, the cerebral aqueduct is narrowed or blocked, the result may be an *obstructive hydrocephalus,* often with severe brain damage. If absorption is interfered with, for example, by meningeal infections, the fluid can still leave the ventricular system and enter the subarachnoid space. The result is often termed a *communicating hydrocephalus.* Hydrocephalus is a common feature in many congenital abnormalities of the brain and spinal cord; the causes are often unknown.

The normal functions of the cerebrospinal fluid are still uncertain. The fluid undoubtedly cushions the brain and spinal fluid and minimizes damage that might otherwise result from sudden movements or from blows to the head and spine. The fluid plays a role in the diffusion of materials into and away from the brain, and it might well transport specific substances, such as neurohormones, from one part of the central nervous system to another.

SUMMARY

The central nervous system includes the brain and spinal cord. It is surrounded by the meninges, which are, from without inward, the dura mater, arachnoid, and pia mater. The subarachnoid space lies between the arachnoid and the pia mater and contains cerebrospinal fluid.

The brain includes the convoluted cerebral hemispheres, the brain stem, and the cerebellum. The hemispheres (comprising the frontal, temporal, parietal, and occipital lobes) have a surface layer, or cortex, composed of gray matter. They contain the lateral and third ventricles, and the internal masses of gray matter known as the basal ganglia. The internal capsules lie between portions of the basal ganglia and emerge at the base of the hemispheres as the cerebral peduncles.

The brain stem is composed of diencephalon, midbrain, pons, and medulla oblongata. The cerebellum is connected to the brain stem by three pairs of peduncles. Between the cerebellum and the pons and medulla oblongata lies the fourth ventricle. The fourth ventricle communicates with the third through the cerebral aqueduct, which runs through the midbrain. The interior of the brain stem is composed of gray and white matter in varying proportions. The cerebellum has an interior of white matter and a surface of gray matter.

The spinal cord is continuous with the medulla oblongata at the foramen magnum. It terminates at the upper border of the second lumbar vertebra. Its interior gray matter is arranged like the letter H, surrounded by white matter arranged into funiculi. Ventral roots of the spinal nerves arise from the anterior column of gray matter, and the dorsal roots terminate in the posterior column of the gray matter. The cord is larger in the cervical and lumbar regions.

The blood supply of the brain and meninges is derived from the common carotid and vertebral arteries; that of the spinal cord and its roots is derived from the vertebral, intercostal, lumbar, and sacral vessels. Diseases of blood vessels are important causes of neurological disorders. Vessels of the brain and spinal cord may be visualized by angiography, a diagnostic procedure that is useful for many neurological as well as vascular disorders.

Blood flow through the brain is high, about 15 to 20 per cent of the cardiac output at rest. Maintenance of constant flow in the face of wide changes in perfusion pressure depends upon autoregulatory mechanisms. The endothelial cells of the capillaries in the central nervous system are united by tight junctions and, together with their basement membrane, compose the blood-brain barrier, which is a major obstacle to the free movement of substances between blood and brain.

Some of the branches of the circulus arteriosus at the base of the brain supply the choroid plexuses of the lateral and third ventricles; branches of the vertebral arteries supply those in the fourth ventricle. Cerebrospinal fluid formed in the plexuses enters the ventricles and circulates through them. Fluid then enters the subarachnoid space and is eventually absorbed into the blood through the arachnoid villi in the dural sinuses. The pressure of this fluid may be measured in the spinal subarachnoid space by introducing a lumbar puncture needle with a manometer attached. Diseases of the brain often change the properties of cerebrospinal fluid, and interference with the circulation of this fluid may result in hydrocephalus.

NAMES IN NEUROLOGY

ALEXANDER MONRO (1733–1817)

In 1700, J. Monro settled in Edinburgh. At the age of 22, he became professor of anatomy, the first of a long line of distinguished anatomists. His son, Alexander Monro, followed in his father's footsteps as professor of anatomy, and it is his name that is attached to the interventricular foramina. The grandson, also named Alexander, held the same chair as professor of anatomy. The three Monros occupied this chair for a period of 126 years (1720–1846), and the first two Monros themselves taught at least 12,800 students.

SYLVIUS (also known as FRANÇOIS DE LA BOË (1614–1672)

Sylvius was a Dutch anatomist whose name is attached to the cerebral aqueduct, although Galen, more than 1000 years before, had seen and described this passage. Another Sylvius, a Parisian teacher also known as Jacques Dubois (1478–1555), named the jugular, subclavian, renal, and other blood vessels, but not the aqueduct of Sylvius.

THOMAS WILLIS (1621–1675)

An English physician, Thomas Willis probably holds first place among the seventeenth-century neuroanatomists. In 1664 he published his famous *Cerebri Anatome*, which classified the cranial nerves and was the most complete description of the anatomy of the nervous system of its day. In this work he described the circulus arteriosus that is now named for him.

REFERENCES

The following three textbooks of anatomy provide differing approaches to the description of the anatomy of the human body.

Gardner, E., Gray, D. J., and O'Rahilly, R.: Anatomy. 4th ed. Philadelphia, W. B. Saunders Company, 1975. A regional approach.
King, B. G., and Showers, M. J.: Human Anatomy and Physiology. 6th ed. Philadelphia, W. B. Saunders Company, 1969. An excellent account on a more elementary level.
Warwick, R., and Williams, P. L. (editors): Gray's Anatomy. 35th British ed. Philadelphia, W. B. Saunders Company; London, Longman Group Ltd., 1973. The classic systemic textbook of anatomy, with an extensive section on the nervous system.

The first five of the following references are excellent neuroanatomical textbooks, each with a different approach. That by Barr is highly recommended for the beginning student. The next five are valuable atlases of the human brain, differing in plane of section and staining method.

Barr, M. L.: The Human Nervous System. 2nd ed. Hagertown, Harper and Row, 1974.
Brodal, A.: Neurological Anatomy. In Relation to Clinical Medicine. 2nd ed. New York, Oxford University Press, 1969.
Crosby, E. C., Humphrey, T., and Lauer, E. W.: Correlative Anatomy of the Nervous System. New York, The Macmillan Company, 1962.
Truex, R. C., and Carpenter, M. B.: Human Neuroanatomy. 6th ed. Baltimore, The Williams and Wilkins Company, 1969.
Willis, W. D., Jr., and Grossman, R. G.: Medical Neurobiology. St. Louis, The C. V. Mosby Company, 1973.
Bossy, J.: Atlas du système nerveux. Aspects macroscopiques de l'encéphale. Paris, Éditions Offidoc, 1971.
Ford, D. H., and Schadé, J. P.: Atlas of the Human Brain. 2nd rev. ed. Amsterdam, Elsevier Publishing Company, 1971.
Miller, R. A., and Burack, E.: Atlas of the Central Nervous System in Man. Baltimore, The Williams and Wilkins Company, 1968.
Roberts, M., and Hanaway, J.: Atlas of the Human Brain in Section. Philadelphia, Lea and Febiger, 1970.
Singer, M., and Yakovlev, P. I.: The Human Brain in Sagittal Section. Springfield, Ill., Charles C Thomas Company, 1964.

The following three references are useful for the normal anatomy of the ventricular system and blood vessels.

Peterson, H. O., and Kieffer, S. A.: Introduction to Neuroradiology. Reprinted from Baker's Clinical Neurology. New York, Harper and Row, Publisher, 1972.
Stephens, R. B., and Stilwell, D. L.: Arteries and Veins of the Human Brain. Springfield, Ill., Charles C Thomas Company, 1969.
Youmans, J. R. (Editor): Neurological Surgery, 3 vols. Philadelphia, W. B. Saunders Company, 1973.

The following references are specialized accounts of cerebral circulation and cerebrospinal fluid.

Davson, H.: Physiology of the Cerebrospinal Fluid. Boston, Little, Brown and Company, 1967.
Katzman, R., and Pappius, H. M.: Brain Electrolytes and Fluid Metabolism. Baltimore, The Williams and Wilkins Company, 1973.
Miller, J. W., and Wollam, D. H. M.: The Anatomy of the Cerebrospinal Fluid. London, Oxford University Press, 1962.
Pease, D. C., and Schultze, R. L.: Circulation to the brain and spinal cord. C. Submicroscopic anatomy. In Abramson, D. I. (editor): Blood Vessels and Lymphatics, New York, Academic Press, 1962.
Purves, M. J.: The Physiology of the Cerebral Circulation. Cambridge, at the University Press, 1972.

Chapter **8**

THE HUMAN PERIPHERAL
NERVOUS SYSTEM

The peripheral nervous system includes the cranial nerves, the spinal nerves with their roots and rami, the peripheral nerves, and the peripheral components of the autonomic nervous system. In common usage, the term *peripheral nerve* ordinarily refers to the nerves that arise from plexuses formed by spinal nerves. This terminological distinction between spinal and peripheral nerves is important from the standpoint of differences in the distribution of these two types of nerves (p. 168).

A *nerve* is a collection of a variable number of nerve fibers. Thus, according to the number of constituent fibers, a nerve may be as large in diameter as a finger, or so small as to be visible only under the microscope. Whatever their number, the fibers are bound together by sheaths of connective tissue.

The various sheaths, which are illustrated in Figure 8–1, convey the intrinsic blood and lymphatic vessels, and also the sensory and autonomic nerve fibers that supply the connective tissue and blood vessels. The connective tissue sheaths also impart strength, especially against tensile stresses. Spinal nerves have thinner and less well-defined sheaths and are, therefore, more fragile. The individual nerve fibers are somewhat longer than the usual length of nerve in which they occur. Thus, when nerves are stretched, as they are during movement, the individual fibers are straightened out rather than stretched.

With regard to the types of fibers present in the various nerves, the dorsal roots, which are composed of the central processes of spinal ganglion cells, contain thousands of myelinated and nonmyelinated sensory fibers. The nonmyelinated fibers are by far the more numerous.

The fibers in the ventral roots, which are the axons of neurons in the ventral gray matter of the spinal cord, are myelinated. If

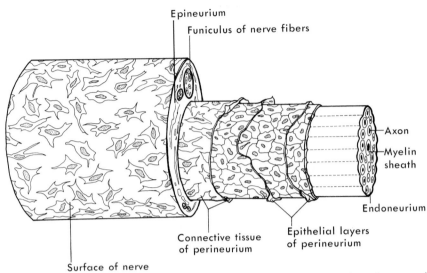

Figure 8-1. Schematic representation of peripheral nerve to show its general arrangement and connective tissue sheaths. Epineurium is the outermost sheath. Its fibroblasts are shown exaggerated in size. Perineurium surrounds smaller bundles of fibers (funiculi). One such funiculus is enlarged to show that the perineurium is composed of an outer connective tissue part, with fibroblasts, and inner layers of flattened epithelial cells. Perineurium constitutes a selective barrier to diffusion. It can be traced centrally, where it is comparable to the pia-arachnoid, and distally it appears to form the outermost parts of the capsules of nerve endings. Endoneurium is the connective tissue that surrounds individual fibers, external to the neurilemma; the details of its arrangement are not shown. (Based on Shanta, T. R., and Bourne, G. H.: The perineural epithelium—a new concept. In Bourne, G. H., editor: The Structure and Function of the Nervous System, vol. I, 379-459. New York, Academic Press, 1968.)

these fibers are grouped according to their diameters, there will be found one group that averages 2 to 8 μm (with a peak of 2 to 3 μm), and another group that averages 12 to 20 μm. The first group includes preganglionic autonomic fibers (p. 338), and *gamma* fibers to neuromuscular spindles (p. 201). The second group is formed by the large *alpha* fibers that are motor to striated muscles (p. 201).

Spinal and peripheral nerves are mixed nerves, containing both sensory and motor fibers. A major peripheral nerve such as the sciatic may contain more than a million fibers.

The functional components of nerves and their branches are discussed in Chapter 2, and also in Chapters 13 and 14 on the spinal cord and brain stem.

Blood Supply of Peripheral Nerves. In general, each nerve receives branches from the arteries in each of the different regions through which the nerve runs. For example, the sciatic nerve with its branches extends from the sacrum to the toes. In so doing, it receives small branches from an artery in the pelvis, and from others in the thigh, in the back of the knee, in the calf of the leg, and in the ankle and foot. These small branches enter the connective tissue sheaths and run longitudinally, often for many centimeters. There is usually significant anastomosis between various branches, thereby providing a considerable protection to nerves against loss of blood supply.

CRANIAL NERVES

Cranial nerves differ significantly from spinal nerves, especially in the way they develop and in their relation to the special senses, and also because some cranial nerves supply pharyngeal arch structures. They are attached to the brain at irregular intervals; they are not formed of dorsal and ventral roots; some have more than one ganglion, whereas others have none; and the optic nerve is a fiber tract and not a true peripheral nerve. Cranial nerves do not emerge from plexuses, but are attached directly to the brain. Some, notably the glossopharyngeal, vagus, and accessory nerves, are closely connected or are interconnected near their origins, and the vagus throughout its peripheral distribution contributes to the formation of autonomic plexuses. Cranial nerves exhibit few of the features of segmental distribution described later (p. 168). Finally, some cranial nerves contain functional components not present in spinal nerves (p. 306).

Cranial nerves follow complicated paths to the peripheral structures they serve. Detailed descriptions of their distributions can be found in anatomical textbooks. The usual method of description groups the cranial nerves into twelve pairs (but see p. 20).

1. Olfactory Nerve. The small filaments composing this nerve arise in the olfactory mucous membrane of the upper part of the nasal cavity. They ascend through openings in the front part of the floor of the cranial cavity and end in the *olfactory bulb.* The *olfactory tract* runs backward from the bulb and ends at the base of the brain near the optic chiasma (Fig. 12–26, p. 283). The olfactory nerve and its central connections are associated with the sense of smell (p. 281).

The *nervus terminalis* (p. 21) is also present in the adult human being; its significance is obscure. The *vomeronasal nerve* is present in human embryos.

2. Optic Nerve. This nerve arises from the *retina* of the eye (p. 249). It leaves the orbit through the *optic canal* and joins the opposite optic nerve to form the *optic chiasma* (Fig. 12–13, p. 265, and Fig. 8–2). Two bundles, the *optic tracts,* extend posteriorly from the chiasma, proceed around the cerebral peduncles, and end near the superior colliculi. The various optic pathways are concerned with visual mechanisms (p. 246). The optic nerves and tracts are not true peripheral nerves, but are fiber tracts of the central nervous system, connecting the retina and the brain. The retina is a part of the central nervous system.

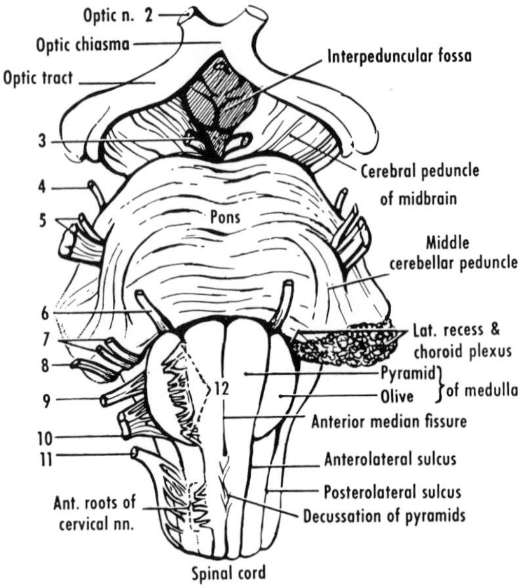

Figure 8-2. The brain stem, anterior aspect, showing the cranial nerves (indicated by numerals). (From Gardner, E., Gray, D. J., and O'Rahilly, R.: Anatomy. 4th ed. Philadelphia, W. B. Saunders Company, 1975.)

3. Oculomotor Nerve. After its origin from the front of the midbrain (Fig. 7–16, p. 140, and Fig. 8–2), the oculomotor nerve runs anteriorly into the orbit, where it ends in muscles that attach to the eyeball and move it in various directions. A portion of the nerve is distributed to certain smooth muscles within the eye (p. 342).

4. Trochlear Nerve. The trochlear nerve is a bundle of fibers that arises from the back of the midbrain, around which it winds to run anteriorly into the orbit (Fig. 8–3). Here it ends in a single muscle attached to the eyeball.

5. Trigeminal Nerve. The trigeminal nerve (Figs. 8–2, 8–3) has a *motor root* and a *sensory root,* both attached to the side of the pons. Near the pons, the sensory root has an enlargement, the *trigeminal* (or *semilunar*) *ganglion,* from which three large branches arise to be distributed to various muscles (chiefly the muscles of mastication), to the skin of the face and part of the scalp, to the mucous membrane of the mouth and nasal cavity, to the eye (especially the cornea), to the teeth, and to the dura mater. The motor root joins the branch that is distributed to the muscles of mastication, and provides both motor and proprioceptive fibers for those muscles.

6. Abducent Nerve. The abducent nerve arises from the front of the pons, just above its junction with the medulla oblongata (Fig. 8–2). It enters the orbit, where it supplies a single muscle attached to the eyeball.

7. Facial Nerve. This nerve is attached laterally, just at the junction of the pons and medulla oblongata (Figs. 8–2, 8–3). Its main distribution is to the muscles of expression (the facial muscles), located around the mouth, nose and eyes, and on the forehead and scalp. Some fibers are also distributed to the mucous membrane of the anterior two-thirds of the tongue (for taste), and some to certain of the salivary glands and to the lacrimal gland (p. 342). The *geniculate ganglion* is found on the nerve in its course through the skull.

8. Vestibulocochlear Nerve. Formerly called auditory or acoustic, the new term better reflects its function, but for simplicity it can be called the *eighth nerve.* It is attached, laterally, at the

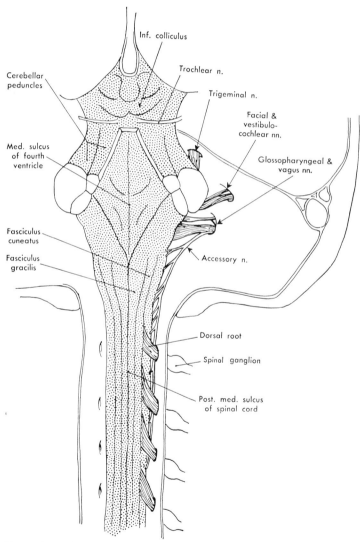

Figure 8–3. Diagram of the posterior aspect of the brain stem, spinal cord, and certain cranial and spinal nerves. The cerebellum has been removed to expose the floor of the fourth ventricle. The glossopharyngeal, vagus, and accessory nerves leave the skull through the same foramen (jugular foramen). The upper one or two filaments constitute the glossopharyngeal nerve.

junction of the pons and medulla oblongata (Figs. 8–2, 8–3, and 12–14, p. 266). It has *cochlear* and *vestibular* divisions, each of which arises in the inner ear. Each has a small ganglion along its course in the inner ear, called *spiral* and *vestibular ganglia*, respectively. These nerves are associated with the sense of hearing and of balance or equilibrium.

9. Glossopharyngeal Nerve. This nerve is closely associated with the vagus nerve. There is a series of nerve rootlets attached to the lateral surface of the medulla oblongata (Figs. 8–2, 8–3), between the olive and the inferior cerebellar peduncle. The upper one or two of these rootlets form the glossopharyngeal nerve, which supplies the mucous membrane and a muscle of the throat (pharynx), a salivary gland, and the mucous membrane of the posterior third of the tongue (for taste). There are two ganglia along its course, the *superior* and the *inferior.*

10. Vagus Nerve. The majority of the rootlets just mentioned form the vagus nerve, which supplies the mucous membrane of the pharynx and larynx and also the muscles of these organs. In addition, it has a complex distribution to viscera in the thorax and abdomen. It has two main ganglia, the *superior* and the *inferior,* which are found on the nerve within and just below its foramen of exit. The position of the vagus is shown in Figures 8–2 and 8–3.

11. Accessory Nerve. The lower of the nerve rootlets from the medulla oblongata joins others that have ascended through the foramen magnum from the cervical spinal cord. The accessory nerve formed by this mingling of fibers (Figs. 8–2 and 8–3) then divides. One division, which is composed of fibers arising from the medulla oblongata, joins the vagus nerve and is distributed with it to the muscles of the pharynx and larynx. The other division, which is composed of fibers arising from the spinal cord, ultimately supplies two muscles, the *trapezius* and the *sternocleidomastoid.*

12. Hypoglossal Nerve. This nerve is formed from a number of rootlets attached to the ventrolateral surface of the medulla oblongata, between the pyramid and olive (Fig. 8–2). It supplies the muscles of the tongue.

SPINAL AND PERIPHERAL NERVES

The dorsal and ventral roots are attached to the spinal cord by a series of filaments. Ordinarily a pair of dorsal roots and a pair of ventral roots can be traced to the foramina between adjacent vertebrae (Figs. 8–4, 8–5), each root entering a dural pouch and then a dural sheath. Near or in each foramen is an ovoid swelling of each dorsal root, the *spinal ganglion.* Just beyond the ganglion, corresponding dorsal and ventral roots joint to form a spinal

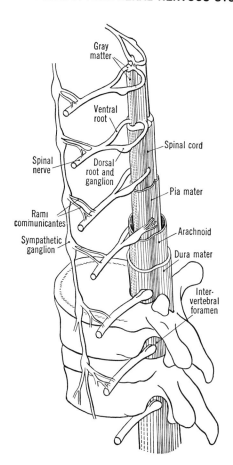

Gray matter
Ventral root
Spinal cord
Spinal nerve
Dorsal root and ganglion
Pia mater
Rami communicantes
Arachnoid
Sympathetic ganglion
Dura mater
Inter-vertebral foramen

Figure 8–4. The spinal cord and meninges within the vertebral canal. The layers of meninges and then the white matter are shown as if successively cut away, leaving the columns of gray matter. The rami communicantes join the ventral rami of spinal nerves; the dorsal rami are not shown.

nerve. Their dural sheaths become confluent and merge with the epineurium of the spinal nerve. The spinal nerve then makes its exit through the foramen and shortly divides into dorsal and ventral rami. The first pair of spinal nerves leaves between the first cervical vertebra and the base of the skull; consequently the remaining cervical spinal nerves leave above the corresponding vertebrae, with the exception of the eighth cervical nerve. Since there are but seven cervical vertebrae, the eighth nerve leaves above the first thoracic vertebra. Below this level the spinal nerves leave below the corresponding vertebrae. There are, then, seven cervical vertebrae and eight pairs of cervical spinal nerves; twelve thoracic vertebrae and twelve pairs of thoracic nerves; five lumbar vertebrae and five pairs of lumbar nerves; one sacrum but five pairs of sacral nerves, because embryologically there are five sacral vertebrae; and for the coccyx, usually one pair of coccygeal nerves. The remainder, if any, are rudimentary.

The dorsal rami supply the back; the ventral rami supply the limbs and the ventrolateral parts of the neck and body wall. In the cervical and lumbosacral regions, the ventral rami intermingle and

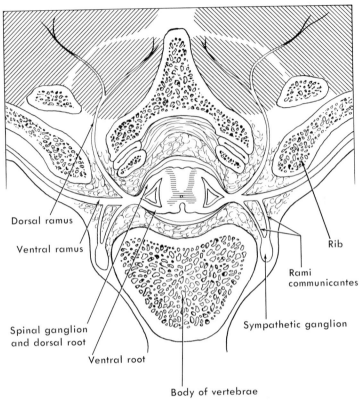

Figure 8–5. Drawing of a horizontal section through a thoracic vertebra and the spinal cord.

form plexuses (*cervical, brachial,* and *lumbosacral,* Fig. 8–6),
from which major peripheral nerves emerge. The ventral rami of
the second to the twelfth thoracic nerves do not form plexuses.
The details of distribution of the spinal and peripheral nerves are
given in the anatomical textbooks cited on p. 159.

PATTERNS OF DISTRIBUTION

Each spinal nerve has a pattern of (ultimate) distribution referred to as segmental or dermatomal, at least as far as its cutaneous fibers are concerned. The term "segmental" refers to the fact
that the longitudinal extent of spinal cord to which a pair of right
and left spinal roots is attached comprises a *segment* of the cord.
The term "dermatome" refers to skin, and a *dermatome* is the area
of skin supplied by the sensory fibers of a single dorsal root
through the dorsal and ventral rami of its spinal nerve.

The *intercostal* and *subcostal* nerves (the ventral rami of the
twelve thoracic nerves) are mostly segmental in distribution.
However, when a ventral ramus enters a plexus (cervical, brachial,

or lumbosacral) and joins other such rami, its component funiculi ultimately enter several of the peripheral nerves emerging from the plexus. Thus, as a general principle, each ramus entering a plexus contributes to several peripheral nerves and each such peripheral nerve contains fibers derived from several ventral rami (Fig. 8–7). The distribution of such peripheral nerves is not segmental; each has its characteristic area of supply (Figs. 8–8, 8–9).

The mixture of nerve fibers in plexuses is such that it is difficult, if not impossible, to trace their course by dissections, and dermatomal distribution has been determined by physiological experimentation and by studying disorders and surgical sections of spinal roots and nerves. The results of such studies have yielded

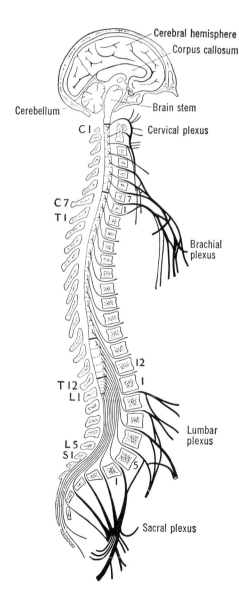

Figure 8-6. Drawing of the brain and cord in situ. The brain is shown sectioned in the median plane (see Figure 7–9, p. 134). Although not illustrated, the first cervical vertebra articulates with the base of the skull. The letters along the vertebral column indicate cervical, thoracic, lumbar, and sacral. Note that the cord ends at the upper border of the second lumbar vertebra.

Figure 8–7. Schematic representation of peripheral nerve
distribution from a plexus
formed by spinal nerves. Spinal
nerve *A* enters a plexus and
reaches an area of skin by way
of peripheral nerves *X* and *Y*.
Spinal nerve *B* also enters the
plexus and reaches a different
area of skin by way of peripheral
nerves *X* and *Y*. Peripheral
nerves *X* and *Y*, therefore, each
contain parts of the two spinal
nerves.

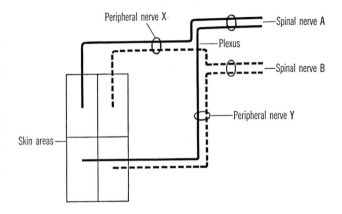

complex maps, chiefly because of variation, overlap, and differences in method. Variation results from intrasegmental rootlet
anastomoses adjacent to the cervical and lumbosacral spinal cord
and from individual differences in plexus formation and peripheral
nerve distribution. Overlap is such that section of a single root
does not produce complete anesthesia in the area supplied by that

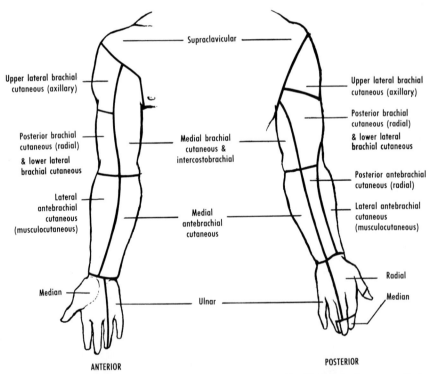

Figure 8–8. Approximate areas of cutaneous nerve distribution to the upper limb,
in contrast to the dermatomes of Figures 8–11 and 8–12. These cutaneous nerve
areas do not show overlap or variation. (From Gardner, E., Gray, D. J., and O'Rahilly,
R.: Anatomy. 4th ed. Philadelphia, W. B. Saunders Company, 1975.)

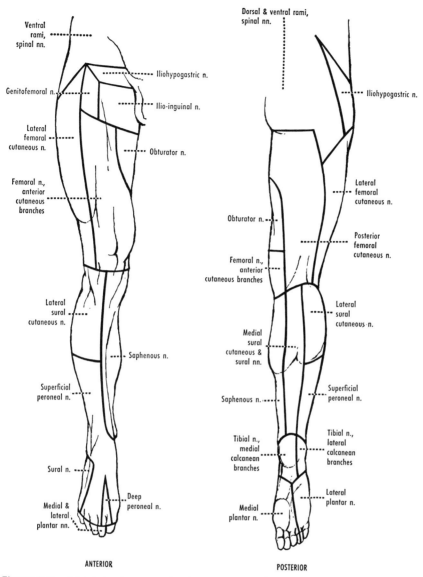

Figure 8-9. Approximate areas of cutaneous nerve distribution to the lower limb, in contrast to the dermatomes of Figures 8–11 and 8–12. Neither overlap nor variation is shown. (From Gardner, E., Gray, D. J., and O'Rahilly, R.: Anatomy. 4th ed. Philadelphia, W. B. Saunders Company, 1975.)

root (Fig. 8–10); at the most, some degree of hypalgesia may result. Overlap is greater for touch than for pain; hence the more common occurrence of hypalgesia rather than hypaesthesia after section of a single root. By contrast, when a peripheral nerve is cut, the result is a central area of total loss of sensation surrounded by an area of diminished sensation. The last is due to overlap from adjacent peripheral nerves and is often less for touch than for pain. The

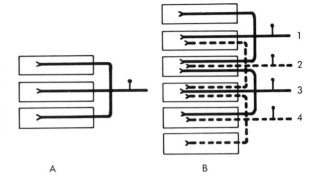

Figure 8–10. Overlap, *A:* The distribution of a single spinal nerve (3) is schematically represented as sending branches to three dermatomes. *B:* The distribution of four spinal nerves is schematically represented. Note that if spinal nerve 3 were cut, the area it supplies would still receive branches from spinal nerves 1, 2, and 4 (also 5, not shown).

A   B

effect on muscles of spinal and peripheral nerve section is discussed below.

Perhaps the most accurate dermatomal maps (Figs. 8–11 and 8–12) are those derived from studies on human patients, based on physiological methods that were possible because of surgical procedures necessary for managing neurological or neurosurgical disorders. Those physiological methods are:

(1) *Method of residual sensitivity.* A single dorsal root is left intact, as contiguous roots above and below are divided. This gives the total distribution of the intact dorsal root. (2) *Constructive method.* A series of contiguous dorsal roots are divided; consequently the superior border of the resulting anesthesia represents the inferior border of the dermatome corresponding to the next higher intact root and the inferior border of the anesthetic area represents the superior border of the next lower intact root. (3) *Stimulation of dorsal roots.* Electrical stimulation yields vasodilatation in areas of skin which are smaller than the dermatomes determined by the residual method, but which are similar in shape and location.

It must be emphasized that these results relate to the *normal,* full dermatome; the maps derived from them do not show the sensory change resulting from section of a single root or spinal nerve. This must be deduced from the normal maps or else depicted in separate maps dealing specifically with sensory losses. Moreover, as discussed on pp. 227 and 296, the role of central gray matter must be considered. The excitability of transmission neurons is changed when roots are sectioned, and the change in excitability can affect the transmission from intact roots and thereby affect the size (not the location) of dermatomes.

Muscles. There is little specific correspondence between dermatomes and underlying muscles. The general arrangement is that the more rostral segments of the cervical and lumbosacral enlargements supply the more proximal limb muscles, and that more caudal segments supply the more distal muscles. Tables have been published showing the muscles usually supplied by each spinal cord segment. Such tables often do not take variation into account. A muscle usually receives fibers from each of the spinal nerves which contribute to the peripheral nerve supplying it (although one spinal nerve may be its chief supply). Section of a single spinal nerve weakens several muscles but does not usually paralyze them. Section of a peripheral nerve results in severe weakness or total paralysis of the muscles it supplies. Moreover, autonomic dysfunction occurs in the area of its distribution.

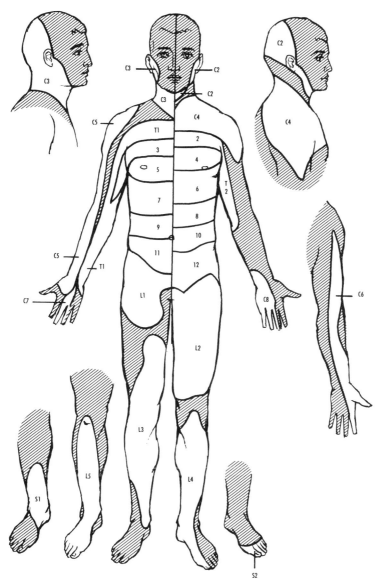

Figure 8–11. Anterior view of normal dermatomes. The right and left halves show the total distribution of alternating dermatomes, thereby illustrating the degree of overlap. In some regions, however, overlap is great and more than two or three dermatomes may overlap. Hence, additional figures (above, at the right side, and below) are necessary to show the total distribution of certain dermatomes. (From Gardner, E., Gray, D. J., and O'Rahilly, R.: Anatomy. 4th ed. Philadelphia, W. B. Saunders Company, 1975.)

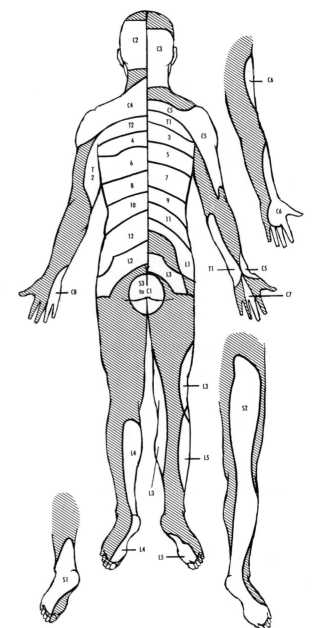

Figure 8–12. Posterior view of normal dermatomes. See legend of Figure 8–11.

AUTONOMIC NERVOUS SYSTEM

Certain general principles of organization are presented here to clarify the relationship of spinal and peripheral nerves with the peripheral portions of the autonomic system. This system is covered in much more detail in Chapter 15.

By classic anatomical definition, the autonomic nervous system is that system of motor nerve fibers that supplies cardiac muscle, smooth muscle, and glands. In its simplest form it consists of a pathway of two succeeding nerve cells. However, as presented in Chapter 15, the autonomic nervous system is far more complex, anatomically and functionally, than the simplistic definition just given would indicate.

The autonomic pathway begins with certain nerve cells in the brain stem and spinal cord. The axons of these cells, termed *preganglionic* fibers, leave the brain stem over certain cranial nerves and ventral roots, and synapse in peripheral autonomic ganglia (including the suprarenal medullae and certain chromaffin cells). The axons of the ganglion cells are termed *postganglionic fibers* and are distributed to the heart, smooth muscle, and certain gland cells. The locations, arrangements, connections, and patterns of distribution of the autonomic fibers form the basis for an anatomical classification into *sympathetic* and *parasympathetic systems* or *divisions.*

Sympathetic Division. There is a long nerve trunk on each side of the vertebral bodies that extends from the base of the skull to the coccyx. Each is known as a *sympathetic trunk.* Ganglia are present at fairly regular intervals along these trunks. Three or more pairs of ganglia occur in the neck, usually ten to twelve in the thorax, and a variable number of pairs in the abdomen and pelvis. Branches of the trunks are distributed to the organs of these areas and form extensive prevertebral plexuses. Ganglia also occur in the plexuses; they are of the same structure and function as those in the sympathetic trunks. Branches to and from the sympathetic trunks connect the trunks with the ventral rami of each spinal nerve. These branches are called *rami communicantes* (Figs. 8–4 and 8–5); they contain pre- and postganglionic fibers (Fig. 15–1, p. 330). Branches of the sympathetic trunks to adjacent viscera likewise contain pre- and postganglionic fibers.

Parasympathetic Division. Part of this division includes those cranial nerves supplying visceral structures. These are the oculomotor, facial, glossopharyngeal, vagus, and accessory nerves. There is also a sacral portion composed of branches of the second and third (sometimes third and fourth) sacral nerves that supply viscera in the pelvis. Numerous ganglia occur in the parasympathetic division, but are not located in a definite trunk. Instead, they are scattered, being found in or near the organs supplied; hence the postganglionic fibers are short.

SUMMARY

Attached to the base of the brain are twelve pairs of cranial nerves, which have complex distributions to cranial, cervical, thoracic, and abdominal structures.

Thirty-one pairs of dorsal and ventral roots are attached to the spinal cord at regular intervals. Each dorsal root joins the ventral root of the corresponding side and from the same cord segment to form a spinal nerve. Each spinal nerve leaves the vertebral canal and divides into a dorsal and a ventral ramus. The dorsal rami supply the skin and muscles of the back. Ventral rami supply the limbs and the sides and front of the body. In the cervical, brachial, lumbar, and sacral regions they enter into plexuses from which peripheral nerves emerge. These nerves have pattterns of distribution that are fundamentally different from the segmental pattern characteristic of spinal nerves. The peripheral nerves receive their blood supply from the main arteries in the regions through which they pass.

Certain branches of spinal nerves, plus sympathetic trunks and associated ganglia, supply motor fibers to viscera, and constitute the sympathetic division of the autonomic nervous system. Branches of certain of the cranial nerves, plus branches of the second and third sacral nerves to the pelvis, form the parasympathetic division. During the course of their distribution, sympathetic and parasympathetic fibers become intermingled. This is especially true in the thorax, abdomen, and pelvis.

REFERENCES

The textbooks cited on p. 159 contain descriptions of the anatomy of the peripheral nervous system and also contain sections dealing with the segmental distribution of spinal nerves and the anatomy of the autonomic system. In addition, the following reference provides a short account of the peripheral nervous system and a useful bibliography.

Gardner, E., Gross Anatomy of the Peripheral Nervous System. In Dyck, P. J., Thomas, P. K., and Lambert, E. H. (editors): Peripheral Neuropathy. Philadelphia, W. B. Saunders Company, 1975.

The first two of the following three references deal with dermatomes; the last is a superb account of peripheral nerve injuries.

Foerster, O.: The dermatomes in man. Brain, *56*:1–39, 1933.
Foerster, O.: Symptomatologie der Erkankungen des Rückenmarks und seiner Wurzeln. In Bumke, O., and Foerster, O.: Handbuch der Neurologie. Vol. 5, 1–403. Berlin, J. Springer, 1936.
Seddon, H.: Surgical Disorders of the Peripheral Nerves. Edinburgh, Churchill Livingstone, 1972.

The following references deal with various aspects of the connective tissue sheaths of nerves.

Burkel, W. E.: The histological fine structure of perineurium. Anat. Rec., *158*:177–189, 1967.
Causey, G.: The Cell of Schwann. Edinburgh, E. and S. Livingstone, Ltd., 1960.
Shanta, T. R., and Bourne, G. H.: The perineural epithelium—a new concept. In Bourne, G. H. (editor): The Structure and Function of the Nervous System, Vol. I, 379–459. New York, Academic Press, 1968.

Chapter 9

THE DEVELOPMENT OF THE HUMAN NERVOUS SYSTEM

In considering the structure of the adult nervous system, questions arise that may be answered more easily by studying the embryo and the fetus. For example, how does the adult nervous system become cavitated? How do nerves and ganglia form? Is there a timetable of development? Moreover, there are broader questions of major importance—namely, when does function begin, when do patterns of behavior appear, and what are the respective roles of heredity and environment in determining and influencing development? These and other questions are being studied on nearly every level of experimental, morphological, behavioral, and clinical approaches.

BASIC FEATURES OF NEURAL DEVELOPMENT

Development commences with fertilization, which is a process of events that begins when a *spermatozoon* makes contact with an *oocyte* and ends with the intermingling of maternal and paternal chromosomes at metaphase of the first mitotic division of the *zygote.* A series of cell divisions then follows, a process that eventuates in the billions of cells that make up the infant at birth.

In human beings, pregnancy usually lasts an average of about 266 days (9 calendar or 10 lunar months). This time is usually divided into the *embryonic period* and the *fetal period,* and clinicians often divide it into first, second, and third trimesters.

The human embryonic period is composed of about the first 8 weeks after fertilization. At the end of this time most embryos are usually 27 to 31 mm in crown-rump length, differentiation is nearly completed, and the embryo in many respects is like a miniature adult. Reflexes are present, the circulation is well established; muscles, vessels, nerves, and skeleton are present in a form and arrangement like that of the adult; and the brain stem, spinal cord, and some of the subcortical structures are present in a highly organized form.

The human fetal period, which is characterized by growth and maturation and by preparation for the change to an external environment, is from the end of the embryonic period until term.

In clinical practice it is customary to date the beginning of pregnancy from the last menstrual period. Ovulation usually occurs about two weeks before the menstrual period, and if pregnancy occurs, menstruation ceases until some time after the infant is delivered. Hence, true age (since fertilization) is about two weeks less than age estimated in weeks since the last menstrual period.

Early in the embryonic period the primitive streak appears, the germ layers (*ectoderm, mesoderm, endoderm*) differentiate, and the notochord forms. The dorsal sheet of embryonic cells, the ectoderm, soon shows a higher metabolic rate in the median plane, evidenced as more pronounced cellular proliferation. As a result there appears first a *neural plate* and then a slight deepening termed the *neural groove* (Fig. 9–1). The plate is the first morphological indication of the nervous system; it is present a little over two weeks after fertilization. At three weeks a deep neural groove is present and the forebrain, midbrain, and hindbrain can be distinguished. The neural groove then begins to close in the region of

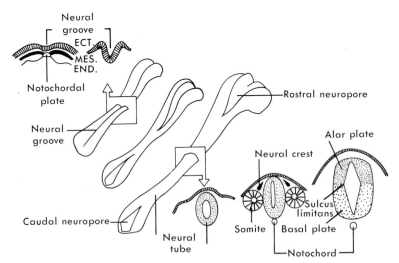

Figure 9–1. The formation and closure of the human neural tube. ECT.: ectoderm; MES.: mesoderm; END.: endoderm. (Courtesy of Dr. Ronan O'Rahilly.)

the neck. The process of closure, which forms a *neural tube,* extends rostrally and caudally. The opening in the neural tube that temporarily remains at the rostral end is termed the *rostral neuropore;* it closes at about three and a half weeks. The *caudal neuropore* closes about two days later. The nervous system is now a complete tube, with a fluid-filled cavity.

Reflexes begin to appear before the end of the embryonic period, at about seven weeks. At this time, stimulation of the skin around the mouth leads to reflex muscular contractions in the head and neck. Thereafter, the number of reflex responses increases rapidly and involves more parts of the body, and motor activity becomes more and more complex as descending tracts from forebrain areas begin to influence the lower centers. However, the nervous system should not be thought of as the development of level upon level of stereotyped reflex responses. Reflexes are local, highly differentiated mechanisms; the study of them affords little insight either into other early neural functions, or into higher functions, evidences of which are present very early in development. The appearance of reflexes involving the brain stem should be regarded as being associated with the rapid development of neural systems which, before pregnancy is over, can insure viability. These systems include the cardiac, circulatory, respiratory, and alimentary centers.

GENERAL DEVELOPMENTAL PROCESSES

In all vertebrates, the early development of the nervous system is characterized by certain general processes that in turn depend upon specific morphogenetic processes. These general processes include the following: The *induction* of one tissue or organ by another. For example, the segmented part of the neural tube (that part from the midbrain caudally) is induced by the notochord (i.e., its differentiation is initiated). The nonsegmented part of the nervous system (forebrain) is induced by the cephalic mesoderm. The neural arches of the vertebrae are induced by the neural tube. Another process is *differentiation.* This is related to differential cellular proliferation and is represented, for example, by local areas of cellular differentiation and proliferation that bring about the appearance of the cephalic flexure that separates the midbrain and forebrain. It is also represented by the early appearance in the brain of local areas of increased mitotic activity termed *neuromeres. Tubulation* is a process whereby a fluid-filled tube is formed from an ectodermal groove. *Cephalization* is a process characterized by greater activity in the developing brain than in the spinal cord; it includes the replacement of the neuromeres by the forebrain, midbrain, hindbrain, and their derivatives.

SPECIFIC MORPHOGENETIC PROCESSES

These comprise a variety of changes that bring about the general processes cited above and lead to the definitive formation of the nervous system.

Differential Cellular Proliferation. The cells of the neural plate and groove form a pseudostratified layer in which there occurs a to-and-fro nuclear movement related to mitosis (Fig. 9–2). The daughter cells remain in this layer, termed the *ventricular* (or *matrix* or *germinal*) *zone* or *layer.* Soon a cell-free *marginal layer* (Fig. 9–3) appears (this layer is the forerunner of white matter). Zones of greater mitotic activity, leading to the neuromeres in the rostral portion of the neural tube, can soon be detected. The cells of the ventricular zone are the forerunners of all central nervous system neurons and all neuroglial cells except microglia. However, the cells which will form neurons cannot now be distinguished from those which will form neuroglia.

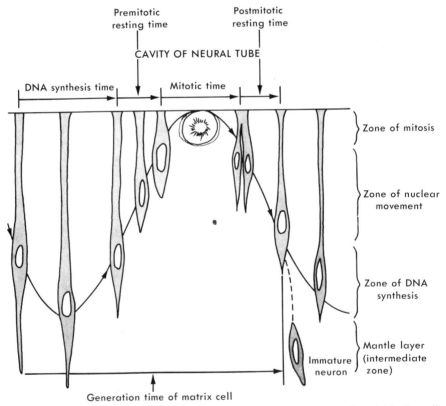

Figure 9–2. Schematic representation of the to-and-fro movement of nuclei in the cells of the ventricular layer. Note that migration out of this layer occurs after mitosis. (Based on Sauer, F. C., in J. Comp. Neurol., *62*:377–405, 1935, and Fujita, S., in J. Comp. Neurol., *120*:37–42, 1963.)

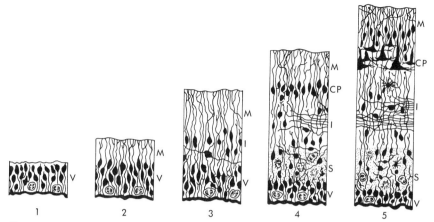

Figure 9–3. Schematic drawing of five stages (1–5) in the development of the vertebrate central nervous system. V, ventricular zone or matrix; M, marginal layer; I, intermediate zone or mantle layer; S, subventricular or subependymal zone; CP, cortical plate. (From Boulder Committee, Anat. Rec., *166*:257–262, 1970. By permission of the authors and publisher.)

As the cells of the neural groove proliferate, they change in shape so that the ends facing the potential lumen become narrower. These changes in cell shape, together with associated morphogenetic movements of the somites, are major factors in helping to bring about the closure of the neural tube. Of equally critical importance are specific cellular relationships, including adhesiveness, tight junctions, and terminal bars, because interference with these features may lead to disruption and disorganization of the neural tube.

In each lateral part of the neural groove there is a group of cells destined to become *neural crest cells* (Fig. 9–1). However, they cannot be distinguished morphologically until the neural groove is about ready to close. These two groups come together and then separate, forming two longitudinal columns of cells. The constituent cells then migrate peripherally and form the spinal ganglia, some of the cranial ganglia, neurilemmal cells, parts of the autonomic system, and parts of the pharyngeal arch skeleton, as well as smooth muscle of the eye and pigmented cells (melanophores) in the skin.

Ectodermal cells other than those that form the neural tube and neural crest also contribute to the nervous system (see placodes, pp. 188 and 189).

Migration. At about the time that the neural groove closes, or shortly thereafter, some of the daughter cells in the ventricular zone migrate peripherally and begin to form the *intermediate zone* or *mantle layer* (Fig. 9–3). Having migrated, they no longer divide and are now immature neurons which will form part of the gray matter of the spinal cord and brain stem. Shortly thereafter, other daughter cells from the ventricular zone migrate and begin to form the *subventricular* or *subependymal zone,* between the ventricular and intermediate zones. Two types of cells can be distinguished in the subventricular zone. One type is presumably the forerunner of neuroglial cells; they continue to divide. The other type is the forerunner of nerve cells; in some regions, notably the cerebral hemispheres, they continue to divide and give rise to small nerve cells (sometimes termed microneurons), even after birth.

Also, as the cerebral hemispheres form, migrating immature nerve cells move outward past the intermediate zone and form a *cortical plate,* the forerunner of cerebral cortex. Successive waves of migration occur, the later cells moving past the earlier ones to more superficial positions.

In the hindbrain, migrating cells in a special area termed the *rhombic lip* (the edge of the alar plate) begin to form the cerebellum. Some of the cells form a special layer, the *external granular layer,* which persists for some time after birth and gives rise to cells that migrate and form deeper layers of the cerebellar cortex.

Eventually, throughout the nervous system, the matrix becomes exhausted in terms of the mitotic activity of its constituent cells (Fig. 9–4) and the remaining cells differentiate into ependyma.

Growth and Maturation. As immature nerve cells form, beginning in the intermediate zone, they begin to develop processes, first axons and then dendrites (Fig. 9–5). The axons soon form tracts; those that will supply muscles or go to autonomic ganglia grow out of the spinal cord and brain stem. The full maturation of dendrites, however, often takes many years.

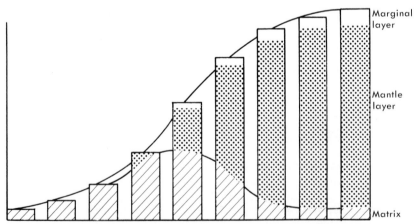

Figure 9–4. Schematic representation of the sequential development of the layers of the neural tube (spinal cord part). The matrix (ventricular zone) thickens as cell division proceeds, the mantle layer (dotted portion) forms as daughter cells migrate, and the marginal layer comprises a peripheral zone of cellular processes. The matrix is finally exhausted, becomes thinner, and forms ependyma. (Based on Keyser, A.: Acta Anat., 83 [Suppl. 59], 1972.)

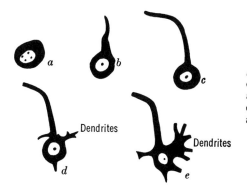

Figure 9–5. Simplified representation of neuronal differentiation of multipolar cell from an immature apolar neuron. *a*: Apolar neuron; *b* and *c*: With differentiation into a neuron, an axon appears. *d* and *e*: Dendrites appear and increase in number.

The neural crest cells that will become ganglion cells commonly develop two processes, but quickly become unipolar cells through eccentric growth (Fig. 9–6). One process grows into the spinal cord or brain stem and the other grows peripherally and forms a sensory receptor.

Interaction. Specific and important intercellular relationships are a feature of normal development. For example, growing axons will extend for long distances and nevertheless reach and connect with the appropriate nerve cells. These events are genetically determined and programmed.

If a muscle is absent, the corresponding motor cells of the spinal cord will not develop properly. If the nerve cells are absent, the muscles and joints will not develop properly.

Cell Loss. Genetically programmed cell death is a characteristic feature of normal development. For example, the continuous column of neural crest cells is soon regularly interrupted by the death of cells so that definitive spinal ganglia appear. Likewise, continuous columns of cells in the intermediate zone become broken up to form nuclei, especially those supplying the limbs. The caudal part of the spinal cord dedifferentiates and becomes the filum terminale.

THE DEVELOPMENT OF THE SPINAL CORD

When the neural tube that will form the spinal cord is fully closed, it has thick lateral walls and a thin roof and floor, termed

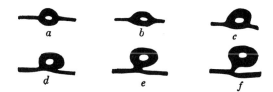

Figure 9–6. Illustration of the manner in which eccentric growth (more rapid growth on one side of the cell) transforms a bipolar cell into a unipolar one.

roof plate and floor plate, respectively. These plates are ependymal in structure; only later will nerve fibers cross in them and form commissures. Each lateral wall is marked on its interior by a longitudinal groove, the *sulcus limitans,* which delimits the *alar* and *basal plates* (Fig. 9–7). These plates become prominent as cells form and migrate into the mantle layer (the future gray matter of the spinal cord). This growth, coupled with selective cell loss, results in the formation of the characteristic nuclei of the gray matter by the third or fourth prenatal month. This is correlated with the onset and development of increasingly complex motor activity. By the end of the fourth month, movements of the fetus are usually so marked that the mother feels them.

The cells in the basal plate become associated with motor systems. As they differentiate, the axons of many of them grow out of the neural tube into developing muscles, forming ventral roots as they grow out. Also, at many levels outgrowing fibers are autonomic, being directed toward autonomic ganglion cells.

The cells in the alar plate become associated with sensory mechanisms and receive the ingrowing fibers from the differentiating neural crest cells. As the latter grow in, they form dorsal roots.

At the end of the embryonic period, the spinal cord extends the whole length of the vertebral canal. The vertebral column now begins to grow faster than the spinal cord so that, by full term, the cord only reaches to about the level of the third lumbar vertebra. The usual adult level is reached during the next year or two. As a result of this disproportionate growth, the spinal nerves below the cervical segments descend in an increasingly oblique fashion.

The absence of the spinal cord from the caudal part of the vertebral canal is contributed to by the dedifferentiation of the caudal part of the embryonic cord. During the embryonic period, more than 40 pairs of somites and more than one pair of coccygeal nerves develop. As a result of selective cell death, the most caudal structures begin to disappear and the caudal part of the spinal cord persists only as the filum terminale. The caudal part of the central canal ends as the *ventriculus terminalis,* which occupies the conus medullaris and the upper part of the filum terminale.

THE DEVELOPMENT OF THE BRAIN

The part of the neural tube within what will be the cranium becomes the brain. Even before the neural tube is closed, however, the major subdivisions (forebrain, midbrain, and hindbrain) can be distinguished, partly because of the early appearance of the cephalic flexure, which separates the forebrain and midbrain. The notochord, the sulcus limitans, and the basal and floor plates extend only to about the region of the cephalic flexure. The roof plate, however, extends to the rostral end of the neural tube, to the region of closure of the rostral neuropore. It exhibits character-

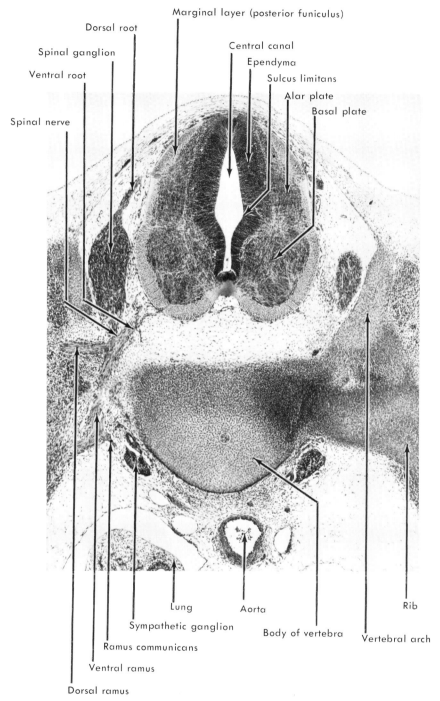

Figure 9-7. Transverse section through the developing thoracic spinal cord of a human embryo about seven weeks old. Note that the spinal ganglion is an enlargement of the dorsal root, that the dorsal and ventral root join to form a spinal nerve, and that the nerve almost immediately divides into a dorsal and a ventral ramus. Magnification 55×. (From the Carnegie Embryological Collection.)

istic local features. In the hindbrain it forms the roof of the fourth ventricle and is related to the formation of the cerebellum. In the midbrain it becomes covered by the tectum as the cerebral aqueduct forms. In the forebrain it becomes the roof of the third ventricle and, rostrally, the *lamina terminalis*. This lamina in turn is the path for the major commissures of the cerebral hemispheres.

In terms of external appearance, the various flexures and the general form of the prenatal brain are shown in Figure 9–8. The divisions and derivatives of the neural tube are given in Table 9–1.

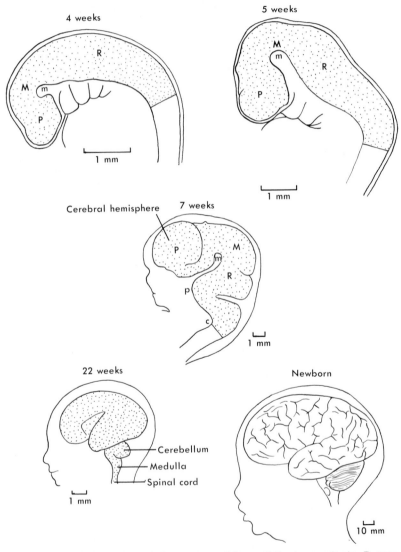

Figure 9–8. The development of the external form of the human brain. P, prosencephalon; M, mesencephalon; R, rhombencephalon; m, mesencephalic (cephalic) flexure; p, pontine flexure; c, cervical flexure. (Courtesy of Dr. Ronan O'Rahilly.)

Table 9-1. Neural Tube Divisions and Derivatives

Divisions	Subdivisions	Derivatives Walls	Derivatives Lumen
Forebrain (Prosencephalon)	Telencephalon (Endbrain)	Cerebral hemispheres; Telencephalon medium	Lateral ventricles; Rostral end of third ventricle
	Diencephalon (Interbrain)	Thalamus; Hypothalamus; Neurohypophysis; Pineal body	Most of third ventricle
*Midbrain (Mesencephalon)	No subdivision	Tectum; tegmentum; Basis pedunculi	Cerebral aqueduct
*Hindbrain (Rhombencephalon)	Metencephalon (Afterbrain)	Pons; Cerebellum	Upper part of fourth ventricle
	Myelencephalon (Marrowbrain)	Medulla oblongata	Lower part of fourth ventricle; Upper part of central canal
*Remainder of neural tube (Medullae spinalis)	No subdivision	Spinal cord	Most of central canal

*Cells migrating from these parts of the neural tube, together with neural crest cells, give rise to autonomic ganglion cells, the suprarenal medullae, chromaffin cells, neurilemmal cells, and pigment cells.

MIDBRAIN AND HINDBRAIN

In the midbrain, the rapid growth of the *tectum* dorsal to the cerebral aqueduct foreshadows the appearance of the colliculi. Ventral to the aqueduct, the *tegmentum* and *basis pedunculi* develop during the embryonic period. However, the pyramidal tracts, which comprise much of the basis pedunculi, do not appear until during the third month.

In the hindbrain, as soon as the neural tube closes, the lateral walls begin to spread apart, like the opening of a book. Accompanying this is a widening and a thinning of the roof plate, which becomes the roof of the fourth ventricle. Sometimes at the end of the embryonic period, but usually during the fetal period, the caudal part of the roof plate develops an opening, the median aperture, by which the fourth ventricle communicates with the subarachnoid space. The lateral apertures also open during the fetal period, but somewhat later than the median.

During the embryonic period, the hindbrain becomes subdivided into the metencephalon (pons and cerebellum) and the myelencephalon (medulla oblongata). The cerebellum first appears as an outgrowth from the rhombic lip, which is the line of attachment of the roof plate to the alar plates of the neural tube. The two *cerebellar plates,* one on each side, grow dorsally and medially, over the roof plate. They fuse in the median plane early in the fetal period. The two cerebellar plates differentiate first into the caudal part of the vermis of the cerebellum and the adjacent hemisphere (the archicerebellum, p. 358). The remainder of the cerebellum forms throughout the fetal period and its differentiation is not completed until after birth.

Cranial nerves. The olfactory and optic nerves are considered with the forebrain. The motor and sensory nuclei of the third to the twelfth cranial nerves are derived from the basal and alar plates of the midbrain and hindbrain. They form more or less continuous columns which occupy typical positions in the brain stem and which correspond to the functional components of the cranial nerves (Fig. 14–4, p. 308). The axons of the motor cells grow out of the brain stem; some axons are directed to parasympathetic ganglion cells, but most supply muscles of the head and neck.

The ganglia of the trigeminal, glossopharyngeal, and vagus nerves are derived in part from neural crest cells, just as are the spinal ganglia. However, some of the ganglion cells are derived from *placodes,* which are groups of neuroectodermal cells near the neural tube and neural crest that form sense organs as well as ganglion cells. Placodal cells (the *otic placodes*) are also a source of ganglion cells for the facial and vestibulocochlear nerves, as are neural crest cells. These placodes, which form on each side of the hindbrain, also give rise to the internal ear. The various cells that contribute to the ganglion of the facial nerve (geniculate ganglion) become unipolar, whereas the cells that form the vestibular and cochlear ganglia remain bipolar.

FOREBRAIN

The forebrain is nonsegmented and lacks a floor plate; the roof plate becomes specialized, as indicated above. Lateralization of the forebrain occurs throughout the embryonic period. The optic primordium can be recognized in the prosencephalic neural folds by about the end of the third week. Shortly thereafter, with the rostral neuropore just closed, cells have begun to form an optic vesicle on each side. This marks the subdivision of the forebrain into a telencephalon and a diencephalon, with the *optic vesicles* arising as evaginations of the diencephalon. The proximal portion of each optic vesicle becomes constricted to form the *optic stalk.* The more dilated distal portion of the stalk lies adjacent to thickened ectoderm that constitutes the *lens disc.* The optic vesicle then invaginates to form the double-layered *optic cup.* The walls of the optic cup give rise to the retina, which even in the adult retains a tendency to separate between layers that correspond to the embryonic two layers (Fig. 12–3, p. 249). The optic cup also forms the epithelium of the ciliary body and the iris. Because of the nature of their diencephalic origin, the retinae and optic nerves are extensions of the central nervous system. The optic nerves are fiber tracts, not peripheral nerves, and contain neuroglia, not neurilemma.

Cerebral hemispheres. By four and a half weeks the dorso-lateral walls of the forebrain become "domed." This change indicates the beginning of the *cerebral vesicles.* These shortly become evaginations that comprise chiefly the primordia of the cerebral cortex (the primordia of the basal ganglia and the olfactory structures appear somewhat earlier). Moreover, the cerebral hemispheres mark the appearance of lateral ventricles, with the interventricular foramina being present at the site of the evaginations. Connecting the two evaginations across the rostral median plane is the *telencephalon medium.* This extends from the optic chiasma to the roof plate of the third ventricle. It becomes the *lamina terminalis* in the adult and is the site of the major commissures of the hemispheres (anterior, hippocampal, and corpus callosum).

Within the evaginating hemispheres, the first cortex to become recognizable is that of the hippocampus (*archicortex*), followed by that of the piriform cortex (*paleocortex*). The *neocortex* is then distinguished by the appearance of the cortical plate (Fig. 9–3). The cerebral hemispheres develop rapidly, growing backward and downward. Choroid plexuses appear, the basal ganglia and limbic system continue to differentiate, and before the end of the embryonic period a lateral sulcus is beginning. By term, most gyri and sulci are present (Fig. 9–8).

In late somite embryos two ectodermal thickenings, the *olfactory* or *nasal placodes,* form just below and lateral to the forebrain. These become depressed to form *olfactory pits* from which the nasal cavities arise and which form the olfactory epithelium. Some of the ectodermal cells differentiate into bipolar nerve cells which remain in the epithelium and whose axons grow toward the forebrain, forming the filaments of the *olfactory nerves.* These nerves end in the *olfactory bulbs,* which also form in the embryonic period.

Diencephalon. The thalamus and hypothalamus begin to differentiate during the embryonic period, as does the pineal body. The adenohypophysis is differentiated early (by about the end of the third week) and from its inception is in contact with the brain; the area of contact indicates the region of the infundibulum, from which the neurohypophysis develops.

THE PERIPHERAL NERVOUS SYSTEM

The peripheral nervous system develops from the neural crest and the basal plate, and is also closely related to the alar plate.

SPINAL AND PERIPHERAL NERVES

Many of the neuroblasts that lie in the ventral portion of the basal plate become motor neurons and send their axons out of the spinal cord, where, at regular intervals, they are collected into ventral roots. The fibers of these roots grow into body areas which may be thought of as transversely oriented "embryo segments" (these are more clearly defined in lower vertebrates). The muscles that the ventral root fibers will supply develop from tissue which at first lies but a millimeter or less from the neural tube. The first axons traversing this distance establish a path which fibers developing later seem to follow. The factors that determine the growth and termination of fibers are not well understood. Certain general relationships are obvious. For example, there is a general relationship between the region in which a limb bud is developing and the spinal cord at that level so that nerves from this portion of the cord grow into the region. But there is no initial specific relationship between the axons of the spinal nerves and the muscle fibers developing within the limb bud. It may be predetermined that a certain axon enters a given embryo segment, but within that segment the axon may vary in the exact site of its termination. This is because the direction of its growing tip is influenced by the physical nature of the non-nervous environment, such as obstructions, changes in consistency, or stresses and strains. These are prominent in regions of attachment of limb buds, where they probably influence the formation of plexuses. Once a path is established by the first fibers, however, growth of later axons is much less haphazard. Although growth is somewhat nonspecific, variation is not as marked as it might be, because of the short distances traversed and because of the pattern formed by the earliest fibers. It cannot be denied, however, that there is some specificity which determines that motor and sensory fibers form their proper endings once they have grown into their region of supply. Moreover, limbs will not develop properly if nerves are absent, and if limbs or portions of limbs are absent, the corresponding portions of the nervous system may not develop properly.

Spinal ganglion cells develop from neural crest cells, as mentioned previously. The peripheral processes (dendrites) of the unipolar cells in each segment of the neural crest accompany corresponding ventral root fibers to form a spinal nerve. The central processes (axons) of the cells grow into the spinal cord, toward the dorsal portion of the alar plate, thereby forming a dorsal root. The cell bodies in each neural crest segment are collected together and form a spinal ganglion.

AUTONOMIC GANGLION CELLS

Many neural crest cells, and perhaps additional cells from the basal plate, migrate peripherally to positions along the vertebral column and near thoracic, abdominal, and pelvic viscera. In these positions, they differentiate into autonomic ganglia. The cells that migrate from the thoracic and upper lumbar portions of the neural crest and neural tube form the ganglia of the sympathetic trunk and the prevertebral plexuses. They also form accessory ganglia (p. 340) and the cells of the chromaffin system, namely, the supra-renal medullae and the para-aortic bodies. Parasympathetic ganglion cells form after similar migration from neural crest and basal plate in the brain stem and in the sacral region.

It is of considerable importance that developing sympathetic nerve cells in birds and mammals are sensitive to the growth-promoting effects of a protein termed the *nerve growth factor*. This protein is a normal constituent of sympathetic cells and blood and body fluids. Its presence suggests the possibility that there may be other growth factors for other cells of the developing nervous system.

BLOOD SUPPLY AND CEREBROSPINAL FLUID

With the definitive formation of the vascular system in the embryo, blood vessels soon invade the central nervous system (shortly after the migration of neurons from the matrix) and, in so doing, carry with them a small amount of connective tissue, some of the cells of which may contribute to the formation of microglia (p. 57). These are said to be the only mesodermal elements of the central nervous system.

After the neural tube is formed and until the neuropores are closed, the tube contains amniotic fluid. With complete closure of the tube, cerebrospinal fluid begins to form, even before choroid plexuses are present. The plexuses begin to appear near the end of the embryonic period.

A GENERAL VIEW OF PRENATAL NEURAL DEVELOPMENT

By the end of the embryonic period, the spinal cord and brain stem are highly organized and are present in a form and arrangement like that of the adult, as are the cranial and spinal nerves and their autonomic components. By this time also, organized head and neck movements occur in response to cutaneous stimulation in the trigeminal area.

By contrast, although certain major diencephalic and olfactory structures are present and the cerebral hemispheres exhibit recognizable divisions into certain major components (neocortex; basal ganglia and lateral olfactory structures; septum and medial olfactory structures; hippocampus), the neocortex has no significant intrinsic differentiation. However, synapses begin to appear in the cortical plate early in the fetal period, and by term the basic organization of the neocortex is well-developed.

The extraordinary complexity and timing of these phenomena are indicated first by the fact that many structures do not appear until well along in the fetal period (e.g., corpus callosum, pyramidal tracts). Second, as mentioned above, the cerebral cortex differentiates throughout the prenatal period but even at birth its cells are "immature" with respect to numbers and arrangement of dendrites and synaptic junctions. These elements continue to increase in size and number for many years. There is considerable evidence that lack of afferent input to cortical neurons interferes with proper dendritic and synaptic maturation.

The brain as a whole undergoes a major growth spurt that begins during the third trimester and lasts until well into the second year of postnatal life. This growth is due chiefly to proliferation of glial cells and is therefore associated with the onset of myelination. During this growth spurt, the brain is susceptible to a variety of influences that may retard growth.

It is clear that a genetically controlled time table brings about the basic organization of the nervous system and the development of that part of the brain which is necessary for survival, i.e., vital centers and reflex mechanisms. The continued maturation of these centers leads rapidly toward the time when the fetus can survive in an air-breathing environment (about 26 weeks, plus or minus a few weeks). From this time on, muscular activity becomes more and more complex, swallowing and respiratory movements occur, electrical activity of the brain develops, and the special sensory systems become functional (e.g., the fetus begins to hear). About the time that the fetus becomes viable in terms of air breathing, it has been noticed that there appears what might be called an alertness, in which there is a kind of "affect" that alternates with "sleep." However, the morphological and physiological correlations with the onset of such physiological states are still unknown.

Finally, it should be emphasized that although the basic patterns and organization of the brain, and therefore the pattern of behavior, are genetically determined, both the early development and the subsequent maturation are dependent upon various hormones. For example, the thyroid hormone is important in the formation of synapses and, together with corticosteroids, influences cell proliferation and differentiation. Androgens seem to bring about a permanent "masculinizing" effect on central neurons concerned with neuroendocrine regulation. Prenatal hormone deficiencies can cause severe disorders, including neurological deficiencies. The classical example is cretinism resulting from thyroid deficiency and which is associated with severe mental retardation.

DEVELOPMENTAL DEFECTS

Congenital anomalies and malformations range from minor variations to a variety of major defects. These are exemplified by *anencephaly* (absence of much of the head and brain) and by *myelomeningocele* (extensive open portions of the spinal cord, meninges, and vertebrae, resulting from failure of the neural tube to close). These two groups of defects, together with associated *hydrocephalus,* comprise most of the major congenital malformations of the nervous system and a significant number of all major congenital malformations recognizable at or shortly after birth. Thus they represent an important cause of morbidity and mortality.

These defects, with their grossly apparent abnormalities, are to be contrasted with a congenital disease entity in which there is severe mental retardation but no morphological abnormality of the brain. This is Down's syndrome (trisomy 21), with its characteristic mental deficiency, physical defects in many non-nervous systems, and probability of an early death. Individuals born with this disorder nearly always have 47 chromosomes, with trisomy 21.

CAUSES, MECHANISMS, PATHOGENESIS

The causes of developmental defects are many. Genetic transmission is the chief one in about 20 per cent of cases. Environmental factors (e.g., radiations, infections, metabolic disturbances, drugs, and chemicals) are the major causes in the remainder. Even so, the specific environmental causes are usually unknown. Whatever the causes, they operate through certain mechanisms. The term "mechanism of teratogenesis" is applied tentatively to the earliest recognizable event thought to have played a primary role in abnormal development. There are a number of such mechanisms, examples of which are chromosomal aberrations (Down's syndrome, cited above), mitotic interference, and enzyme inhibition and dysfunction.

Whatever the mechanisms, they lead to certain pathogenic changes such as cell death, failed cellular interaction, impaired morphogenetic movement, or mechanical disruption. The final defect is intrauterine death, malformation, growth retardation, or functional deficit.

Certain additional features of the foregoing causes, mechanisms, and pathogenesis need to be emphasized.

1. The causes of a specific defect are often multifactorial and, depending upon conditions, a specific cause may initiate different mechanisms, and a specific mechanism may bring about different pathogenic changes. Hence, it is a general principle that a final teratogenic defect may be brought about by a variety of sequences of events.

2. Tissues and organs have critical periods of development during which they are especially susceptible to teratogenic agents; these are usually just preceding and during differentiation, when protein synthesis is especially important. For example, the critical period for the production of polydactylism (the presence of extra fingers or toes) by environmental factors is from just before the appearance of limb buds to definitive differentiation, a period extending from about the third week to about the sixth week after ovulation.

3. The effect of a teratological agent depends upon: (a) The time during which it acts (Thalidomide taken during critical periods of skeletal development may cause severe limb defects; taken later it will have no teratogenic effect). (b) The nature of the agent (Thalidomide has different effects from other teratogenic agents). (c) The species involved (Thalidomide is more teratogenic for humans than for any of the other species studied, and seems not to be teratogenic at all for some species).

4. The critical periods of one organ system often coincide with those of another, and a single teratogenic agent may, therefore, involve more than one system, for example, both the skeletal and neurological systems. Hence, the existence of one congenital defect indicates the possible presence of others.

SUMMARY

Development begins with fertilization, when a spermatozoon makes contact with an oocyte. Prenatal development is divided into an embryonic period (the first eight weeks after fertilization) and a fetal period (from the embryonic period until term). Cell division leads to the formation of three cellular germ layers — ectoderm, mesoderm, and endoderm. A dorsal invagination of the ectoderm forms first a neural groove and then a neural tube. Before the neural tube closes, the forebrain, midbrain, and hindbrain are indicated. The remainder of the neural tube forms the spinal cord.

The general developmental processes include induction, differentiation, tubulation, and cephalization. The specific morphogenetic processes comprise different cellular proliferation, migration, growth and maturation, interaction, and cell death.

Differential cellular proliferation leads to the formation of various layers comprised of immature neurons and glial cells derived from the matrix or germinal layer of the neural tube. The neurons soon develop dendrites and then an axon.

In addition to the neural tube, ectodermal cells lateral to the tube on each side comprise neural crest cells that migrate peripherally and form spinal ganglia, some of the cranial ganglia, neurilemmal cells, parts of the autonomic system, parts of the pharyngeal arch skeleton, smooth muscle of the eye, and melanophores. In addition, some of the special sense organs and some of the cranial ganglion cells develop from ectodermal placodes. The neural crest and placodal neurons become either unipolar or bipolar.

Soon after neural tube closure, the spinal cord, hindbrain, and midbrain exhibit roof and floor plates, alar (sensory) and basal (motor) plates, separated by a sulcus limitans. The forebrain soon becomes subdivided into the diencephalon and telencephalon as the optic system and cerebral hemispheres develop.

By the end of the embryonic period, the spinal cord and brain stem are present in a form and arrangement like that of the adult, organized reflexes are present, and major centers are functioning. The cerebral hemispheres exhibit divisions into their major components, but the cerebral cortex has no significant intrinsic differentiation. The maturation of the brain continues throughout the fetal period as cells grow and synapses and dendritic patterns increase in complexity, with a brain-growth spurt beginning in the third trimester and lasting until the second year. Major physiological processes develop and the fetus becomes viable in an air-breathing environment at about 26 weeks.

Congenital anomalies and malformations are major causes of morbidity and mortality. Genetic transmission is the chief cause in about 20 per cent of cases, with environmental factors being mainly responsible in the remainder. The mechanisms by which these causes operate are many, and these in turn bring about pathogenic changes that result in the final defect.

NAMES IN NEUROLOGY

JOHN LANGDON HAYDON DOWN (1828–1896)

In 1866, John Down, a London physician, published a short description of the syndrome that is still recognized as an entity today and that still bears his name. (Warkany, J.: Congenital Malformations: Notes and Comments. Chicago, Year Book Publishers, 1971.)

REFERENCES

The following references comprise major sources for further, advanced reading.

Hamilton, W. J., and Mossman, H. W.: Hamilton, Boyd and Mossman's Human Embryology. Fourth ed. Cambridge, W. Heffer & Sons Ltd., and Baltimore. The Williams and Wilkins Company, 1972. The best modern textbook of human embryology.

Holmes, L. B., Moser, H. W., Halldórsson, S., Mack, C., Pant, S. S., and Matzilevich, B.: Mental Retardation. New York, The Macmillan Company, 1972. An atlas of diseases with associated physical abnormalities.

Hooker, D.: The Prenatal Origin of Behavior. Reprint of the 1952 edition. New York, Hafner Publishing Company, 1969. The classic work on the development of reflex behavior in living human embryos and fetuses.

Jacobson, M.: Developmental Neurobiology. New York, Holt, Rinehart and Winston, Inc.,

1970. An excellent monograph on the basic principles of the main processes of morpho-
genesis.

O'Rahilly, R.: A Color Atlas of Human Embryology. Philadelphia, W. B. Saunders Company,
1975.

Tobach, E., Aronson, L. R., and Shaw, E. (editors): The Biopsychology of Development. New
York, Academic Press, 1971. Contains some especially good, critical reviews of the major
questions and hypotheses.

Volpe, E. P.: Human Heredity and Birth Defects. New York, Pegasus, 1971. A short, well-
written account that is a biological sciences curriculum study book.

Warkany, J.: Congenital Malformations: Notes and Comments. Chicago, Year Book Publishers,
1971. A massive source book.

Wilson, J. B.: Environment and Birth Defects. New York, Academic Press, 1973. A first-rate,
extremely valuable presentation of causes, mechanisms, and pathogenesis.

The following are papers, reviews, and chapters of selected important topics.

Bartelmez, G. W., and Dekaban, A. S.: The early development of the human brain. Contrib.
Embryol., *37*:13–32, 1962.

British Medical Bulletin. Development and Regeneration in the Nervous System. Vol. 30.
London, Medical Department, The British Council, 1974. This comprises a number of excellent short reviews.

Dobbing, J.: Vulnerable periods of brain development. In: Lipids, Malnutrition and the Developing Brain. CIBA Foundation and Nestle Foundation Symposium. Amsterdam,
Elsevier, Excerpta Medica, 1972.

Gottlieb, G.: Conceptions of prenatal behavior, and Lehrman, D. S.: Semantic and conceptual
issues in the nature-nurture problem. *In* Aronson, L. R., Tobach, E., Lehrman, D. S., and
Rosenblatt, J. S. (editors): Development and Evolution of Behavior. Essays in memory of
T. C. Schneirla. San Francisco, W. H. Freeman Co., 1970.

Levi-Montalcini, R.: Events in the developing nervous system. Progr. Brain Res., *4*:1–29,
1964.

O'Rahilly, R., and Gardner, E.: The timing and sequence of events in the development of the
human nervous system during the embryonic period proper. Z. Anat. Entw., *134*:1–12, 1971.

Straus, W. L., Jr.: The concept of nerve-muscle specificity. Biol. Rev., *21*:75–91, 1946.

Chapter 10

THE CONTROL OF MUSCULAR ACTIVITY

The pattern of muscular activity is controlled by the central nervous system, but this does not mean that one first thinks of movements to be performed in a particular activity and then initiates the nerve impulses that bring about the movements. On the contrary, most movements are complex, almost automatic patterns. Walking exemplifies such a pattern. Once walking is learned (it has to be learned laboriously), it is carried out according to fairly definite sequences and patterns of muscular activity that are "voluntarily" initiated and controlled. This control resides mainly if not entirely in the cerebral cortex and is mediated by groups of fibers that leave the cortex and project to the basal ganglia, cerebellum, brain stem, and spinal cord. These projection fibers are loosely termed *pyramidal* and *extrapyramidal*. The pyramidal fibers (or pyramidal system) comprise those that project from the cerebral cortex directly to motor neurons in the brain stem and spinal cord. In the latter instance, they form the pyramids of the medulla oblongata as they descend to the spinal cord, hence the term pyramidal. The extrapyramidal fibers (none are present in the medullary pyramids) comprise a heterogeneous system that involves cortical projections to the basal ganglia and cerebellum, with these in turn projecting to brain stem motor mechanisms and thence to motor neurons.

It should be emphasized that the term "voluntary" (or "voluntary control") is somewhat misleading; there is a large element of "involuntary" mechanisms in all movements. Moreover, pyramidal and extrapyramidal functions are not sharply distinguished. For example, suppose that one reaches out and picks up something on a table. The use of the fingers is the element of this motion of which one is mainly conscious; the muscles concerned are

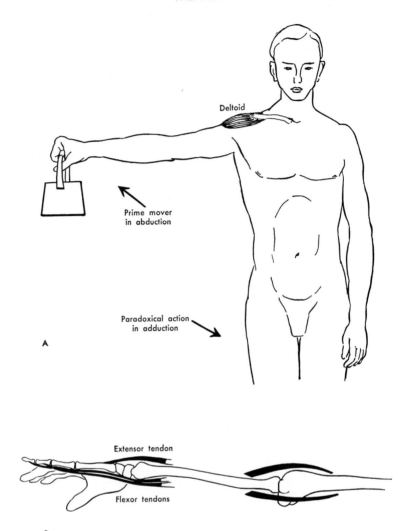

Figure 10-1. *A,* the deltoid muscle, which is an abductor of the arm, is shown as a prime mover in lifting a pail of water (other muscles stabilize elbow and hand). It also does negative work in controlling the lowering of the pail (adduction) — a paradoxical action. The adductors are inactive unless resistance is offered to the movement. *B,* if the flexor muscles, which are shown inserting into a finger, contract so as to flex the fingers, the wrist would also flex were it not that the extensor muscle contracts and acts as a synergist, preventing undesired action at intermediate joints. The elbow joint can be fixed or stabilized in the desired position by simultaneous contraction of flexors and extensors.

the *prime movers* (Fig. 10-1). But in order to get the fingers to the object that is to be picked up, the forearm is extended as the forearm flexors relax. Furthermore, as one reaches out, other muscles stabilize the shoulder. At the same time, the body leans forward, the center of gravity shifts, and compensatory stabilizing muscle actions in the trunk and lower limbs insure that posture is maintained.

The various patterns of muscular activity that coexist with the prime movements involve *synergists,* which prevent undesired movements at intermediate joints when a prime mover crosses two or more joints. They also involve *fixators,* which stabilize certain joints, and *antagonists,* which act directly opposite to the movement or movements under consideration. Antagonists may either relax completely during movement (this occurs when a movement is carried out against resistance) or they may relax gradually as they lengthen, thereby controlling or modifying the action of the muscle bringing about the movement. This gradual lengthening of an active muscle is an example of paradoxical action in which the muscle controls a movement in a direction opposite to that in which it usually operates (Figs. 10–1, 10–2). In this capacity, it does negative work. It is to be noted that in some instances, gravity acts as the prime mover. Finally, the role of a muscle or a group of muscles may shift. A prime mover in one instance may become an antagonist in another. Also a synergist may become a prime mover.

Thus, an apparently simple act involves many muscles in a complex procedure. We pay little attention, if any, to the individ-

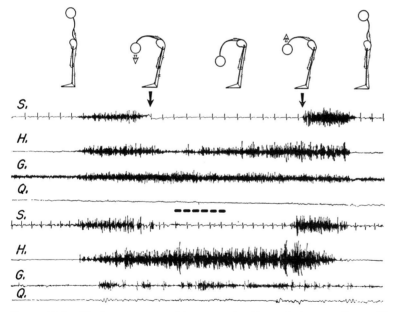

Figure 10–2. Electromyograms of two normal subjects during standing and bending down. In standing, no activity is recorded from sacropinalis (S), hamstrings (H), or quadriceps femoris (Q). The short vertical deflections in S are the electrocardiogram. As the subject leans forward, activity appears in S (negative work; the muscles control the leaning forward as they lengthen), in hamstrings (same reason) and gastrocnemius (G). Activity stops in sacrospinalis at full flexion (ligaments now are the support of the back), to reappear as the subject extends and returns to standing. These records show the lack of muscular activity in an easy standing position, and the complicated activity during movement. The upper four records are from one subject, the lower four from another subject. (Based on Figure 2, from Portnoy, H., and Morin, F., Am. J. Physiol., *186*:122–126, 1956. By permission of authors and publisher.)

ual elements of the act, only to the prime movement. Speaking, walking, running, dancing, using a typewriter, playing a piano, fielding a baseball, are examples of skilled acts that we usually take for granted to the extent that we lose sight of their enormous complexity and forget the months or years of learning or practice they require. How learning occurs and how practice maintains and improves performance are essentially unknown. Moreover, some individuals can never do some things well, or as well as others, no matter how much they practice.

Both in movement and in posture, muscles may act against the influence of gravity, and the muscles most concerned are often called antigravity muscles. It is held that reflexes involving neuromuscular spindles are prominent in antigravity muscles during standing. Most experiments, however, have been made on four-footed animals, and one must be cautious in applying such findings to human beings. In an easy standing position, little if any muscular contraction or tone can be detected in the so-called antigravity muscles of human beings (Fig. 10–2); intrinsic muscle tone is due to elastic and viscous properties; it can be enhanced or decreased by neural actions. The human skeleton and human joints are arranged so that one can stand upright with a minimal expenditure of energy (unless one is overweight, or has poor posture).

LEVELS OF CONTROL

It is convenient (if not strictly accurate), in the study of motor pathways and their role in the control of muscular activity, to consider the nervous system as being made up of a series of levels. These levels may be represented by the cerebral cortex, the basal ganglia, the cerebellum, the brain stem, and the spinal cord. In general, the lowest level is the most specific in function and the highest the least specific. That is, a motor cell in the spinal cord or brain stem supplies certain muscle fibers and no others. Its activity cannot directly cause any other muscle fibers to contract. The cerebral cortex represents the highest degree of control and the greatest degree of lability. It controls activity through an almost infinite variety of combinations.

The regions of the cerebral cortex from which the pyramidal and extrapyramidal motor paths arise are called *motor areas.* Most of them are located in the frontal lobes. The nerve cells of the neocortex are arranged in six layers. In the motor areas the fifth layer is thick and many of its constituent cells are the sources of motor pathways (p. 400). The axons of these cells leave the cortex and enter the white matter of the hemispheres. They then descend in the internal capsule and reach motor cells in the brain stem and spinal cord by a variety of pathways. Some pathways are direct, as mentioned above, and comprise the pyramidal system. The others are indirect and comprise the extrapyramidal system in which the cortical projections reach the basal ganglia and cerebellum, which are inextricably interrelated with the cerebral cortex in the control of muscular activity.

The basal ganglia and the cerebellum project, directly and indirectly, to the reticular formation of the brain stem, which can be considered to be the next lower level of control. The reticular formation is a mixture of white and gray matter concerned with many different functions. Some of the constituent cells, including those forming the *red nuclei* and certain *vestibular* and *reticular nuclei,* are important in the control of muscular activity. Their axons descend as *rubrospinal, reticulospinal,* and *vestibulospinal* tracts to the gray matter of the spinal cord, which represents the lowest level of control. This level is capable of organized activity on a reflex level.

The normal contraction of a muscle is initiated only by impulses reaching motor endings by way of axons of specific motor cells in the brain stem or spinal cord. This motor pathway from the central nervous system to muscles is the *final common path.* All motor tracts in the central nervous system, no matter what their origin, are directed toward motor cells in the brain stem and spinal cord.

Alpha Motor Fibers. The extrafusal fibers in skeletal muscles are supplied by nerve fibers that range from 8 to 20 μm in diameter, and which are termed *alpha* fibers; they form motor endings as described on p. 50. Each *alpha* fiber supplies a number of skeletal muscle fibers. The nerve cell, its axon, and the muscle fibers supplied by it form a *motor unit* (Fig. 10–3). A nerve impulse along the parent fiber of a motor unit can initiate the contraction of all the muscle fibers of that unit. The number of units in any one muscle depends upon the number of muscle fibers in the whole muscle, and upon the number of muscle fibers in a motor unit. In human beings, some muscles have fewer than 100 muscle fibers per motor unit, whereas others may have between 1500 and 2000. It follows that a muscle with many motor units for a given number of muscle fibers is capable of more precise work than is a muscle with fewer motor units for the same given number of muscle fibers. Thus, the muscles of the thumb have many small units, each with only a few fibers, whereas antigravity muscles are characterized by relatively fewer motor units, each of which has a large number of muscle fibers.

Gamma Motor Fibers. The intrafusal muscle fibers of *neuromuscular spindles* are supplied by *gamma* motor fibers. These fibers, which are small myelinated axons that range from 2 to 8 μm in diameter, arise from a number of small motor cells in the brain stem and spinal cord. The neuromuscular spindles (Figs. 10–4, 10–5) are the best known and most widely studied of the proprioceptive receptors. They are present in nearly all muscles, generally near musculotendinous junctions. Each spindle is usually

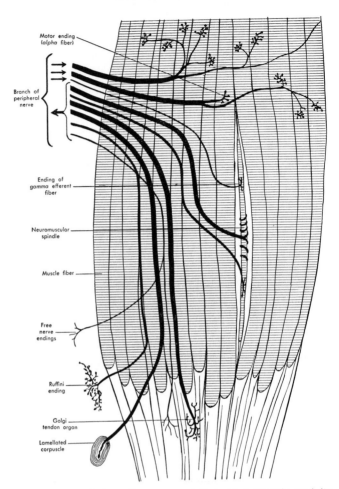

Figure 10-3. Schematic representation of a muscle and its
nerve supply. Arrows indicate direction of conduction. Each
muscle fiber has a motor ending from a large myelinated (*alpha*)
fiber. The muscle fibers within a spindle have motor endings from
small myelinated (*gamma*) fibers. Muscle nerves contain many
sensory fibers. Some are large myelinated fibers from primary
(annulospiral) endings in spindles, from neurotendinous spindles
(Golgi tendon organs), and from pacinian corpuscles in the connective tissue within and external to the muscle. Smaller myelinated and nonmyelinated fibers arise from Ruffini endings in the
connective tissue in and around muscle, and in joints. Finally
there are small myelinated and nonmyelinated fibers that form
free endings in the connective tissue in and around muscle.

several millimeters long and consists of several specialized muscle
fibers and associated nerve endings. The entire spindle is fusiform
in shape, and is contained within a fluid-filled capsule of connective tissue. Its muscle fibers, termed intrafusal, are of two kinds, *nuclear-bag* and *nuclear-chain.* The middle of the nuclear-bag fiber
contains an aggregation of nuclei; here the striations are less
marked. The nuclear-chain fiber has only a single row of nuclei.
Each type of intrafusal fiber receives a large afferent nerve fiber

Nerve fiber   Intrafusal fiber

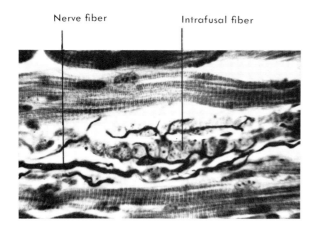

Figure 10–4. Photomicrograph of a nuclear-bag fiber and primary ending from a neuromuscular spindle (mouse). The lack of cross-striations in the bag region is evident. (Reproduced from Gardner, E.: Anat. Rec., *83*:401–409, 1972. Courtesy of Wistar Institute of Anatomy and Biology.)

Figure 10–5. Schematic representation of a neuromuscular spindle. Parts of three skeletal muscle fibers are shown (cross-striated, nuclei at edge). Inside the connective tissue sheath of the spindle are three muscle fibers (thinner than regular skeletal muscle fibers, with central nuclei, and striations minimal or absent in region of sensory endings). Sensory nerve fibers form primary (annulospiral) and secondary (flower-spray) endings, the primary arising from the large fibers. (The form of primary and secondary endings varies according to species. In some, such as rabbit and man, the primary endings of the large fiber may be flower-spray in type, not winding around the muscle fiber.) Small nerve fibers (*gamma* efferents) form motor endings at each end of the spindle muscle fibers. Motor discharges over *gamma* efferents cause the spindle muscle fibers to contract at each end, thus stretching the intervening, non-contractile, sensory region and activating the sensory endings. Arrows indicate direction of conduction. (Based on Barker, D., Quart. J. Micr. Sc., *89*:143–186, 1948; Boyd, I. A., Phil. Trans. Royal Soc. Lond., Ser. B., *245*:81–136, 1962; and Matthews, P. B. C., Physiol. Rev., *44*:219–288, 1964.)

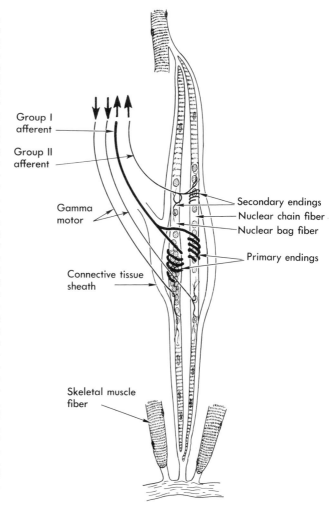

Group I afferent

Group II afferent

Gamma motor

Connective tissue sheath

Skeletal muscle fiber

Secondary endings

Nuclear chain fiber

Nuclear bag fiber

Primary endings

that forms a spiral ending (*primary ending*) around it at its middle. Smaller afferent fibers form *secondary endings* on the chain fibers, and occasionally on the bag fibers also. Each type of intrafusal fiber also has small motor endings formed by a *gamma* fiber. These motor endings are located chiefly at each pole of the bag fibers, but tend to be scattered along the length of the chain fibers.

Intrafusal muscle fibers sometimes receive a motor supply from branches of adjacent *alpha* motor fibers; such branches are termed *beta* fibers.

Neuromuscular spindles are sensitive to changes in tension caused by an increase in muscle length, that is, by stretching, and are therefore often called stretch receptors. When the muscle is stretched, the primary spindle endings signal both the length of the muscle and the velocity of stretch, whereas the secondary endings signal mainly the length. The sensitivity of the spindle to stretch depends upon the tension in the intrafusal fibers, and the tension in turn depends upon the contraction resulting from *gamma* fiber activity. When impulses over *gamma* motor fibers activate the intrafusal fibers, the latter contract at each end and stretch the intervening non-contractile portions where the sensory endings are located. The sensory endings are mechanically distorted by this stretch, just as they are by the stretch produced by an external pull on the muscle, and their firing or discharge threshold is lowered. Hence, an increased number of nerve impulses reaching intrafusal fibers over *gamma* motor fibers results in increased sensitivity to tension in the muscle as a whole. A decreased *gamma* discharge results in decreased sensitivity.

When a spindle is activated, the resulting nerve impulses reach the spinal cord and activate motor neurons (see two neuron reflex, p. 116), which then discharge impulses to the stretched muscle, causing it to contract and regain its former length. This reflex action is probably the chief basis of tendon jerks, that is, the deep reflexes mentioned on p. 123.

On a reflex level, the neuromuscular spindle and its nerve fibers comprise a system that functions in the reflex control of muscular activity. The sensory impulses from the spindle also reach the brain stem, cerebellum, and cerebral hemispheres by a variety of ascending pathways. Moreover, a number of descending pathways influence the excitability of *gamma* motor neurons and, therefore, the frequency of impulses reaching the intrafusal fibers. Changes in the functions of this descending control are undoubtedly a factor in disorders of central control of muscular activity (p. 214).

Muscles have other kinds of sensory endings, as shown in Figure 10–3. Also, there are encapsulated endings termed *Golgi tendon organs* or *neurotendinous endings* that are located in tendons or in the muscles near the musculotendinous junctions. A Golgi tendon organ is stimulated by the tension produced in the tendon during contraction of the motor units related to the ending, or during contraction of the whole muscle, or by passive stretch of the whole muscle (these last two are less effective). The impulses arising from the endings inhibit the motor neurons supplying the muscle.

When a muscle is suddenly stretched, as by tapping the tendon, the tendon jerk (phasic reflex) depends upon a monosynaptic reflex pathway from primary spindle afferents (Ia fibers; see below). However, steady stretch of a muscle elicits a steady afferent barrage over three different kinds of fibers: the primary and secondary spindle fibers (Ia and II), and the fibers from Golgi tendon organs (Ib). The stretch reflex that results is far more complicated, and the precise roles of the various muscle afferents are still uncertain. Undoubtedly the stretch reflex is involved in the automatic adjustment of postural contractions, but its role in voluntary movement is uncertain, and whether or to what degree the afferent impulses from spindles are involved in the perception of position and movement is open to question (see p. 236).

The afferent fibers from neuromuscular spindles and Golgi tendon organs are often classified according to diameter and in relation to function. The large afferent fibers, those that range from 12 to 20 μm in diameter, are called Group I fibers. Those from spindles are designated Group Ia, and those from tendon organs, Group Ib. The smaller afferent fibers, those from 4 to 12 μm in diameter, and which form the secondary endings in neuromuscular spindles, are termed Group II fibers. Group III fibers are the smallest of the myelinated fibers in muscle nerves, and Group IV comprises the nonmyelinated fibers.

GENERAL FEATURES OF CONTROL

A few general rules can be cited that hold for the normal control of muscular activity.

The body is represented mostly upside down in the motor areas of the cerebral cortex. As a result, pathways concerned with movements of the lower limbs originate in the cortex of the upper parts of the motor areas and on the medial aspects of the hemispheres. Pathways dealing with movements of the head and neck tend to originate in the lower and more anterior portions of the motor areas, just above the beginning of the lateral sulcus.

The limbs are represented mainly contralaterally, that is, the pathways for the right upper and lower limbs originate chiefly in the left cerebral hemisphere, and vice versa.

The head, neck, and trunk tend to be represented bilaterally, that is, the motor neurons supplying the muscles in these regions, with certain exceptions, usually receive descending fibers from both cerebral hemispheres.

The pyramidal system seems to be chiefly excitatory in function, and is largely responsible for the voluntary control of skilled movements involving the head, neck, and limbs. The cerebellum, which is considered further in Chapter 16, seems to be particularly responsible for coordinating the timing of activity in various groups of muscles, both in postural and in locomotor mechanisms. In so doing, it appears to enhance muscle tone. The basal ganglia, which are considered further in Chapter 17, are especially important in inhibitory mechanisms, in the "suppression" of muscle tone, and in the coordination of the activity of muscles by groups. All three systems (cortical, cerebellar, and ganglionic) are integrally involved in every type of muscular activity.

PYRAMIDAL SYSTEM

This is a direct path from the cerebral cortex to the brain stem and spinal cord, and is most prominent in primates. It is concerned especially with many of the muscles supplied by cranial nerves (e.g., those that bring about phonation), and with those of the limbs and particularly the hands. However, all other muscles are under the influence of the pyramidal system, though to a lesser extent.

The pyramidal system can be subdivided into the fibers that project to the spinal cord and those that project to the brain stem.

CORTICOSPINAL TRACTS

The direct path to the spinal cord consists of corticospinal fibers that originate from fairly extensive areas of the cerebral cortex, especially the sensorimotor cortex (precentral and postcentral gyri). A substantial number of the fibers arise from the precentral gyrus (area 4, p. 400). The fibers descend in the internal capsule and cerebral peduncle, and then in bundles in the anterior portion of the pons. These bundles then come together and form the pyramids of the medulla oblongata, one on each side of the anterior median fissure. Just above and at the junction of the medulla oblongata and spinal cord, many of the fibers (estimated roughly at 70 to 90 per cent) in each pyramid cross to the opposite side, interlacing as they do so and forming the *decussation of the pyramids*. The fibers that cross then descend in the lateral funiculus of the spinal cord as *lateral corticospinal tracts* (Figs. 10–6, and 13–2, pp. 207 and 289). Of those fibers that remain uncrossed, most descend in the ventral funiculus as *anterior corticospinal tracts;* some descend in the lateral funiculus as lateral corticospinal fibers.

It should be noted that, in common usage, the term *pyramidal tract* is synonymous with *corticospinal tract*.

As the corticospinal tracts descend, they become smaller and smaller as constituent fibers turn into the gray matter and end. In

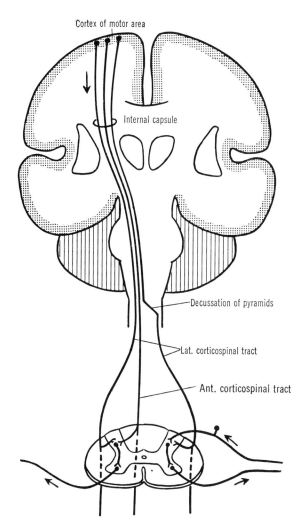

Figure 10-6. Diagram of cortico-spinal tracts.

primates, many fibers end by synapsing directly with motor cells (the anterior corticospinal fibers may cross to the opposite side before synapsing). Others synapse with interneurons. There is evidence that in both situations the endings are in relation to neurons concerned with muscles that have many motor units per unit number of muscle fibers. This makes for greater precision of movement.

There is good evidence that the pyramidal system is primarily excitatory to the neurons with which its fibers synapse, and that the excitation can be manifested in a variety of ways. Impulses descending over corticospinal fibers may activate interneurons and motor neurons. Or they may facilitate these cells, that is, lower their thresholds without causing them to discharge.

Some of these features can be demonstrated in human beings. For example, in many normal people it is difficult to obtain tendon reflexes, such as a knee jerk. If, just before the patellar tendon is tapped, the subject clenches his fists, the knee jerk may then be obtained and it may be marked. Presumably this enhancement or *reinforcement* results from the fact that impulses from the cerebral cortex reach not only the motor cells to the muscles involved in clenching the fists, but probably reach other motor cells, including those supplying the leg extensors. In addition, the *gamma* efferents to the neuromuscular spindles may be activated. Hence, facilitation of the appropriate motor cells coupled with more sensitive neuromuscular spindles enables the reflex knee jerk to occur.

A concept that has been widely held views the pyramidal system as primarily inhibitory. This is probably based chiefly on the interpretation of certain motor disorders and views the presence of hyperactive and abnormal reflexes as resulting from a loss of inhibition. This concept of pyramidal function may not be entirely incorrect, but it is inadequate to explain most features of pyramidal function.

Finally, it is likely that those pyramidal fibers that synapse with interneurons may modulate transmission cells of sensory pathways (see p. 227).

CORTICOBULBAR TRACTS

Corticobulbar tracts are tracts that arise chiefly from the lower and anterior portions of the motor areas (p. 401), descend through the internal capsule, and project directly to various brain stem nuclei, including the motor nuclei of cranial nerves. Functionally, they belong to the pyramidal system even though none of their fibers ever descends through the medullary pyramids. They have similar physiological properties, and some of the fibers end in various sensory relay nuclei which they modulate. The term corticobulbar is derived from the older term "bulb" applied to the brain stem. *Corticobulbar fibers* are further distinguished by being named according to the part of the brain stem they end in, e.g., *corticomesencephalic, corticopontine,* and *corticomedullary tracts.* Although these various fibers are given different names, in no instance is there a clear-cut tract that can be distinguished. Rather, after the fibers leave the internal capsule and enter the cerebral peduncle, they descend in a diffuse fashion throughout the brain stem.

From the standpoint of organization, it is convenient to discuss the various paths according to the muscles they control, namely those of the eye and tongue, and those that develop from pharyngeal arches.

Eye Muscles. Eye movements are nearly always conjugate, that is, the eyes move together. There are two different kinds of associated or conjugate movements. One comprises smooth movements that pursue or follow, and that are continuously regulated, depending on the presence of a moving stimulus. The other pattern consists of rapid search movements called *saccades* that are too fast to be continuously controlled by visual feedback. The supranuclear pathways for these two kinds of eye movements seem to be different.

One pathway, that concerned in horizontal (lateral) gaze in the first kind of eye movement, is shown in Figure 10–7. In the example given of looking to the right, the right lateral rectus muscle, supplied by the abducent nerve, and the left medial rectus muscle, supplied by the oculomotor nerve, act to turn the eyes to the right. At the same time the opposing muscles relax. The motor path originates chiefly in area 8 of the frontal lobe (sometimes known as the *frontal eye field,* p. 400). These corticopontine fibers descend in the internal capsule and there is a question as to whether they relay in the basal ganglia. Somewhere during their descent they cross the median plane and reach a group of nerve cells in the lower pons known as the *center for lateral gaze* (Fig. 10–8). Many consider this center to be one or more of the vestibular nuclei. From this center, axons project to the nucleus of the abducent nerve and others ascend in the opposite medial longitudinal fasciculus to the oculomotor nucleus.

The pathway for saccadic eye movements originates in the occipital cortex and reaches the center for lateral gaze only after leaving the brain stem and relaying in the cerebellum. There is still another type of horizontal gaze in which the eyes are kept fixed on an object as the head turns. The motor path concerned may well be similar to that for saccadic movements.

Smooth pursuit movements in vertical directions appear to be controlled by both the frontal and occipital cortex, especially the occipital. The paths concerned (corticomesencephalic fibers) descend to the tectum (roof) of the midbrain, where they make connections with the nuclei of the oculomotor and trochlear nerves.

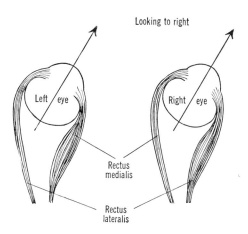

Looking to right

Left eye

Right eye

Rectus medialis

Rectus lateralis

Figure 10–7. Conjugate activity in looking to the right. The right lateral rectus muscle and the left medial rectus contract, while the right medial rectus and left lateral rectus relax.

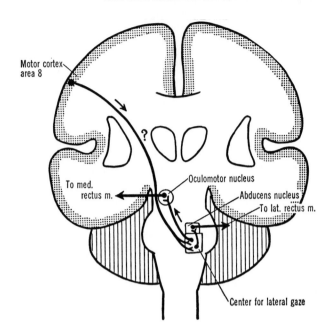

Figure 10-8. Pathway for horizontal (lateral) conjugate gaze. Descending fibers project to the center for lateral gaze in the pons, which in turn relays to eye muscle nuclei. The question mark indicates the possibility that the descending fibers relay in basal ganglia.

Eye movements are rarely confined to strictly horizontal or strictly vertical axes. Consequently, both frontal and occipital lobes and their pathways are coordinated in eye movements. Also, there are probably pathways by which conjugate gaze in a particular direction can be controlled by the ipsilateral hemisphere. Whether these are normally in operation is uncertain. They undoubtedly account for the fact that after destruction of cerebral cortex or pathways on one side, conjugate gaze to the opposite side may be lost only temporarily. During this time, the activity of the unaffected hemisphere may cause spontaneous, maintained conjugate gaze toward the side of the lesion. There are other reflex eye movements of clinical importance, including *nystagmus,* which may be pathological or which can result from vestibular activity (p. 275).

Tongue. Each hypoglossal nerve supplies one half of the tongue and the nucleus of each nerve is often bilaterally controlled, that is, receives fibers from the lower portions of the frontal motor areas of both cerebral hemispheres. These corticomedullary fibers descend in the internal capsule and then proceed diffusely through the brain stem to the hypoglossal nuclei.

Pharyngeal Arch Muscles. The nuclei of the nerves concerned (facial, trigeminal, glossopharyngeal, vagus, and accessory) are each, with one or two exceptions, bilaterally supplied by the cerebral cortex (chiefly the lower portions of the frontal motor areas). These nuclei and their central pathways are of major importance, partly because of their role in facial and jaw movements, breathing, and swallowing, but especially because they carry out the motor aspects of speech. The corticobulbar fibers descend in the internal capsule and cerebral peduncle and then proceed diffusely in the brain stem to the motor nuclei in the pons and medulla oblongata.

The facial nuclei comprise a clinically important exception to the rule of bilateral supply. The motor cells in the upper portion of each facial nucleus, i.e., those which supply the muscles that close the eyes and wrinkle the forehead, receive fibers from both cerebral hemispheres. However, the motor cells in the lower portion of each facial nucleus, those which supply muscles of the lips, nose, and cheek, receive fibers only from the opposite motor area (Fig. 10–9).

Finally, portions of the sternomastoid and trapezius muscles are of pharyngeal arch origin and are supplied by the spinal part of the accessory nerve (the cells of origin are in the intermediate gray matter of the upper cervical cord). Turning the head to one side, a movement in which the sternomastoid takes part, is chiefly controlled by the opposite motor areas.

EXTRAPYRAMIDAL SYSTEM

Although the details of the extrapyramidal system are considered in subsequent chapters on the brain stem, cerebellum, and forebrain, basic concepts need to be presented here so as to permit some correlation with certain disorders of movement.

The extrapyramidal paths originate from a wide extent of cerebral cortex, but especially from motor areas of the frontal

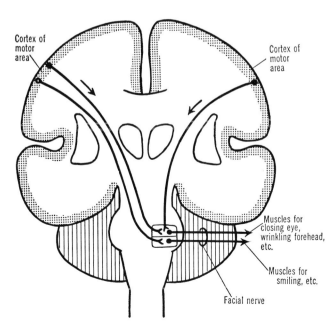

Cortex of motor area

Cortex of motor area

Muscles for closing eye, wrinkling forehead, etc.

Muscles for smiling, etc.

Facial nerve

Figure 10–9. Motor pathway for facial muscles. The upper part of the facial nucleus, which supplies one group of facial muscles, receives fibers from both cerebral hemispheres, whereas the lower part of the nucleus receives fibers only from the contralateral hemisphere.

lobe. Many of the fibers descend in the internal capsule and cerebral peduncles to the pons and are then relayed to the cerebellum, from which projections arise, some to excitatory and inhibitory centers of the brain stem, and others back to the cerebral cortex. Many other fibers from the cerebral cortex descend in the internal capsule to the basal ganglia, and then by a variety of paths to excitatory and inhibitory centers of the brain stem (Fig. 10–10). These centers project to motor neurons by means of rubrospinal, reticulospinal, and vestibulospinal tracts. Inhibitory fibers (chiefly reticulospinal) seem to descend mostly in the lateral funiculus, adjacent to or intermingled with lateral corticospinal fibers. Excitatory fibers (all three types of tracts) probably descend mostly in the ventral funiculus. These various descending tracts end in the gray matter of the spinal cord, either by synapsing with motor neurons directly or with interneurons. Moreoever, the descending

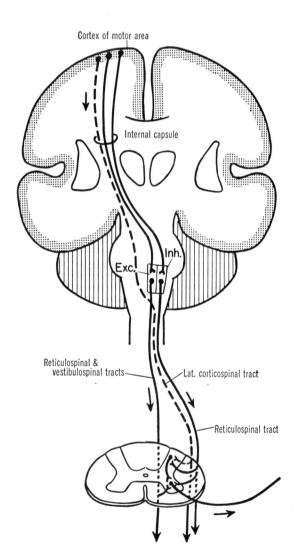

Figure 10–10. Simplified representation of a few of the extrapyramidal pathways. The brain stem excitatory and inhibitory mechanisms are indicated schematically, and the lateral corticospinal tract is included to show its relationship to the reticulospinal tract.

extrapyramidal tracts may influence the *gamma* efferents and thereby the sensitivity of neuromuscular spindles.

CLINICAL CORRELATIONS

The functions of motor areas and their pathways have been studied in a variety of ways. Motor areas have been removed surgically, both in experimental animals and during surgical procedures in humans. The electrical activity of normal and abnormal motor areas has been recorded and analyzed. In experimental animals, fibers descending in the internal capsule, cerebral peduncle, pyramid, and spinal cord have been studied under many different conditions, including degeneration and loss of function after surgical section. Comparable defects (Fig. 10–11) resulting from disease or injury in humans have been observed and studied

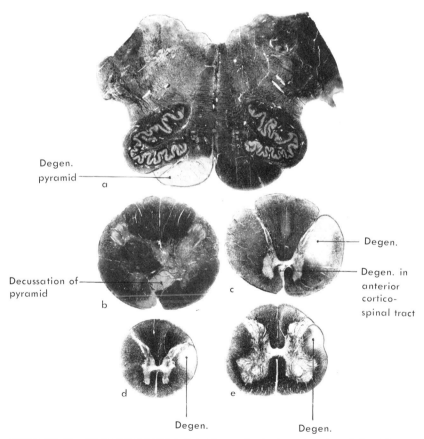

Figure 10–11. Photomicrographs of sections of spinal cord and medulla oblongata from a case of thrombosis of the arterial supply of the left internal capsule. Weigert stain. The degenerating fibers lie in the unstained areas, and at the indicated levels are corticospinal fibers. In *a*, the left pyramid is involved. In *b*, the degenerating fibers are crossing to the right side. Some remain on the same side, as shown in *c*, cervical cord. In *d*, thoracic cord, and *e*, lumbar cord, the lateral corticospinal tract decreases in size as it descends in the lateral funiculus.

for centuries. It is the study of clinical disorders which has yielded the information that is the basis of much that we know today about motor pathways.

As a general rule, any interruption of connections between the cortex or subcortical levels and the motor cells in the brain stem or spinal cord is said to be an *upper motor neuron lesion.* Such a lesion usually interrupts both corticospinal and extrapyramidal fibers (the term "upper motor neuron lesion" is usually not applied to disorders affecting only extrapyramidal fibers).

UPPER MOTOR NEURON LESIONS

In the internal capsule, cerebral peduncle, and lateral funiculus of the spinal cord, corticospinal and extrapyramidal fibers are so closely intermingled that whatever affects one system also affects the other. The chief effects of such lesions are as follows.

Paresis or Paralysis.   There is paresis (weakness) or paralysis on the opposite side of the body, to a varying degree depending upon the number of descending fibers destroyed. The closer the destruction is to the spinal cord, the more chance there is of destroying all descending fibers.

The limbs are predominantly affected, the trunk muscles being much less influenced owing to their bilateral cortical control (unless the lesion is bilateral).

Weakness in muscles supplied by cranial nerves is variable and may be virtually absent, except for the lower facial muscles.

Reflexes.   One of the basic features of upper motor neuron lesions is that reflex arcs remain anatomically intact. Another feature is that the loss of extrapyramidal inhibitory mechanisms predominates. The normal action of gravity against the weight of the body may initiate stretch reflexes. Since inhibitory mechanisms are diminished or lost, reflex contractions are exaggerated and may be evidenced clinically as hyperactive tendon jerks. Increased reflex activity may be such as to lead to repetitive phasic jerks following a single stretch. Such repetitive response is known as *clonus.*

Since the extrapyramidal excitatory mechanisms may still be functioning, or may be removed from cortical control, the combination of loss of inhibition and maintenance of excitation, together with afferent impulses and an altered state of sensitivity of neuromuscular spindles, all lead to significant increases in muscle tone, especially in antigravity muscles. These muscles are said to be *spastic* and the combination of spasticity and loss of voluntary motion is known as *spastic paralysis,* a synonym for upper motor neuron lesion. Spasticity can be detected when the examiner bends the joint of a patient; the stretch thus put on the muscle leads reflexly to an increase in tension which resists the flexion of the joint.

Abnormal reflexes may appear, such as the Babinski reflex

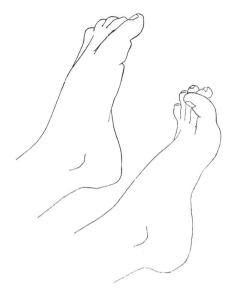

Figure 10–12. *Upper:* The normal response to scratching the sole of the foot. *Lower:* Pathological or Babinski response.

(Fig. 10–12), which is one of the most significant reflex signs in clinical neurology. Some reflexes may be lost, notably the superficial abdominal reflexes.

It must be emphasized that the signs and symptoms are not invariable, but depend upon the nature of the disorder, the suddenness of onset, the age of the patient, and a host of other clinical considerations. It should also be pointed out, in connection with earlier concepts of the pyramidal system as inhibitory in function, that it was widely held that upper motor neuron disorders were entirely the result of lesions to only the pyramidal system. Consequently, the terms "pyramidal signs" or "pyramidal lesions" are still widely used and must be considered synonymous with the terms "spastic paralysis" or "upper motor neuron lesions."

Localization. (Fig. 10–13) Upper motor neuron lesions are common in the internal capsule and lesions here result in signs mainly in the opposite half of the body. Weakness in the opposite half is known as *hemiparesis;* more severe loss or a paralysis is often termed a *hemiplegia.* A clue to the level of the lesion may be afforded if descending fibers to the facial nucleus are involved. In such instances, the opposite lower facial muscles are weak or paralyzed, but the patient can still wrinkle his forehead and close his eyes. Interference with conjugate eye movements may also afford a clue.

Localization at brain stem levels may be possible if the lesion also affects one or more cranial nerves. For example, a destructive lesion of a cerebral peduncle is likely to involve the emerging oculomotor nerve and thus give an ipsilateral third nerve palsy and an opposite hemiplegia.

If motor fibers are destroyed after they have crossed in the lower medulla oblongata, and when they lie in the lateral funiculus of the upper cervical cord, the result will be a hemiplegia on the same side as the lesion. More distal lesions may affect but one limb, a *monoplegia.* The exact location of a lesion may be more accurately determined if sensory tracts, motor or sensory cells, or spinal roots are also involved. Bilateral lesions in the upper part of the spinal cord may involve all descending motor tracts and result in a *quadriplegia.*

It should be noted that with a lesion on one side below the pyramidal decussation, trunk muscles below the lesion and on the same side are not always affected to the degree expected. A possible explanation is that anterior corticospinal fibers, which descend uncrossed and then cross before they enter gray matter, may supply motor cells to trunk muscles below the lesion.

Lesions of Only the Pyramidal System

In experimental work carried out in nonhuman primates, destruction of only corticospinal fibers (by cutting a medullary pyramid or by destroying a small portion of a precentral gyrus) is followed by weakness on the opposite side of the body, especially in the hands; sometimes it is accompanied by limpness (even flaccidity) of muscles and the appearance of abnormal reflexes, such as Babinski's. However, voluntary control is still largely retained and a remarkable degree of recovery may occur over a period of months.

A comparable lesion in human beings is rare. However, there is some evidence which tends to indicate that when it does occur the defects are similar to those produced experimentally.

LOWER MOTOR NEURON LESIONS

The pathway from the cortical motor areas is completed by the final common path. Destruction of these motor neurons or their axons is followed by a characteristic clinical picture, whether the destruction is in the spinal cord, the ventral roots, or in spinal or peripheral nerves. In any case, impulses cannot reach the muscle fibers supplied by the destroyed nerve fibers, and voluntary control of these muscles is completely lost. For the same reason, reflexes involving such muscles are impossible. Muscle fibers deprived of their nerve supply eventually shrink or atrophy, and during the course of this change the degenerating fibers show fibrillary twitchings. The characteristics of strength-duration curves are also changed (p. 84). If there is no regeneration, the muscles eventually are replaced by connective tissue and fat. Because the nerve impulses necessary for muscle tone are lost, muscles become limp or *flaccid.* This lower motor neuron type paralysis is, therefore, frequently referred to as a *flaccid paralysis.*

Flaccid paralyses are not the only disorders in which reflexes are lost. For instance, if one or several dorsal roots are cut, sensation in the areas supplied by these roots is diminished or lost. The afferent impulses cannot reach the spinal cord, and reflexes depending upon them are lost. Paralysis is not present, however, because ventral roots are still intact, and motor impulses for voluntary activity can still reach the muscles. A diagnosis of dorsal root involvement can be made because the areas in which sensation is diminished or lost conform to the embryological distribution of segments in which each spinal nerve supplied its own dermatome.

Lesions involving spinal nerves result in both motor and sensory losses in segmental areas. Lesions of major peripheral nerves, such as the sciatic, cause flaccid paralyses of the muscles supplied by that nerve, accompanied by loss of cutaneous sensations. Differentiation can be made from spinal nerve lesions because the motor and sensory losses are in areas characteristic of peripheral nerve distributions rather than segmental distributions (p. 168).

Figure 10–13 is a composite diagram illustrating the paths involved in the various motor disabilities.

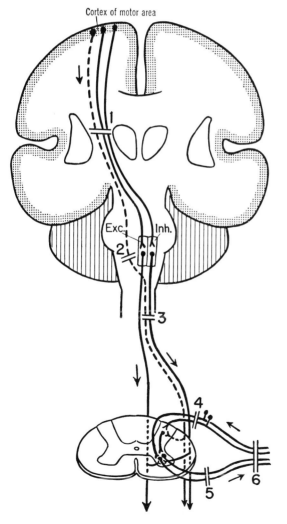

Figure 10–13. Diagram illustrating lesions of motor and reflex paths. *1:* A lesion here (internal capsule) causes an upper motor neuron defect, the severity of which depends on the extent of the lesion. *2:* A lesion here (near decussation of pyramids) affects only corticospinal fibers. *3:* A lesion here (lateral funiculus of cord) causes an upper motor neuron defect more severe than that at *1* because more descending fibers are cut (this feature is not actually illustrated). *4:* Section of dorsal root or roots causes diminution or loss of reflexes, sensation, muscle tone and coordination, but no paralysis. *5:* Section of a ventral root or roots causes a lower motor neuron defect. *6:* Section of a spinal or peripheral nerve results in combined motor and sensory losses.

SUMMARY

The control of muscular activity can be considered as if the nervous system involved a series of levels. These are the cerebral cortex, the basal ganglia, the cerebellum, the brain stem, and the spinal cord. All muscular activity is ultimately mediated by impulses leaving the brain stem and spinal cord by the final common path.

Within the brain stem are excitatory and inhibitory mechanisms that project to the spinal cord and which in turn are influenced by the cerebellum, basal ganglia, and cerebral cortex. Direct projections from the cerebral cortex to the brain stem and spinal cord comprise the pyramidal system of corticobulbar and corticospinal tracts. Indirect projections to motor nuclei by way of cerebellum and basal ganglia and the brain-stem excitatory and inhibitory centers comprise the extrapyramidal system. The pyramidal system is primarily excitatory and is concerned especially with head, neck, and limb muscles. The extrapyramidal system is concerned with timing and coordination of muscle groups, and with the modulation of muscle tone.

Muscles in the limbs are mainly controlled by the contralateral cerebral hemisphere, while muscles near the median plane of the body are under bilateral cerebral control.

Interruption of connections between the cortex and motor neurons causes upper motor neuron lesions. Such lesions mostly involve both extrapyramidal and corticospinal fibers, and are characterized by a varying degree of paralysis, spasticity of antigravity muscles, exaggerated deep or tendon reflexes, and abnormal reflexes.

Interruption of the pathway from motor neurons to muscles causes a lower motor neuron lesion. This is followed by paralysis of voluntary motion with limpness or flaccidity of the involved muscles, muscular atrophy, loss of reflexes, and fibrillary twitching. When the lesion is in spinal or peripheral nerves, the flaccid paralysis is accompanied by sensory losses.

NAMES IN NEUROLOGY

JOSEF FRANÇOIS FÉLIX BABINSKI (1857–1932)

Babinski, born in Paris of Polish parents, was an outstanding clinical neurologist. He was the first to realize the significance and importance of the abnormal extensor reflex (and associated fanning of the toes) that now bears his name. His many papers on the subject form a series which began in 1896.

REFERENCES

See the references cited on pp. 327 and 419 for physiological and clinical aspects of muscular activity.

The following books deal with muscle functions in human beings. The accounts by Duchenne and Beevor are classics. Duchenne used electrical stimulation of muscles, and Beevor, palpation of active muscles, to determine functions. Both Basmajian and Joseph used electromyography in their studies, which are excellent examples of modern experimental and anatomical research. The account by Carlsöö is a first-rate treatment of kinesiology.

Basmajian, J. V.: Muscles Alive. 3rd ed. Baltimore, Williams and Wilkins Company, 1974.
Beevor, C.: The Croonian Lectures on Muscular Movements, 1903, and Remarks on Paralysis of the Movements of the Trunk in Hemiplegia, 1909. Ed. and repr. London, Macmillan and Co., Ltd.
Carlsöö, S.: How Man Moves. London, Heinemann, 1972.
Duchenne, G. B.: Physiology of Motion. Translated and edited by E. B. Kaplan. Philadelphia, W. B. Saunders Company, 1959.
Joseph, J.: Man's Posture. Springfield, Ill., Charles C Thomas, 1960.

The following references comprise an excellent short review, a book of major importance, and a detailed physiological review.

Evarts, E. V.: Brain mechanisms in movement. Sci. Amer., *229*:96–103, 1973.
Matthews, P. B. C.: Mammalian Muscle Receptors and Their Central Actions. London, Edward Arnold (Publishers) Ltd., 1972.
Stein, R. B.: Peripheral control of movement. Physiol. Rev., *54*:215–243, 1974.

During his lifetime, the eminent clinical neurologist Sir Francis Walshe wrote a number of superb reviews on neurological problems. The major ones, including studies of the origin of the pyramidal tract and of the Babinski response, are collected in the following volume.

Walshe, F.: Further Critical Studies in Neurology and Other Essays and Addresses. Edinburgh, E. & S. Livingstone Ltd., and Baltimore, The Williams and Wilkins Company, 1965.

Chapter 11

THE GENERAL SENSES
AND THEIR PATHWAYS

Sensation and perception depend upon processes that begin with the detection by receptors of changes in the environment. The resulting nerve impulses are carried by fibers in peripheral and cranial nerves to the spinal cord and brain. The number, frequency, and pattern of the impulses comprise a first-order coding of messages. Within the central nervous system, the impulses are transmitted over pathways that begin in gray matter in which further coding and modification occur. The final processes in sensation and perception are the functions of forebrain "centers." All the coding processes are subject to modulation by efferent impulses to a varying degree. For example, the sensitivity of the neuromuscular spindle is determined by the *gamma* efferent system. To what degree other receptors are subject to efferent modulation is still uncertain, although the presence of efferent fibers in the vicinity of many receptors has long been known. At the central levels, all transmission neurons are subject to control by impulses descending from the brain.

Physiologists have generally tried to separate sensation from perception, and have dealt with different sensory modalities in terms of certain specific features, such as receptor mechanisms, anatomical pathways, and psychophysical processes. The term "modality" refers to any one of several sensations that are thought to be "primary." According to the traditional lay concept, the primary senses are vision, hearing, smell, taste, and touch. This concept is reflected in the division of senses into general and special categories. The *general senses* include touch, temperature, pressure, position, a few sensations from viscera, and that unique experience termed pain. The *special senses* include vision, hearing, balance, taste, and smell.

The above classification is useful in many respects, but it does not deal with what is actually perceived, namely, properties such as shape, size, weight, distance, depth, texture, the tonal qualities of sound, wetness, smoothness, and a host of other perceptual phenomena. Nor does it take into account those even more important and pervasive phenomena that affect the total organism. For example, pain, like pleasure, can be so profound a phenomenon in terms of impact upon affective behavior, motivation, and action, that it can scarcely be correlated with the physiological mechanisms involved. For none of these perceptual phenomena are there any well-established neural correlates, other than general relationships to certain brain stem and forebrain structures and pathways. Nevertheless, the beginning elucidation of these relationships is proving to be of enormous psychological and clinical importance.

RECEPTORS

It should be emphasized again that receptors and their parent fibers code the information that is transmitted to the brain. The pattern that comprises the code consists of the number, frequency, and grouping of impulses over a given period of receptor stimulation. The pattern varies according to the nature of the stimulus and the receptor.

One of the major questions is whether receptors and their connections are functionally specific. That is, does the same type of sensation always result when a specific receptor is stimulated? It may when simple stimuli are used and when highly specialized receptors are tested. But it must be emphasized that what is coded peripherally is again coded centrally, and that pathways to "higher centers" exist not just as conduction mechanisms but as integral components of complex sensory and perceptual phenomena. Finally, it should be pointed out that only two of the "general sense receptors" have been studied rigorously. These are the pacinian corpuscle and the "dome" receptor of skin (the neuromuscular spindle has been more extensively studied, but whether or to what degree it contributes to sensory and perceptual mechanisms is uncertain).

CUTANEOUS AND SUBCUTANEOUS RECEPTORS

The skin is an impermeable protective membrane that is extraordinarily sensitive to changes in the outside world, as well as to certain changes in the internal environment. It contains many receptors (Fig. 11–1), only a few of which can be related directly to a kind or quality of sensation. When skin is lightly stroked with a wisp of cotton, or is touched with a fine hair or probe (common methods in clinical testing), what is felt is called *touch,* or *light*

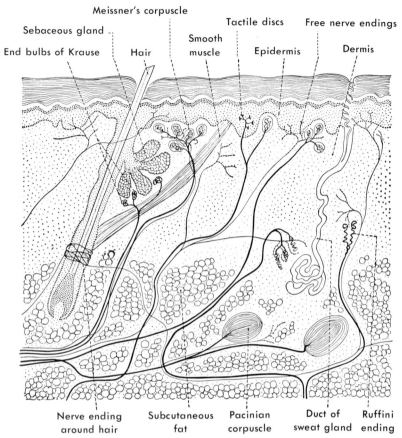

Figure 11-1. Schematic representation of the nerve supply of skin with sparse hair. Not all the endings shown are to be found in any one skin area and some of the endings (e.g., Meissner's corpuscle) are found chiefly in glabrous skin. The functions of the end bulbs of Krause are unknown. The highly schematic representation of tactile discs is shown more accurately in Figure 11-2. The heavy lines are myelinated fibers, the light lines, nonmyelinated fibers. (Modified after Woollard et al.: J. Anat., 74:441-458, 1940.)

touch (the term says nothing about quality, or that the sensation is sometimes *tickle,* and under certain conditions may be painful). What is felt can be localized to a particular part of the body, often to a small area termed a *touch spot.* Moreover, two such spots can be distinguished when touched simultaneously (two-point discrimination), provided that they are sufficiently far apart. The necessary distance depends upon the region of the body. In the skin of the back, two such spots must be several cm apart before they can be distinguished as two; in areas such as the thumb and fingers, two spots a few mm or less apart can be recognized separately.

Touching or bending a hair can usually be identified very precisely, and it seems likely that a stimulus so slight as to produce but one nerve impulse can be felt. Stimuli sufficient to affect subcutaneous tissue may result in a sense of *pressure (deep touch).* Changes in skin temperature are readily perceived. Finally, the skin is acutely sensitive to various noxious stimuli that are usually painful.

The receptors in skin and subcutaneous tissues can be categorized as mechanoreceptors, thermoreceptors, and nociceptive receptors. All of these are sometimes grouped under the term *exteroceptive,* because they are usually stimulated by changes in the external environment.

Receptors in mucocutaneous junctions (e.g., lips) and in various mucous membranes of the respiratory, digestive, and genitourinary systems have receptors that resemble those in skin, but none has been studied in any detail.

Mechanoreceptors. All of the readily identifiable endings in skin and subcutaneous tissues are mechanoreceptors, i.e., they are sensitive to mechanical deformation. They are usually more sensitive to one kind of deformation than another, and their parent fibers fall into the A group. The structure, arrangement, pattern, and location of some of the receptors differ according to whether they are located in hairy or in glabrous (non-hairy) skin. Some of the cutaneous receptors are sensitive to vibrations at low frequencies, and follow best (i.e., respond to each vibration) at frequencies of about 30 cycles per second (the resulting sensation is best described as flutter); these receptors have not yet been identified.

The mechanoreceptors in hairy skin can be categorized according to whether they adapt slowly or rapidly. A variety of rapidly adapting receptors derived from myelinated fibers of various sizes occur in relation to hair follicles. These receptors are especially sensitive to hair displacement and to the displacement of the skin around the hair follicles. They seem to function as velocity detectors. Their parent fibers fall into the A *beta* group.

At least two types of slowly adapting receptors have been studied in hairy skin. Both discharge more or less steadily to an indentation of skin, both tend to occur in spots, both are derived from the smaller of the A *alpha* fibers, and from the A *beta* fibers, and both possess the sensitivity and dynamic range sufficient to account for much of the sensory capacity of human skin. One of the types of mechanoreceptors is present as a complex "dome" ending whose structure is shown in Figure 11–2. It is extremely sensitive, and discharges up to 1000 times a second when pressed upon vertically. The other slowly adapting mechanoreceptor is also stimulated by skin indentation, but in addition responds when skin is stretched. The receptor has not been identified; it may be a Ruffini ending.

Slowly and rapidly adapting endings are also present in non-hairy skin. The rapidly adapting ones have not been identified; they are probably Meissner's corpuscles. The slowly adapting ones are structurally similar to those in hairy skin.

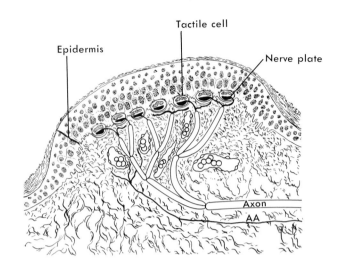

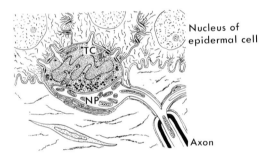

Figure 11–2. Upper: A diagram of a "dome" touch corpuscle in hairy skin. Note that the myelinated axon at the base of the dome gives rise to several branches that end as nerve plates (tactile discs) in relation to a specialized tactile cell. An accessory nonmyelinated axon (AA) is also present. *Lower:* Diagram of a tactile cell and nerve plate based on electron microscopic studies. The tactile cell (TC) is embedded in the epidermis above and bulges into the dermis below. The end of the axon terminal (from the myelinated axon) forms a nerve plate (NP) that invaginates the tactile cell. (Based on Iggo, A., and Muir, A. R.: J. Physiol., *200*:763–796, 1969. By permission of the authors and publishers.)

Pacinian corpuscles are present in the deeper parts of the dermis and throughout the subcutaneous tissue (Fig. 11–1). Their structure is shown in Figure 3–29, p. 55. These are exquisitely sensitive, rapidly adapting mechanoreceptors. They are stimulated by any pressure on the skin of sufficient magnitude to reach and deform the corpuscle (note that any such stimulus will also activate cutaneous receptors). It has been estimated that compression of only 0.5 μm may fire a Pacinian corpuscle. These receptors respond to vibrating stimuli (e.g., from a tuning fork), discharging one spike per stimulus cycle from 40 to 1000 cycles per second; they are most sensitive to frequencies of about 250 to 300 cycles. The resulting sense of vibration is not well localized, and remains even if the skin is anesthetized.

Thermoreceptors. Thermoreceptors comprise certain receptors in skin that have not been identified and which are sensitive to changes in temperature from a slightly variable neutral range. These temperature changes are those that occur in the air and in the blood flowing through the skin. The receptors are also sensitive to infrared radiation.

The "cool" or "cold" receptors occur in spots in both hairy and glabrous skin, and discharge in bursts at temperatures ranging from 18° to 40°C. "Warmth" receptors are much less numerous (in some regions there are few if any warmth receptors), but they also occur in spots, and seem to be maximally sensitive at about 40°C. The parent fibers of thermoreceptors fall in the A *delta* and C groups.

Nociceptive receptors. It is commonly held that cellular and tissue injury, from whatever cause, activates specific "pain receptors," or nociceptive receptors, either by direct damage to the endings or by the release of chemicals that stimulate the endings, and that impulses from these receptors travel centrally and eventually reach a "pain center" in the brain. There is little doubt that injury does activate certain receptors (presumably free nerve endings in the skin and subcutaneous tissue), and that the resulting nerve impulses travel centrally over A *delta* and C fibers. However, it is equally clear that other receptors and fibers may be and often are involved. Nociceptive receptors derived from these slowly conducting fibers are activated only by intense stimuli and often adapt rapidly; yet under certain circumstances, pain may by triggered by stimuli that are too low in intensity to stimulate the nociceptive receptors. Moreover, other stimuli that are usually painful (excessive heat or cold, certain noxious chemicals) do not necessarily activate nociceptive receptors. Finally, there is abundant evidence that central processes play a key role in pain mechanisms (p. 236). It is likely, therefore, that many different kinds of receptors and nerve fibers play a role in pain mechanisms.

MUSCLE, JOINT, TENDON, AND OTHER DEEP TISSUE RECEPTORS

These comprise mechanoreceptors of various kinds, and nociceptive receptors. The mechanoreceptors are sometimes termed *proprioceptive*, because they are often stimulated by energy changes initiated by or in the structures in which they are located.

Mechanoreceptors. These are present in muscles, joints, tendons, ligaments, fascia, and periosteum.

The endings in muscles include neuromuscular spindles and other receptors, as shown in Figure 10–3, p. 202. Their possible role in kinesthesia is discussed later.

The receptors in joint capsules and ligaments include slowly adapting Ruffini endings and rapidly adapting paciniform corpuscles (Fig. 3–28, p. 54). Both types of endings signal joint movement, and the Ruffini endings seem also to signal position. The impulses are transmitted centrally over moderate sized myelinated fibers, and are involved in kinesthetic sensations. There are also Golgi endings in ligaments that are structurally similar to Golgi tendon organs, and which are sensitive to tension and torsion of the ligaments. Like the Ruffini endings, they are slowly adapting. The mechanoreceptors and some free endings in joints, periosteum, and fascia are often arranged in triads of Ruffini endings, lamellated corpuscles (pacinian or paciniform), and free nerve endings. The triad is sometimes termed a proprioceptive triad, although the proprioceptive or mechanoreceptive function of the free endings in these groups has not yet been demonstrated.

The Golgi tendon organs are described on p. 204. Like the muscle receptors, their possible sensory role is discussed later.

The various specialized endings in periosteum and fascia include Ruffini endings and pacinian corpuscles. The latter are often numerous on interosseous membranes, near joints, and in the channels for tendons in the fingers and toes. Ruffini endings are common in the extensor aponeuroses of the digits.

Nociceptive Receptors. What was described for skin holds for the deeper tissues, although the nature of the noxious stimuli may differ (e.g., twisting of joint ligaments or distention of a joint capsule can be especially painful, as can a blow to a bone). Moreover, the quality of deep pain is often significantly different from that of cutaneous pain (e.g., it may be described as "sickening").

RECEPTORS IN VISCERA

The receptors in viscera, which are sometimes termed *enteroceptive* (or *interoceptive*), have been less extensively studied and few of them have been identified. Free nerve endings are present in the walls of many of the viscera (e.g., intestine) and are thought to be activated by distention of the walls. This can be extremely painful, as can inflammation; such pain may be referred (see later discussion of referred pain). Complex receptors that are structurally similar to Ruffini endings occur in the walls of some of the larger arteries and in the venous chambers of the heart, in the lungs, and in other organs such as the urinary bladder. All of these receptors appear to be activated by stretch and are involved in the reflex control of the functions of these organs. Complex receptors in the carotid body (at the bifurcation of the common carotid artery) are sensitive to changes in oxygen tension. Pacinian corpuscles are commonly present in the mesenteries of the abdominal viscera, where they are usually associated with small arteries. It may be that the effective stimulus is a deformation produced by changes in diameter of these vessels with each pulse. It would appear, therefore, that few of the receptors listed above, except the nociceptive receptors, are concerned with sensory mechanisms.

Hunger and thirst are important sensations whose peripheral receptors remain unidentified.

ORGANIZATION OF GRAY MATTER

The parent fibers of receptors enter the spinal cord by way of dorsal roots and the brain stem by way of certain cranial nerves.

In the dorsal roots, the larger fibers tend to collect into a medial division before entering the spinal cord. Immediately after entrance, these fibers divide into descending, local, and ascending branches, most of which end in the gray matter. However, some of the ascending fibers reach the medulla oblongata by way of posterior funiculi, and end in certain nuclei of the gray matter.

The smaller fibers in the dorsal roots, especially the C fibers, form a lateral division. Immediately after entrance, they divide into local, short descending, and short ascending branches, all of which end in the dorsal gray matter.

The cells in the gray matter of the spinal cord, which can be loosely categorized as motor neurons, interneurons, and transmission neurons, tend to be arranged in layers. These layers are discussed in Chapter 13, but are outlined here insofar as they are pertinent to sensory mechanisms. The posterior two-thirds of the dorsal gray matter consists of (1) a portion immediately adjacent to the dorsal root entry zone and which consists chiefly of a light-staining area termed the *substantia gelatinosa* (Fig. 13–1, p. 288), and (2) a fairly well defined area termed the *nucleus proprius.* The substantia gelatinosa includes layers 2 and 3 (layer 1, on the surface of the substantia, can be disregarded), and seems to act as a gate for the transmission of impulses to higher centers (Fig. 11–3). Transmission cells are located in layers 4 to 6, which together comprise the nucleus proprius, and their axons form ascending pathways (Fig. 11–4). These transmission cells receive cutaneous and subcutaneous afferents, those in layer 5 also receive visceral afferents, and those in layer 6 also receive kinesthetic (muscle-joint-tendon) afferents. The excitability of the cells in all these layers is controlled by descending fibers, including some from the pyramidal tracts. Among the outstanding features of these five layers is convergence, that is, a single cell may be activated by impulses from different receptors (e.g., cutaneous and visceral impulses impinging upon the same transmission cells in layer 5). It must be emphasized, however, that the functions of the spinal gray matter can only be tentatively or theoretically assigned, and that cutaneous and deep afferent terminals and transmission cells are present in other layers (see spinocerebellar tracts, p. 365). Nevertheless, the concepts presented in Figures 11–3 and 11–4 have proved to be powerful ones, with significant implications, especially for psychological processes and clinical medicine.

Comparable gray matter in the brain stem is less well understood. The fibers that reach the medulla oblongata by way of the posterior funiculus end in the *nucleus gracilis* or the *nucleus cuneatus* (Fig. 11–5). These two nuclei, which form the gracile and

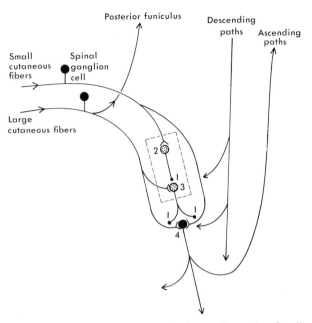

Figure 11-3. The gate control theory for pain. Small cutaneous afferents activate transmission cells in layer 4 by two mechanisms: direct excitation of layer 4 cells, and indirect excitation by way of two successive inhibitory cells (inhibition [I] of inhibition [I]). In layers 2 and 3 (presynaptic inhibition is shown here, but postsynaptic inhibition is probably also present). The area enclosed by the rectangle (interrupted line) includes the neurons that comprise the gate. Thus, the small fibers "open the gate." Large fibers, which give branches that ascend in the posterior funiculus also activate layer 4 cells directly, but by collaterals they activate cells in layer 3 which in turn inhibit layer 4 cells. Thus, the large fibers "shut the gate." (Based on Melzack, R., and Wall, P. D., in Yamamura, H., editor: Anesthesiology and Neurophysiology, Boston, Little, Brown and Company, 1970.)

cuneate elevations on the dorsal aspect of the medulla oblongata, contain transmission cells that tend to have a one-to-one relationship to activating fibers. Convergence is limited, and in primates control by descending fibers is limited. The axons of the transmission cells form the medial lemniscus (see discussion of the lemniscal system, p. 232).

The parent fibers of the receptors in the skin, subcutaneous tissues, teeth, mucous membranes, and joints of the head and neck enter the central nervous system chiefly over the trigeminal nerves and upper cervical dorsal roots. Some fibers enter by way of the facial, glossopharyngeal, and vagus nerves, but then join the central trigeminal connections. Most of the entering trigeminal fibers end in two nuclei on each side. One is the *main sensory nucleus,* which is at the level of entrance (Fig. 11–5). The other is the *nucleus of the spinal tract of the trigeminal nerve,* a long column of gray matter that is continuous caudally with the dorsal gray matter of the upper part of the cervical spinal cord. The fibers that end in this nucleus are trigeminal fibers that turn downward and form the *spinal tract of the trigeminal nerve* (Fig. 11–6). Little is known about the internal organization of either the main sensory nucleus or the spinal nucleus.

Those trigeminal fibers that do not end in either of the two nuclei comprise the parent fibers from neuromuscular spindles in the muscles of mastication. The unipolar neurons whose peripheral fibers form neuromuscular spindles in these muscles are unique in that they are located within the brain stem rather than in the trigeminal ganglion. These neurons and their processes form the *mesencephalic tract* and *nucleus of the trigeminal nerve.*

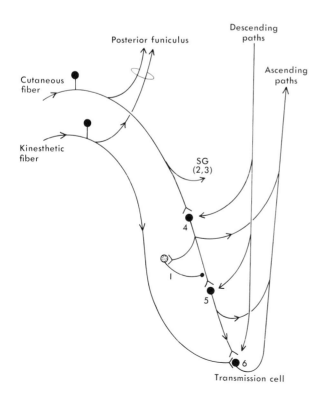

Figure 11–4. A schematic representation of probable arrangements in layers 2 to 6 of the dorsal gray matter. Note that cutaneous (and subcutaneous) afferents activate cells in layers 4 to 6, whose axons form ascending pathways, whereas kinesthetic fibers arise (chiefly) in layer 6 (layer 5 is the chief source of spinothalamic fibers for pain). Note also that a presynaptic control mechanism exists between layers 4 and 5, that cutaneous afferents gave branches to the substantia gelatinosa (SG: layers 2 and 3), and that descending fibers are directed to all the layers. The cells in layers 2 and 3 form a gate control mechanism (Fig. 11–3). (Based on Melzack, R., and Wall, P. D.: Science, *150*:971–979, 1966 and Wall, P. D.: Brain, *93*:505–524, 1970.)

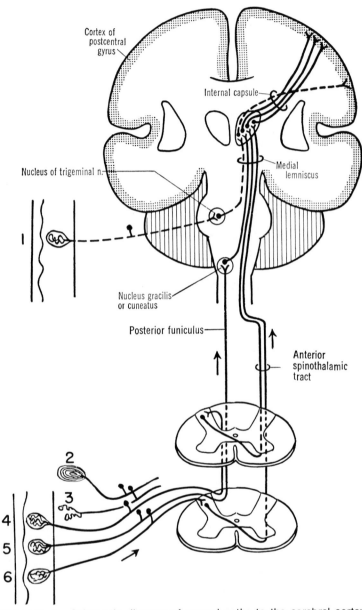

Figure 11-5. Schematic diagram of several paths to the cerebral cortex. 1, 4, 5, and 6 indicate the several cutaneous receptors. The pacinian corpuscle (2) and Ruffini ending (3) have paths which are similar to the path taken by 5, but which, for purposes of simplification, are not shown. Note that the tactile paths have several routes.

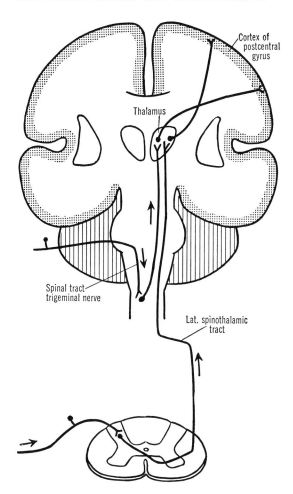

Figure 11-6. Diagram of the traditional concept of the pain and temperature path. Note that secondary fibers from the trigeminal nerve join the lateral spinothalamic tract.

PATHWAYS

The following account of the pathways that originate from transmission cells is not organized according to traditional concepts, which view each pathway as conducting a specific sensory modality. Instead, the pathways are presented as four different kinds, or groups, each of which exhibits certain anatomical and physiological characteristics, and each of which is organized for the transmission of particular kinds of information.

The four groups of central projection pathways are: (1) the lemniscal system, which is involved in the active search for information; (2) the spinothalamic system, which is involved in sensory-discriminative processes; (3) the spinocervicothalamic tract, which seems to have characteristics of both (1) and (2); and (4) a diffuse, multisynaptic ascending system that is of particular importance in drive, motivation, and affect.

LEMNISCAL SYSTEM

This is also called the dorsal column system (or dorsal column-medial lemniscus system.) It is composed of those ascending branches of large fibers which reach the medulla oblongata, where they end in the nucleus gracilis or nucleus cuneatus, as mentioned previously (Fig. 11–5). There is a morphological feature of the posterior funiculus that is the result of lamination of the ascending fibers. The fibers that enter the spinal cord at lower levels and then ascend in the posterior funiculi are displaced medially by those that enter at higher levels. Beginning in the upper thoracic cord and continuing into the cervical cord, each posterior funiculus is separated into a *fasciculus gracilis* and a *fasciculus cuneatus* (Fig. 13–1, p. 288). The fasciculus gracilis contains fibers derived from the lower limb and the lower trunk. It derives its name from its long, slender shape; it is the more medial of the two. The fasciculus cuneatus is shorter, and is wedge-shaped; it contains fibers from the upper trunk and upper limb. The fibers in each fasciculus end in the corresponding nucleus.

The axons that arise from the cuneate and gracile nuclei on each side cross to the opposite side and form a prominent tract, the *medial lemniscus.* The two medial lemnisci ascend to nuclei in the basal and lateral portions of the thalamus, which in turn project to the postcentral gyrus of the parietal lobe by way of the internal capsule. The postcentral gyrus is a *primary cortical receptive area* (see p. 406). During its course, each medial lemniscus is joined by fibers arising in the main sensory and spinal trigeminal nuclei from the opposite side.

As is true for the motor area, the body is represented upside-down in the postcentral gyrus. Impulses beginning in the head and neck end in the lower part of the gyrus, whereas those from the lower limb end in the upper portion, and those from the upper limb end in intermediate areas.

The lemniscal system includes fast conducting fibers from mechanoreceptors (especially the rapidly adapting ones) in skin, subcutaneous tissues, joints, and ligaments; the modalities involved are touch, pressure, vibration, and movement. This system traditionally has been considered to be responsible for sensory discriminative processes, with precise somatotopic localization of stimuli. This view is now being questioned, because section of posterior funiculi results in surprisingly little sensory deficit, and two-point discrimination and perception of weight and texture are unaffected. The chief deficits are motor, with profound inability to identify objects by exploration with the hand and fingers. It may well be that the lemniscal system (including central trigeminal fibers), with its rapidly acting components and precise peripheral localization, is more concerned with getting information and exploring and manipulating external objects.

There is substantial evidence that the information it transmits to higher centers triggers control mechanisms that in turn initiate the motor activities involved in external manipulation and exploration. Moreover, transmission mechanisms at lower levels are monitored and modulated by descending impulses.

SPINOTHALAMIC SYSTEM

This comprises a system in which the ascending fibers originate from transmission cells, chiefly in layers 4 to 6, and cross mostly to the opposite anterolateral portion of the white matter from which they ascend to the ventral and lateral portions of the thalamus (Figs. 11–5, 11–6). These are the same portions of the thalamus in which the medial lemnisci end. During their ascent in the brain stem they are joined by fibers from transmission cells in the spinal nucleus of the trigeminal nerve.

The spinothalamic system is activated by mechanoreceptors (chiefly the slowly adapting cutaneous, subcutaneous, and joint endings), by thermoreceptors, and by nociceptors. Those spinothalamic fibers concerned with the transmission of thermal and nociceptive information tend to ascend in the lateral funiculus and comprise the *lateral spinothalamic tract.* Those spinothalamic fibers concerned with mechanoreceptors tend to ascend in the more anterior portions of the spinal cord and comprise the *anterior spinothalamic tract.*

The spinothalamic system, whose transmission cells are subject to powerful modulation by descending fibers, appears to be primarily involved in sensory-discriminative mechanisms, in the precise relationships of stimuli to the areas or parts stimulated, and in the initiation of perceptual mechanisms.

SPINOCERVICOTHALAMIC TRACT

Some of the local branches of the large fibers that enter the spinal cord synapse with transmission cells, chiefly in layers 4 and 5, whose axons ascend ipsilaterally in the dorsal part of the lateral funiculus as the *spinocervicothalamic tract* (Fig. 11–7). Its axons end in the *lateral cervical nucleus,* which is located in the dorsal part of the lateral funiculus of the upper cervical cord. The axons arising in the nucleus cross and ascend to the thalamus with the medial lemniscus.

The spinocervicothalamic tract has been identified only relatively recently and little is known about its functions. It is present in primates, including humans, although its arrangement in humans may be somewhat different than that in lower forms. The tract is activated by mechanoreceptors in large peripheral fields, and to some extent by thermoreceptors and nociceptors. Many of

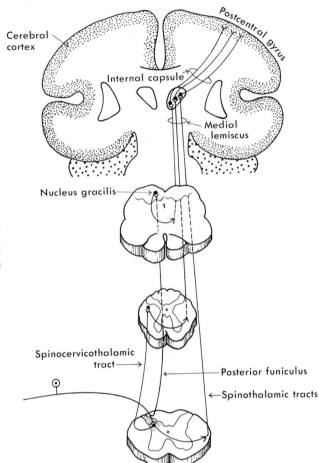

Figure 11-7. Schematic representation of the spinocervicothalamic tract in relation to other ascending systems. Details of the organization of the gray matter (stippled area) are shown in Figures 11-3 and 11-4.

its fibers are rapidly conducting and could therefore function similarly to those of the lemniscal system. However, its origin from spinal transmission cells, that are subject to descending modulation, indicates a possible functional grouping with the spinothalamic system.

MULTISYNAPTIC ASCENDING SYSTEM

The major feature of this system, which is also called the "paramedial ascending system," or the "diffuse ascending system," is a centrally placed, longitudinally disposed "core" that begins in the reticular formation of the lower brain stem. It is composed successively, from below upward, of the reticular formation, the limbic midbrain area, the medial portion of the thalamus, and the limbic forebrain system (Fig. 11-8). This core, whose functional characteristics are described in Chapters 14, 15, and 17, includes chains of neurons, hence the term multisynaptic applied to it. Its input from the spinal cord is by way of collaterals from the spinothalamic tracts, and by way of fibers that originate from transmission cells and ascend bilaterally, adjacent to the gray matter. The specific fibers have not been completely identified; it is likely that they are spinoreticular and spinomesencephalic.

This ascending "core" system is of particular importance in psychological processes, especially in connection with pain (see discussion below).

SENSATION AND PERCEPTION

Much of the research on sensory mechanisms has been concerned with developing quantitative relationships between stimulus and sensory process or sensation. Clinical testing for sensory deficits has tended to be based upon this kind of an approach. Valuable as these approaches are, they give no clues to the nature and neural correlates of everyday perception; for example, why and how do objects look like they do, feel like they do, sound like they do. It is not yet possible to correlate the rich feel of a silk fabric, or the tonal quality of a musical instrument, with neuro-

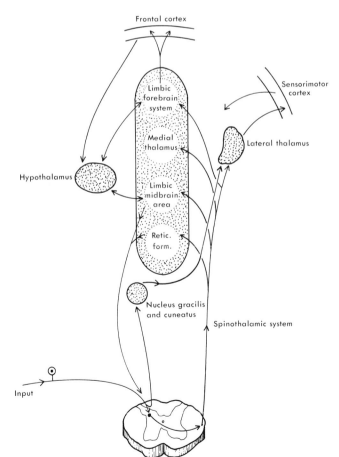

Figure 11-8. Simplified schematic representation of some of the pathways and structures involved in the physiological and psychological processes indicated in Figure 11–9 (based on Casey and Melzack and Wall). The ascending paths to the lateral thalamus and sensorimotor cortex (spinocervico-thalamic not shown) form the sensory-discriminative system. The median core, which includes reticular formation, limbic midbrain area, medial thalamus, and limbic forebrain system (including frontal lobe cortex), is responsible for the motivational and affective components of pain. Input to the core is derived from collaterals of ascending paths and also from special ascending paths (e.g., spinoreticular). The hypothalamus and fibers descending from the core represent some of the central control mechanisms (see text).

physiological or psychophysical processes. For the general senses, the discriminative aspects of these sensory-perceptual phenomena appear to be a function (at least in part) of the postcentral gyri. Each gyrus, which is closely connected with the motor cortex, comprises what is termed, somewhat arbitrarily, the *primary receptive area* for the general senses from the opposite side of the body. The structure of this sensory cortex, which has many entering nerve fibers, especially in its fourth layer, is described in Chapter 17.

The sensory cortex forms one part of a total system. Some of the features of this system, especially those that concern discriminative functions, are discussed later. Others can be illustrated here by reference to two complex processes, kinesthesia and pain.

KINESTHESIA

The term kinesthesia is used to refer to the sense of both movement and position; clinically, it is often referred to as muscle-joint-tendon sense. It deals in part with one's identity, or "body-image." To put it in everyday terms, the right hand knows where the left hand is, and vice versa.

The perception and awareness of the position of the body and its parts depend upon impulses from the inner ear (p. 274) and from receptors in joints and ligaments. Muscle and tendon receptors (presumably neuromuscular spindles and neurotendinous endings) also play a part, but to a degree as yet uncertain. The role of cutaneous receptors is even more indefinite. The kinesthetic sense may be tested by having the subject close his eyes; the examiner then passively moves a finger or toe of the subject to a new position. The subject is then asked to state what the new position is, or to duplicate it with the opposite corresponding member. The passively induced movement stimulates the receptors, including those in muscles and tendons. The impulses arising in joint and ligamentous mechanoreceptors travel centrally by the lemniscal and spinothalamic systems to the postcentral gyrus. The route to the cortex for impulses resulting from stretch of muscles has not yet been determined with any certainty; it appears not to be a part of the lemniscal system to any significant degree.

Little is known about the central mechanisms in kinesthesia. It may well be that interaction between information from muscles and joints is necessary. This same interaction may also be involved in weight discrimination.

PAIN

Pain is considered at some length here rather than in later chapters because clinically pain has been considered in terms of peripheral receptors and nerves and their spinal pathways.

Some of the peripheral receptors described earlier are clearly sensitive to noxious stimuli. However, many aspects of this peripheral sensitivity remain unexplained. In addition, the central control of transmission and the multisynaptic ascending system are of paramount importance (Figs. 11–8, 11–9).

The control of transmission (Figs. 11–3, 11–4) depends upon three important actions: (1) cells of the substantia gelatinosa (and presumably of the spinal trigeminal nucleus also) act as a gate; (2) the output of transmission cells (spinothalamic and perhaps spinocervicothalamic) is controlled by the gate and by descending impulses; (3) the lemniscal system closes the gate locally and through its rostral connections activates descending control

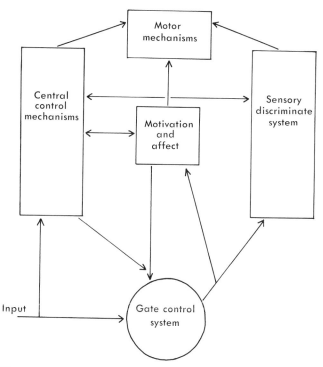

Figure 11–9. Schematic representation of some of the major physiological and psychological processes in pain. The neural correlates are as follows: the lemniscal system activates the central control mechanisms; the spinothalamic system (and perhaps the spinocervicothalamic tract also) is the input for sensory-discriminative mechanisms; and the median core (Fig. 11–8) determines motivational aspect, aversive drive, and unpleasant affect, and monitors central intensity. Central control systems involve a variety of brain stem and forebrain areas, and motor mechanisms range from anterior horn cell to motor cortex output. (Based on Melzack, R., and Casey, P. L., in Kenshalo, D. R., editor: The Skin Senses. Charles C Thomas, Publisher, Springfield, Illinois, 1968.)

mechanisms. It seems likely that pain phenomena are initiated by interactions of these three processes.

Figures 11–8 and 11–9 illustrate the events "beyond the gate." The sensory-discriminative features of pain (e.g., localization) are a function of the spinothalamic system, whereas the powerful motivational drive, unpleasant aspects, and aversive reactions are related to the multisynaptic ascending system. It is this system that appears to determine the "quality" of pain. For example, deep pain (arising from bones, joints, tendons, fascia) and visceral pain have qualities that are often quite different from those of cutaneous pain, as anyone who has had an intestinal cramp or a severe blow to a bone or joint will testify. Such pain is usually diffuse, it tends to radiate, and it is difficult to localize precisely. In addition, it is often severe, even sickening, with major reflex effects upon blood pressure and respiration, and may persist for hours or days.

Referred Pain. Visceral disorders often cause pain that is felt in skin as well as in viscera. The skin pain occurs in regions supplied by nerves originating from the segment of the cord in which the impulses from the involved viscera enter. For example, if the diaphragm, which is supplied by the fourth cervical segment of the spinal cord (phrenic nerve), is inflamed or abnormally stretched, pain may be felt in the skin and subcutaneous tissue supplied by the fourth cervical segment (e.g., the tip of the shoulder). Referred pain is frequent enough to be valuable as a diagnostic sign. For example, heart disease may be associated with pain in the left arm. In the early stages of appendicitis, pain may be felt just below the sternum. The pain of a kidney stone passing down the ureter may be referred to the back and groin. Physicians are able to localize internal disorders more accurately when referred pain is present.

The mechanisms of referred pain are not completely understood, but an important feature is the fact that cutaneous and visceral impulses converge upon transmission cells, especially those in layer 5, from which some of the spinothalamic fibers arise. Hence, the increased input barrage that occurs when impulses from visceral nociceptors arrive probably increases transmission firing and leads to a perception of pain in both skin and viscera. That it is not merely a case of misinterpretation is indicated by the fact that the skin and subjacent tissues are directly painful, and that an anesthetic injected into the skin relieves the referred pain.

Projected Pain. Projected pain, like projected sensations in general, results from the fact that a stimulus applied to a peripheral nerve anywhere along its course causes impulses that are indistinguishable from those that originate at the receptors formed by fibers of that nerve. The cortex interprets them as coming from the receptors. Striking the ulnar nerve at the elbow ("hitting the funny bone") is an example. Although many different kinds of fibers are stimulated, those concerned with nociceptive impulses often predominate. The pain that results appears to radiate down the forearm and hand; i.e., it is a projection of sensation. A classical example is found in tabes dorsalis, which is one of the manifestations of syphilitic infection of the nervous system. The inflammatory process involves dorsal roots. The irritation of the nerve fibers initiates impulses that reach the brain, but, since the impulses are the same as those caused by stimulation of the receptors at the ends of the same fibers, they are interpreted as coming from receptors. The patient, therefore, complains of severe pains in his limbs and viscera, the exact location depending upon the dorsal roots involved.

Even more striking are *phantom limb sensations.* Patients who have had a limb amputated subsequently feel as if that limb were still present. The phantom limb may even become painful. Apparently some type of irritation of the ends of the nerve fibers in the stump initiates nerve impulses. When these reach the brain, they are interpreted as coming from receptors in the absent limb, that is, the areas normally supplied by the fibers. In other words, during the lifetime of the person, previous to the amputation, there has been built up a body scheme in which the brain has become used to the fact that impulses arriving from certain nerves were coming from certain portions of the body. Impulses initiated anywhere along the path are identical with those starting at the peripheral receptors. Sensations due to stimuli at portions of afferent paths other than receptors may be termed referred, projected, or spontaneous. It is apparent that when a person complains of pain somewhere in his body, the cause may be anywhere along the pain pathway.

Occasionally, the predominating sensation in a phantom limb is pain. It is interesting that in medical history and in folklore there are references to the practice of digging up amputated parts which had been buried, in order to straighten out the fingers or toes in the belief that this would relieve painful spasms of the absent limb. These spasms were attributed to the devil.

Pharmacological Control of Pain. Drugs are commonly used to control pain. Aspirin, for example, may be extremely effective and probably acts on peripheral mechanisms, especially as an anti-inflammatory agent. Anesthetics are of major clinical importance and, depending on their nature, can act against receptors and nerve fibers (e.g., local anesthetics), against the gate and transmission mechanisms (e.g., barbiturates), against the reticular formation (e.g., barbiturates, nitrous oxide), or against all central levels (e.g., some of the gas anesthetics). Still other drugs, for example, opiates, have profound effects upon pain mechanisms.

Surgical Control of Pain. Various portions of the pain pathways may be surgically cut in an effort to relieve pain, a therapeutic measure in cases of severe, intractable pain, such as might be present in the terminal stages of cancer or after a severe injury. One such surgical procedure is to cut the lateral spinothalamic tract (Figs. 11–10 and 11–11). This procedure, which

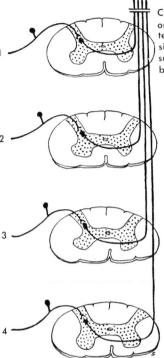

Cut here causes decrease
or loss of pain and
temperature on opposite
side in skin areas
supplied by numbered
branches

Figure 11–10. Diagram illustrating that if the lateral spinothalamic tract is cut, the sense of pain and temperature is decreased or lost on the opposite side (the more discriminative functions are those affected).

probably helps by decreasing the number of ascending impulses, may fail, undoubtedly because it does not affect the diffuse ascending system. In more recent years, surgical attack on the limbic system has often proved effective.

Sensory and Central Control of Pain. Certain kinds of sensory stimulation may relieve pain (e.g., pressing on a painful area, scratching to relieve itch, acupuncture). Moreover, potentially painful injuries may go unnoticed during a game or in the heat of battle. The gate theory is more than a plausible explanation, because large fiber stimulation (especially posterior funiculus stimulation) is being used successfully to relieve pain.

Control may be attempted, often successfully, by a variety of drugs that act on the multisynaptic ascending system (e.g., tranquilizers, relaxants), by hypnosis, and by suggestion (areas of the cerebral cortex may control the diffuse and the sensory-discriminative systems). Surgical attack on the limbic system for the relief of pain has been undertaken with some success. In such instances, perception and discrimination remain, but the effect is altered. Pain is felt but it is of no concern; it doesn't "bother" the patient.

CLINICAL IMPORTANCE OF THE AFFERENT PATHWAYS

Because of the anatomical differences in the afferent pathways, symptoms resulting from lesions of these paths will differ according to the location of the lesions (Fig. 11–12).

Suppose that the posterior, lateral, and anterior funiculi (one half of the cord) are destroyed on the left side of the thoracic cord. Pain and temperature perception may be diminished or lost over the right lower limb because of the destruction of the left lateral spinothalamic tract. Pressure and position sense are diminished in the left lower limb due to the destruction of the left posterior funiculus and left spinocervicothalamic tract. Touch is only slightly affected, because of the multiple ascending pathways. Such a lesion, of course, causes a spastic paralysis of the left lower

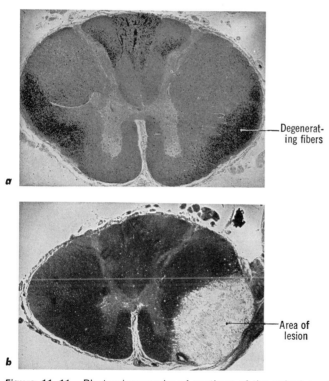

Degenerating fibers

a

Area of lesion

b

Figure 11–11. Photomicrographs of sections of the spinal cord from a patient in whose cord two incisions, right and left, had been made to relieve intractable pain. *a*, Thoracic cord above both incisions. Note dark degenerating fibers (Marchi stain) in both lateral funiculi. Compare this appearance of degeneration with that of Figure 10–11, p. 213. Degeneration in the posterior funiculi is a result of the disease that caused the pain. *b*, Section through one of the incisions in the midthoracic portion of the spinal cord. Note how extensive is the area sectioned.

limb because of destruction of corticospinal and extrapyramidal fibers. If this lesion were in the upper cervical cord, there would be similar signs in the upper limbs as well. The symptoms resulting from hemisection of the spinal cord constitute the *Brown-Séquard syndrome.*

Suppose, however, that the lesion is in the brain stem, above the level of entrance of fibers from the head and face, and that it destroys one of the medial lemnisci. Since the pathways by now are largely crossed and grouped with or near the medial lemniscus, virtually all input to the brain is lost. Hence, there will be anesthesia of the skin and deeper tissues in the opposite side of the trunk and head; position sense will also be lost. If the lesion is large enough to include the lateral spinothalamic tract, pain and temperature perception are decreased or lost over the same areas. If the lesion is extended to include the descending motor fibers, spastic paralysis of the opposite limbs occurs. Of course, any brain stem lesion often involves one of the cranial nerves, in which case there are signs and symptoms relating to its destruction.

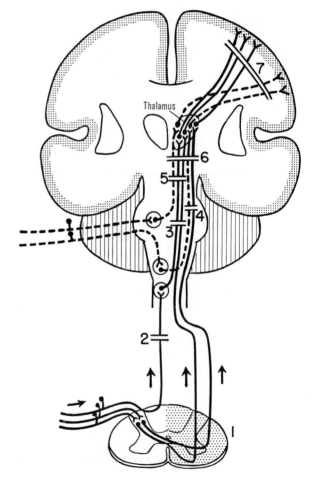

Figure 11–12. Diagram illustrating lesions of sensory paths. 1: The shaded area represents a hemisection of the cord (Brown-Séquard syndrome, described in text). 2: Section of fibers in the posterior funiculus, causing little sensory deficit (see text). 3: Section of the medial lemniscus here causes decreases or loss of general senses (except pain and temperature) in opposite side of the body. 4: Section of the lateral spinothalamic tract causes decrease or loss of pain and temperature in the opposite side of the body and face. 5: Section of the medial lemniscus similar to 3, except that the loss includes the opposite face as well. 6: Lesion of all sensory fibers with decrease or loss of all general senses in the opposite side of the body and face. 7: This represents a lesion in the internal capsule or cortex. The signs are quite variable, but the characteristic feature is that some perception of pain and temperature often remains (see text).

It should be emphasized that although the term "lost" is used, losses are based on the results of simple testing. Detailed, comprehensive examinations reveal that it is rare for any sensation to be totally lost following a lesion that destroys pathways on only one side of the brain stem or spinal cord.

SUMMARY

The number, frequency, and pattern of impulses arising in peripheral receptors comprise a first-order coding of messages to the central nervous system. Second-order coding occurs in various areas of gray matter in the spinal cord and brain stem, from which ascending pathways transmit the information required for sensory-perceptual phenomena. These phenomena may be classified as general and special senses, but such a classification is arbitrary and simplistic.

The receptors involved are those in skin and subcutaneous tissues, muscles, joints, tendons, and viscera. The skin and subcutaneous receptors include: (1) mechanoreceptors (rapidly and slowly adapting endings that are activated by touch or pressure, or in hairy skin by moving a hair, and the rapidly adapting pacinian corpuscles in subcutaneous tissue, which are activated by pressure or vibration); (2) thermoreceptors, which respond to changes in skin temperature; and (3) nociceptive receptors, which respond to noxious stimuli. Mechanoreceptors in muscles, joints, tendons and other deep tissues include: (1) neuromuscular spindles and other receptors in muscles; (2) Ruffini endings and paciniform corpuscles in joints; (3) Golgi tendon organs; and (4) Ruffini endings and pacinian corpuscles in periosteum and fascia. Nociceptive receptors are also present. Various receptors, including nociceptive receptors, are present in viscera. Those associated with sensory-perceptive mechanisms have not been specifically identified.

The parent fibers of receptors enter the spinal cord over dorsal roots and the brain stem over certain cranial nerves. The larger fibers that enter the spinal cord divide into descending, local, and ascending branches; some of the latter reach the medulla. The smaller fibers that enter the spinal cord divide into short descending, local, and ascending branches. The branches that enter the gray matter, in addition to synaptic connections with motor neurons, synapse with cells in the dorsal gray matter, especially those in the first six layers. Layers 2 and 3, the substantia gelatinosa, form a gate that controls transmission cells. The gate is closed by large fibers, opened by small fibers, and is modulated by descending fibers. The cells in layers 4 to 6 are transmission cells that form ascending pathways.

The fibers that ascend in the posterior funiculus end in the nucleus gracilis and nucleus cuneatus, from which axons ascend as the medial lemniscus. The parent fibers of receptors in the head and neck enter over cervical dorsal roots and several cranial nerves, chiefly the trigeminal. The central gray matter of the trigeminal nerve is organized into a mesencephalic, main sensory, and spinal nucleus.

The transmission cells of the spinal cord and brain stem form four central projection systems: (1) the lemniscal system, which is involved in the analysis and control of events; (2) the spinothalamic system, which is involved in sensory-discriminative processes; (3) the spinocervicothalamic tract, which has characteristics of both (1) and (2), above; and (4) a diffuse, multisynaptic system which is of special importance in drive, motivation, and affect.

Although there are as yet no specific neural correlates for perceptual phenomena, it is known that the postcentral gyrus is a primary receptive area for the general senses, dealing with sensory-discriminative processes, including pain. Other aspects of pain, especially the aversive drive, motivational dimensions, and unpleasant nature, are related to the diffuse ascending system, especially its limbic system components. Treatment of pain may be pharmacological, surgical, sensory, or psychological.

NAMES IN NEUROLOGY

CHARLES-ÉDOUARD BROWN-SÉQUARD (1817–1894)

Born of an American father and a French mother, on British soil (Mauritius), Brown-Séquard studied medicine in Paris and published a thesis on experimental studies of the nervous system. Before taking the chair of experimental physiology at the Collège de France in 1878, he held appointments in Paris, Richmond (Virginia), Boston, and London. His experimental studies on the nervous system included that on hemisection of the spinal cord, first reported in his thesis as a medical student, and in more detail in 1849. He defined the clinical entity of cord hemisection in 1860. (Olmsted, J. M. D.: Charles-Édouard Brown-Séquard. Baltimore, The Johns Hopkins Press, 1946.)

REFERENCES

The following books, monographs, and symposia include critical reviews, specialized accounts, and clinical features.

Iggo, A. (editor): Somatosensory System. Vol. II, Handbook of Sensory Physiology. Berlin, Springer-Verlag, 1973.

Kenshalo, D. R. (editor): The Skin Senses. Springfield, Ill., Charles C Thomas, 1968.

Mountcastle, V. B. (editor): Medical Physiology. 13th ed. St. Louis, The C. V. Mosby Company, 1974.

Neil, E. (editor): Enteroceptors. Handbook of Sensory Physiology. Vol. III/1. Berlin, Springer-Verlag, 1972.

de Reuck, A. V. S., and Knight, J. (editors): Myotatic, Kinesthetic and Vestibular Mechanisms. CIBA Foundation Symposium. London, J. & A. Churchill, Ltd., and Boston, Little, Brown and Company, 1967. See also Touch, Heat and Pain. The CIBA Foundation, Boston, Little, Brown and Company, 1966.

Sinclair, D.: The Nerves of Skin. In Jarrett, A. (editor): The Physiology and Pathophysiology of Skin. Vol. II. New York, Academic Press, 1973.

Somjen, G.: Sensory Coding in the Mammalian Nervous System. New York, Appleton-Century-Crofts, 1972.

White, J. C., and Sweet, W. H.: Pain and the Neurosurgeon. A 40-year experience. Springfield, Ill., Charles C Thomas, 1969.

The following are scientific papers and reviews.

Goodwin, G. M., McCloskey, D. I., and Matthews, P. B. C.: The contribution of muscle afferents to kinaesthesia shown by vibration induced illusions of movement and by the effects of paralyzing joint afferents. Brain, 95:705–748, 1972.

Harrington, T., and Merzenich, M. M.: Neural coding in the sense of touch: human sensations of skin indentation compared with the responses of slowly adapting mechanoreceptive afferents innervating the hairy skin of monkeys. Exp. Brain Res., 10:251–264, 1970.

Iggo, A.: Electrophysiological and histological studies of cutaneous mechanoreceptors. In Kenshalo, cited above.

Iggo, A.: Cutaneous thermoreceptors in primates and subprimates. J. Physiol., 200:403–430, 1969.

Iggo, A., and Muir, A. R.: The structure and function of a slowly adapting touch corpuscle in hairy skin. J. Physiol., 200:763–796, 1969.

Melzack, R., and Wall, P. D.: Pain mechanisms: a new theory. Science, 150:971–979, 1966. A powerful concept of major importance, with further considerations and modifications given in the following: Melzack, R., and Casey, K. L., in Kenshalo, cited above; Melzack, R., and Wall, P. D., in Anesthesiology and Neurophysiology, (Yamamura, H., editor), Boston, Little, Brown and Company, 1970; and Casey, K. L., Amer. Scientist, 61:194–200, 1973.

Talbot, W. H., Darian-Smith, I., Kornhuber, H. H., and Mountcastle, V. B.: The sense of flutter-vibration; comparison of the human capacity with response patterns of mechanoreceptive afferents from the monkey hand. J. Neurophysiol., 31:301–334, 1968.

Teuber, H.-L.: Perception. In Field, J., Magoun, H. W., and Hall, V. E. (editors): Handbook of Physiology. Sect. 1, Neurophysiology, Vol. III. Washington, American Physiological Society, 1960.

Wall, P. D.: The sensory and motor role of impulses travelling in the dorsal columns toward cerebral cortex. Brain, 93:505–524, 1970.

Chapter **12**

THE SPECIAL SENSES
AND THEIR PATHWAYS

The categorization of senses as general and special was discussed briefly in the previous chapter. The concept of the special senses as "special" probably developed because of the obvious importance of the sense organs involved, particularly the eye and the ear. Nevertheless, the principles of functional organization, for example, with respect to coding, modulation, and transmission, are similar to those for the general senses in many respects, and the difficulties in relating physiological processes to psychological events are just as great.

In humans, the special senses are rather uniformly developed to a high degree. This does not mean that taste is as subjectively important as vision. It means that taste is associated with a system of pathways and cortical areas that allow for functional elaboration, if necessary. Humans, therefore, differ from other animals in which one or more of these senses may be highly developed. Hearing in a bat is certainly more specialized than in humans. A dog has a remarkable olfactory sense. Birds may have extraordinarily keen vision. But in these animals many of the other senses are functionally inferior to those of humans.

VISION

The peripheral stimuli necessary for this sensory quality are radiations in the visible portion of the electromagnetic spectrum varying in wave length from 400 to 700 nm. The receptors are in the retina, which is the visual layer of the eye. The eye is a complex and efficient optical instrument that is designed to gather and focus light upon the retina. If one compares the eye to a camera, the retina would correspond to the light-sensitive plate or film (but in fact, the eye is more like a television camera, the image on the retina being coded and transmitted rather than imprinted). There is a focusing system composed of the *cornea* and the *crystalline lens* (Fig. 12–1). The cornea is composed of connective tissue and is covered on both surfaces by epithelial cells. It is transparent and is devoid of any blood vessels that might interfere with this property. The cornea is curved, with the convexity forward or outward; when viewed from the front, it is the clear portion of the globe, surrounded on all sides by the "white" of the eye, the *sclera*.

Much of the refraction of entering light occurs during its passage through the corneal surfaces. Light undergoes further refraction as it passes through the lens. The total refraction is such that when light from any object reaches the retina, it forms a real and inverted image on the retina. Just behind the cornea is the *iris.* This has an opening in its center, the *pupil.* There are smooth muscle fibers in the iris, some of which are arranged circularly so that the pupil narrows when they contract. Others are arranged radially, spreading out like a fan, and their contraction widens the pupil (Fig. 12–2). Thus, like the variable aperture of a camera, there is a mechanism for regulating the amount of light admitted to the eye.

The color of the eyes is caused by pigment, most of which is

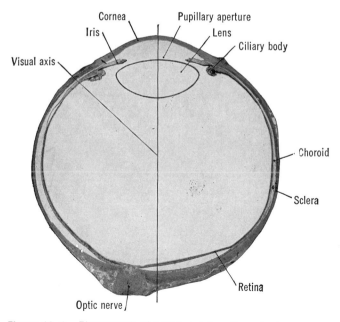

Figure 12–1. Photograph of a horizontal section of a human eye. The lens, which was removed to facilitate making the section, has been drawn in its correct position, but the suspensory strands around it have been omitted. Note that the retina has partially separated from the other coats of the eyeball. The dark line in the posterior part of the iris is due to the presence of pigment.

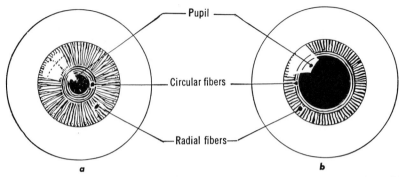

Figure 12-2. Circular and radial fibers in the iris. *a,* Pupillary constriction with contraction of the circular fibers. *b,* Pupillary dilation with contraction of radial fibers and relaxation of circular ones.

concentrated in cells on the posterior surface of the iris. Pigment is also present in the retinal epithelium, which is the outer, non-visual portion of the retina, and in the middle coat of the eye, the *choroid.* The pigment probably serves to prevent blurring or multiplication of images by internal reflection; in the camera this is prevented by painting the interior a dead black.

Sharp pictures at different distances can be taken with a camera by changing lenses or by varying the distance between lens and film. In the eye this is done by changing the curvature of the lens. The structures which make this possible are as follows: Surrounding the outer margin of the lens, and attached to it by fine suspensory strands, are bundles of smooth muscle fibers which form the *ciliary muscle.* When this muscle contracts, the area to which the strands attach is pulled forward. The strands are thus shortened, and the tension which they maintained on the lens is thereby lessened, allowing the elastic lens capsule to bulge forward.

Some fibers in the ciliary muscle are arranged circularly. When they contract, the entire ciliary area moves inward, thereby providing another means of shortening suspensory strands. The resulting increased thickness of the lens refracts the light to a greater degree, thus allowing near objects to be brought into sharper focus. This process is known as *accommodation.* It is accompanied by a narrowing of the pupil, that is to say, by pupillary constriction, and by a medial movement or convergence of each eye.

Between the iris and the cornea is the anterior chamber (Fig. 12–1); between the iris and the lens is the posterior chamber. Both are filled with a thin watery fluid, the *aqueous fluid* or *humor,* which is a filtrate of blood plasma. It circulates through the chambers and after absorption into tissue spaces in the coats of the eye is returned to the venous circulation. Behind the lens is the *vitreous body,* a gelatinous, clear substance that is permanent; that is, it is not undergoing a constant formation, circulation, and absorption.

This complicated structure of the eye may be made somewhat clearer by reference to its formation and development in the embryo and fetus. This is illustrated in Figure 12–3. It can be seen that the retina is an extension of brain substance and that, because of its manner of formation, it is a double layer. The outer layer becomes the pigmented layer (retinal epithelium), and the inner layer the visual or receptive layer of the retina.

THE RETINA

The retina is an extension of the brain, it contains layers of specialized nerve cells, and it is connected to the rest of the brain by a fiber tract called the optic nerve. The retina is the only portion of the nervous system that can be seen directly in the intact living subject by using an *ophthalmoscope.* This instrument is designed so that light from it, when directed into the eye of the subject, is reflected from the retina back to the eye of the observer.

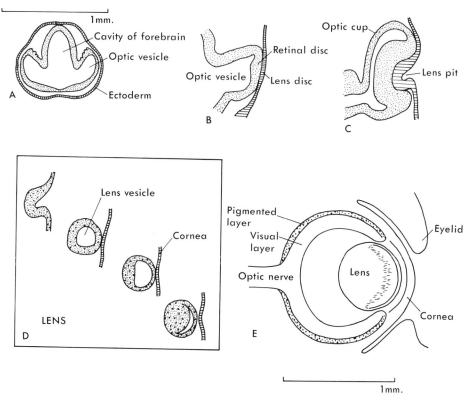

Figure 12–3. The development of the human eye during the embryonic period. A, the optic vesicle as an evagination of the forebrain (diencephalon). B, the appearance of the retinal disc and the lens disc. C, the beginning of the optic cup and the lens pit. D, successive steps in the formation of the lens. E, the major elements of the eye are present. Note the two layers of the retina. Retinal separation in the adult occurs between these two layers. (Courtesy of Dr. Ronan O'Rahilly.)

Light entering the eye along the visual axis (Fig. 12–1) falls upon a portion of the retina known as the *macula lutea,* so called because it is a yellow spot. In the middle of the macula is a depression, the *fovea.* Immediately medial to the macula lutea is a whitish area from which small arteries and veins spread throughout the retina. This is the *optic disc,* the point of exit of the optic nerve. The vessels are the retinal arteries and veins which reach the disc by running in the substance of the optic nerve, and which form a supplementary circulation to the inner portion of the retina. The optic disc and the vessels accurately reflect many pathological changes. Increased intracranial pressure, for instance, may so compress the retinal veins that circulation in the retina is seriously impaired; the resultant swelling is visible during ophthalmoscopic examination. Many other pathological changes (e.g., inflammation or atrophy of the optic disc, vascular disorders) may also be detected. The vascular disorders may be evident here before they are evident elsewhere in the body.

The retina is arranged into layers (Fig. 12–4), which reflect a fundamental organization. The outermost layer is the *retinal epithelium.* The remainder of the retina consists of layers that, from outer to inner, are formed by *photoreceptor cells (rods* and *cones), bipolar cells,* and *ganglion cells,* together with interneurons and glial cells. In general, the photoreceptors, bipolar cells, and ganglion cells are arranged in a somewhat vertical fashion, and light must traverse a number of cells to reach the photoreceptors. Near the optic disc, however, the cells are more obliquely placed, and they are absent in front of the disc. Light striking here does not impinge on photoreceptors; this disc is the *blind spot* of the eye.

Retinal Epithelium. The retinal epithelium consists of a single layer of epithelial cells that develop from the outer layer shown in Figure 12–3. The cavity of the forebrain that intervenes between this layer and the visual layer becomes obliterated, but remains as a potential site of retinal separation in the adult. In many species, including humans, the epithelial cells contain pigment granules, and the layer is then usually called *pigment epithelium* (Fig. 12–4). Processes of these pigment cells usually extend between the photoreceptors. In mammals, they extend for but a short distance (no more than the length of the outer segments); the remainder of the space between the photoreceptors consists of mucopolysaccharide.

The pigment epithelium and the photoreceptors are nourished by diffusion from the capillaries in the choroid (choriocapillary layer, Fig. 12–4). The epithelial cells are secondary storage areas for the precursors of the visual pigment, rhodopsin. The pigment granules in the epithelial cells absorb light not absorbed by the photoreceptors, and therefore probably prevent diffuse stimulation.

Visual Layers of Retina. The cells of these layers are photoreceptors, bipolar and ganglion cells, interneurons, and glial cells.

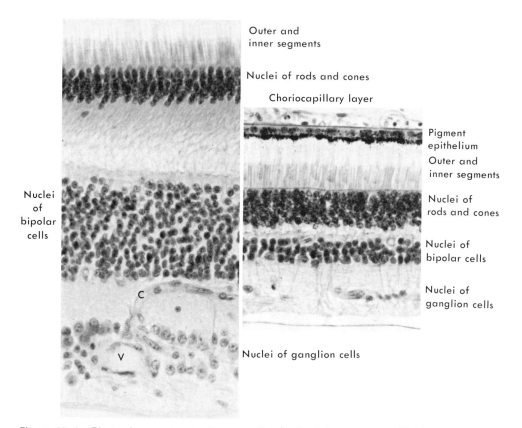

Figure 12-4. Photomicrographs of a human retina, both at the same magnification (about 525x). *Right,* section from the periphery of the retina. Note the sparcity of ganglion cells. The external limiting membrane (not labeled) is visible as a thin, dark line immediately above the nuclei of the rods and cones. The internal limiting membrane (not labeled) is a thin, dark line that forms the inner surface of the retina. *Left,* section near the fovea, where cones predominate (the pigment epithelium separated during processing for microscopic sectioning). Note the thickness of the bipolar and ganglion cell layers, evidence of a much greater tendency to a one-to-one ratio from photoreceptor to ganglion cell in the cone-dominated portions. The layer labeled "Nuclei of bipolar cells" also contains nuclei of glial cells and interneurons (see text). V, venule. C, capillary.

The general arrangement is such that rods and cones synapse with bipolar cells (and with processes of horizontal cells), and these in turn with ganglion cells, whose axons course toward the optic disc where they form the optic nerve. The interneurons form horizontal (lateral) connections, and the glial cells occupy most of the rest of the intercellular space, as they do elsewhere in the central nervous system. A few astrocytes are present, but most of the glial cells are radially arranged, their long processes terminating in relation to the *external* and *internal limiting membranes.* The external limiting membrane (Figs. 12–4, 12–6) is formed mainly by tight junctions between photoreceptor cells and glial cell processes. The internal limiting membrane is a basal lamina that, together with glial cell processes, separates the retina from the vitreous body.

The photoreceptors are the rods and cones, whose character-istic features are shown in Figures 12–5 to 12–7; rods and cones are named because of the shape of their outer segments. The organization of the retina is shown in Figures 12–8 and 12–9. There are 115 to 130 million rods and cones, but, at the most, only one million optic nerve fibers. This necessitates a general con-vergence within the retina. In other words, one or a few ganglion cells receive impulses from a number of bipolar cells, and these in turn from many rods and cones. This means that most ganglion cells are related to hundreds and perhaps thousands of photo-receptors, and that the receptive field of a ganglion cell may be relatively large (Fig. 12–9). All of the retinal connections are synapses. The cells are neurons, though in the rods and cones considerably modified ones. Between the cells, and forming a supporting framework for them, are neuroglial cells, as mentioned previously. The optic nerve, being a fiber tract and not a true peripheral nerve, also contains neuroglial tissue. Its fibers lack neurilemma and are, therefore, incapable of regeneration when once destroyed.

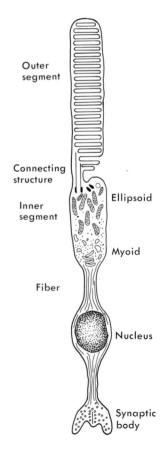

Figure 12–5. Schematic representation of the essential features of a vertebrate photoreceptor. The outer segment contains mem-brane discs on which the photosensitive pigment molecules are concentrated. The inner segment consists of two zones, an ellip-soid, which is a dense aggregation of mitochondria, and a myoid, containing the Golgi complex and granular endoplasmic reticulum. The organelles give way to a fiber, which is succeeded by the nucleus, and the cell ends as a complex synaptic body. (Based on Young, R. W., in Straatsma, B. R., et al. (editors): The Retina. Berkeley, University of California Press, 1969.)

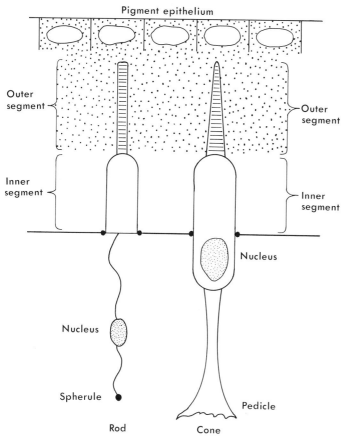

Figure 12-6. Topographical relationships and differences in shape of rods and cones. Portions of the cell membranes of the pigment epithelium are obscured by the pigment, which extends between the outer segments. In mammals the distance varies according to species, and is short in human retinae (see Fig. 12–4). Note the external limiting membrane perforated by the rods and cones; cone nuclei are placed nearer the membrane. The synaptic body in rods is termed a spherule; that in cones, a pedicle.

In the retina as a whole, there are about four times as many rods as cones. In the macula, however, cones predominate, and the fovea is occupied exclusively by them. As one progresses toward the periphery of the retina, the rods become predominant.

The bipolar and ganglion cells are of several different kinds, according to differences in retinal connections (Figs. 12–8, 12–9). Flat bipolar cells receive from cones and connect with ganglion cell dendrites and with amacrine cell processes. Midget bipolar cells receive from one cone only, but flat or diffuse cone bipolars receive from about seven cones (and every cone projects to a flat bipolar). Rod bipolars receive exclusively from rods.

The interneurons of the retina are the *horizontal cells* and *amacrine cells.* Horizontal cells connect cones and rods (Fig.

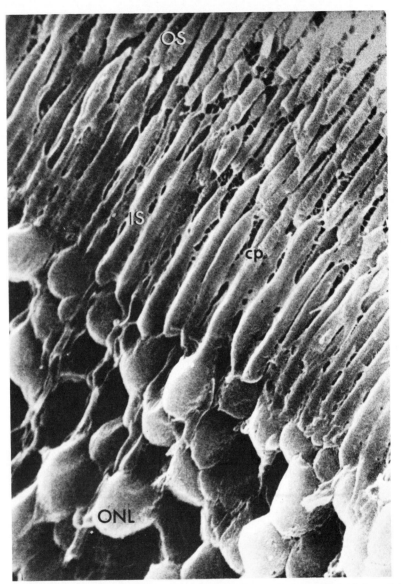

Figure 12-7. Scanning electron microgram of photoreceptor cells (chiefly rods) of rat retina. OS, outer segment. IS, inner segment. CP, connecting piece. ONL, outer nuclear layer (nuclei of rods and cones). Magnification about 4500x. (Figure 11, from Hansson, H.-A., in Z. Zellforsch., *107*:23–44, 1970. By permission of the author and the publishers, Springer-Verlag.)

12–8), and amacrine cells (neurons without an identifiable axon) connect bipolar terminals and ganglion cell dendrites and soma, and other amacrine processes.

The receptive field of a ganglion cell (Fig. 12–9) is that area of the retina which, when stimulated, affects a ganglion cell. In the light-adapted mammalian retina, each field is arranged into two circular and concentric zones that are antagonistic. If the center of a receptive field is illuminated, its ganglion cell fires either when the light goes on or when it goes off. The converse occurs in the periphery of the field, that is, a ganglion cell that fires when the light on the center is turned on, will fire when illumination of the periphery is turned off. From the functional standpoint, it seems likely that a ganglion cell reports more with respect to the degree of light and dark contrast than with light intensity. In animals with color vision (e.g., primates), the antagonistic fields may be color coded, with each zone being maximally sensitive to different wave lengths. The overall size of receptive fields probably does not vary much throughout the retina. However, the fields near the fovea have smaller centers and those in the fovea may correspond to a single cone. It seems likely that the centers of receptive fields may be mediated through direct pathways in the retina, whereas

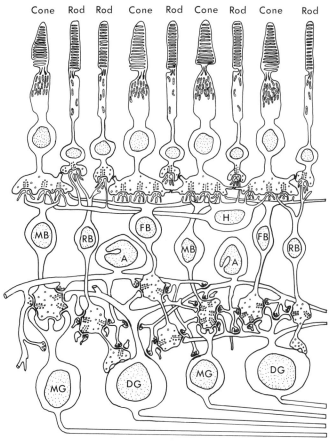

Figure 12–8. A summary diagram illustrating the organization of the primate retina. MB, midget bipolar. RB, rod bipolar. FB, flat bipolar. H, horizontal cell. A, amacrine cell. MG, midget ganglion cell. DG, diffuse ganglion cell. (From Dowling, J. E., and Boycott, B. B., in Proc. Roy. Soc. Lond., B., *166*:80–111, 1966. By permission of the authors and publisher.)

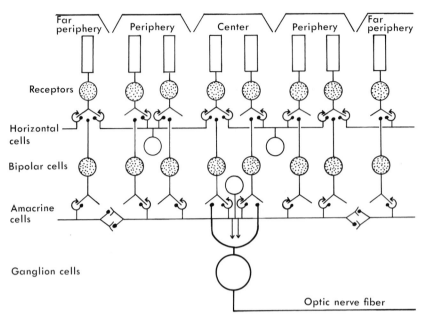

Figure 12–9. A schematic representation of the receptive field of a ganglion cell. ∧, excitatory synapse. →, inhibitory synapse. The synapses between the processes of horizontal cells and receptor terminals, and between amacrine processes and bipolar terminals, are represented as reciprocal contacts. The others are represented as one-way junctions. In this scheme, the ganglion cells connect directly with bipolar cells only in the center of the receptive field. The other bipolars connect by way of the amacrines. (From Dowling, J. E., and Boycott, B. B., in Proc. Roy. Soc. Lond., B., *116*:80–111, 1966. By permission of the authors and publisher.)

the antagonistic surround (periphery of field) is mediated by way of interneurons.

Retinal Functions. When light strikes a photoreceptor, a series of processes is initiated which results in the firing of ganglion cells. The eyes are sensitive to wave lengths in the range from 400 to 700 nm that is, from blue through green to red.

The visual pigment in the outer segments of rods is a lipoprotein complex termed *rhodopsin* or *visual purple.* This is the common pigment in marine fishes and land vertebrates, the various rhodopsins having a characteristic absorption maximum at about 500 nm. Human rhodopsin has an absorption maximum at 497 nm. Many fresh water fishes have porphyropsins rather than rhodopsins, the porphyropsins having absorption maxima at about 522 nm. Both types of pigments are related to the vitamin A complex. Vitamin A (retinol), a carotinoid, is obtained from food and is stored in the liver. It is taken up from the blood stream by the retinal epithelium, which acts as a secondary retinol storage site. Exchange then occurs between the retinal epithelium and the photoreceptors.

Retinol is converted to another compound termed retinal. This combines with opsin to form rhodopsin, which forms the bulk of the outer segments where it is attached to the lamellar membranes that form the discs. When light reaches rod outer segments, it is absorbed by rhodopsin. A photochemical change results, with some of the rhodopsin being bleached in the process. The process is reversible, rhodopsin being resynthesized by a complex series of steps. The velocity at which the photochemical reaction proceeds is proportional to the intensity of light and the concentration of rhodopsin. Only a small part of the total amount of rhodopsin is bleached when exposed to light.

The photochemical changes are accompanied by graded electrical changes that can be recorded as a part of the *electroretinogram* (ERG) (Fig. 12–10). The mechanisms are extra-

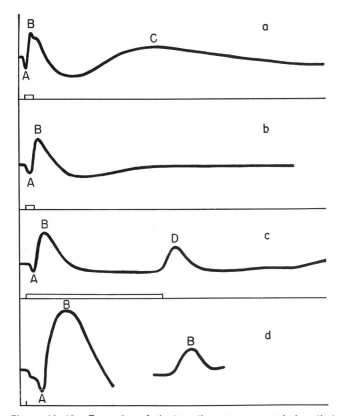

Figure 12–10. Examples of electroretinograms, recorded so that an upward deflection indicates positivity of an electrode in front of the retina, in contrast to an electrode behind or at the side of the retina. *a*, an ERG of a guinea pig (with pure rod retina, or nearly so), in response to a flash of light, the onset and duration of which are signaled on the base line. There is an initial, negative *A* wave, a larger positive *B* wave, and a long-lasting, positive *C* wave. *b*, an ERG of a ground squirrel (with a pure cone retina) in response to a short flash of light, showing *A* and *B* waves. With a long flash of light (*c*), there is a *D* wave or off-effect when the light is turned off. *d*, human ERGs. That on the left is in response to a flash of high-intensity light showing *A* and *B* waves. That on the right shows just a *B* wave when the stimulus is of low intensity. All ERGs are in dark-adapted state, and the human ERGs are based on Armington, J. C., Johnson, E. P., and Riggs, L. A., in J. Physiol, *118*:289–298, 1952.

ordinarily sensitive. It seems likely that one to three quanta of light reaching a rod are sufficient for activation.

The bipolar cells are synaptically activated by photoreceptor cells, but exhibit graded responses rather than action potentials. Ganglion cells do generate action potentials; these are conducted along the axons to the lateral geniculate body (p. 264).

The various electrical changes that accompany retinal activity comprise the electroretinogram, which can be detected by electrodes placed on the surface of the eye. It consists of an *A* wave, due chiefly to late photoreceptor activity, a *B* wave, which represents postsynaptic activity, and a *C* wave, which presumably is generated in the pigment epithelium. There may also be an off-effect termed a *D* wave (Fig. 12–10).

The synaptic transmitters in the retina have not yet been determined. Dopamine, acetylcholine, and GABA have been determined to be present, but their precise retinal functions are unknown.

The nature of the visual pigments in cones is not yet known. Evidently three different kinds are present; at least, three different absorption spectra can be demonstrated for human cones (Fig. 12–11). This fits well with color vision mechanisms (see later discussion).

The eyes of most mammals have both rods and cones. This situation, plus the presence of rod-rich retinas in nocturnal animals and cone-rich retinas in diurnal animals, has led to the duplicity theory of vision. This holds that rods are associated with visual sensitivity (night vision) and cones with visual acuity (day vision) and often with color vision also.

Dark and Light Adaptation. If the eyes have been in complete darkness for forty minutes or more, it will be found that the sensitivity of the eye has greatly increased. The energy of light necessary to stimulate is much less, by about a thousand-fold, than that required in daylight. If the dark-adapted eye is exposed to light of varying wave lengths, of equal energy, it is found that sensitivity is greatest in the green portion of the spectrum, where the greatest absorption by rhodopsin occurs. The light seen is not

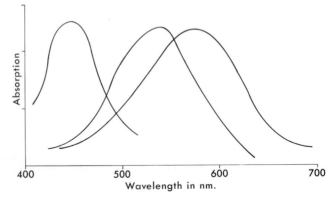

Figure 12–11. Absorption spectra of three cone pigments in human retinae. The absorption spectrum of one pigment peaks at about 445 nm (blue), another at 535 nm (green), and third at 570 nm (yellow). The last absorption spectrum extends into the red wavelengths. (Based on Michael, C. R., in New Engl. J. Med., *288*:724–728, 1973.)

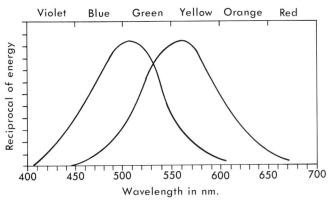

Figure 12-12. Scotopic and photopic luminosity curves, illustrating the Purkinje shift. The scotopic curve shows that the maximum sensitivity of the dark-adapted eye (achromatic vision) is 505 nm. The photopic curve shows that the maximum sensitivity of the light-adapted eye (chromatic vision) is about 560 nm. The two curves, for convenience, are plotted in the same units of sensitivity, although the scotopic eye is much more sensitive.

green, however, but some intensity of gray. The dark-adapted eye cannot distinguish colors. When the dark-adapted eye is stimulated with other wave lengths, it is found that sensitivity decreases according to the manner illustrated in Figure 12–12 (*scotopic curve*). Part of the decrease in sensitivity toward the violet or shorter wave length portion of the spectrum is more apparent than real, because some of the shorter wave lengths are absorbed by the refracting media, such as the lens. Patients who have had lenses removed because of cataracts (*aphakia*) may, by ultraviolet radiation, be able to see objects that are invisible or less visible to others. The dark-adapted eye is quite insensitive at the longer wave lengths, i.e., at the red end of the spectrum. Hence one can dark-adapt by wearing red goggles with the proper transmission characteristics. The red light that gets through stimulates cones, thus enabling one to see. Rods are not stimulated, hence can adapt just as if they were in darkness.

If an eye is exposed to strong light or to daylight, it becomes light-adapted, and the greatest sensitivity is found in the region of 557 nm (*photopic curve,* Fig. 12–12). This shift to the red-green portion of the spectrum is the *Purkinje shift* and represents functional differences between rods and cones. The threshold is at least a thousand times greater than in the dark-adapted retina.

It has been shown that in animals with pure rod and pure cone retinae, there is no Purkinje shift, nor is there one in humans when the stimulating light is so arranged that it falls only on the fovea, where only cones are present. On the basis of the evidence cited, and of other evidence, there is reason to believe that rods are primarily concerned with visual sensitivity, being active in the dark-adapted eye, and that cones are primarily concerned with visual acuity, being active in the light-adapted eye. This, however, is not a clear-cut functional separation. Rods are active in day vision. Nocturnal animals, for example, can see in the daytime. Color vision is supposed to be primarily a cone function, but rods may be concerned to some extent.

Visual Sensitivity. This is the ability to see in dim light and is primarily a function of the rods. There are several reasons for this. As mentioned above, rhodopsin is extremely sensitive to light. Hence, in the dark-adapted eye, less energy is necessary for rod stimulation. Furthermore, convergence is marked between rods and ganglion cells. Therefore, if light of low intensity falls upon each of many rods, the resulting excitation may summate at the succeeding cells and thereby reach the threshold of ganglion cells. Visual sensitivity is aided by reflex widening of the pupil in dim light. This illuminates rods previously unaffected and thereby increases the chances for summation.

Several mechanisms seem to be responsible for the increase in sensitivity during dark adaption. Only a small part of the total amount of rhodopsin is bleached, even in strong light, and the amount resynthesized in the dark accounts only in part for the increase in sensitivity. In dim light, or in darkness, horizontal spread of excitation occurs through interneurons. Probably, in the absence of cone activity, certain inhibitory mechanisms are lost, so that an increasing number of neurons have a lower threshold. Thus, one can speak of both photochemical and neurological components in dark adaption.

Since vitamin A is involved in the metabolism of rhodopsin, vitamin A deficiency may result in night blindness. This vitamin, however, has the general property of being necessary for the maintenance of epithelium, and its role in night blindness may therefore be related to the latter property.

Rods are more numerous in the periphery of the retina. Therefore, in dim light, such as at twilight, objects are best seen from an oblique angle rather than viewed directly ahead, since in the latter case light falls on the macular region where cones predominate.

Visual Acuity. With the light-adapted eye, color sensation becomes possible, as well as an increased sharpness of object contour and detail. One is therefore able to distinguish small objects as entities and to observe them in sharp outline.

Everyone is familiar with the fact that if one moves away from two closely approximated objects, they eventually fuse and appear as one. If the objects are lines, visual acuity may be tested by measuring the least separation by which two lines may be discerned. The smallest visual angle, the angle subserved by the distance separating the two lines, is a minute or less. There are many factors, more than can be discussed here, involved in visual acuity. One is probably the *grain* of the retina or the denseness of receptors within it. That is, if receptors were relatively far apart, light from one or the other of the lines or from the area between might fall on nonsensitive portions of the retina, and this would certainly diminish resolving power. Another factor is undoubtedly the one-to-one type of cone projection of the foveal region. This allows separate paths for impulses due to light from different small sources, such as two lines. The fact that visual acuity is more pronounced in the fovea corroborates the functions of the cones in this matter.

The theoretical conditions for the smallest visual angle may be shown as follows: Suppose two thin black lines on a white background are separated by such a small or narrow distance that the light from the intervening white would illuminate but a single row of cones. It follows that the row of cones on each side would not be illuminated (corresponding to the black lines), but those still farther laterally would be. The brain is thus furnished a means of distinguishing the two separable lines, since there are no nerve impulses from the retinal region corresponding to the lines, in contrast to the impulses arriving from the intervening and neighboring retina. These conditions, however, are not actually found. The focusing and fixation of the eyes are not accurate enough to meet these theoretical demands. Slight movements of the eyeballs result in illumination of the row of cones corresponding to the intervening white background, and in illumination of the row on each side (corresponding to the black lines) as well. Hence impulses from all these cells eventually reach the brain.

There is this difference, however. It was pointed out earlier that receptors respond to increasing intensities of stimulation by higher frequencies of discharges. Accordingly, the row of cones corresponding to the white background is more intensely stimulated, and discharges at higher frequencies than the less intensely illuminated row on each side. Visual acuity thus becomes a matter of intensity discrimination, in which the cerebral cortex is most important.

Visual acuity may also be tested by determining the smallest object which can be seen when viewed against a homogeneous field. The apparent size of a star, for instance, is minute. The angle subtended by it may be much smaller than the minimum visual angle necessary to deal with separable objects. The angle subtended by the minimum visible object has been shown to be a few seconds or less, even one-half second. The extremely fine dark line which may be seen in such tests probably lessens the illumination of a row of cones, the surrounding ones being uniformly illuminated by the homogeneous background.

Critical Fusion Frequency for Flicker.   A flash of light on the eye generally elicits a burst of impulses over the optic nerve. With successive flashes of light, successive bursts of impulses reach the brain, and successive electrical changes can be recorded from the eye. But as the frequency of flashes increases, the ability to distinguish separate flashes decreases. If a sectored disk is rotated in front of a light source, it is found that as the rate of rotation increases, there is a frequency at which the flashes fuse, and give a sensation of continuous brightness. The critical frequency at which such fusion takes place is dependent upon the intensity of the light (a higher frequency for higher intensities), and upon a number of other factors, including attention, the condition of the retina, and the condition of the brain. A familiar example of fusion is that of motion pictures. The number of frames per second is high enough so that individual frames are not seen.

Color Vision.   As mentioned previously, the eyes are sensitive to wave lengths ranging from 400 to 700 nm, from blue through green to red. Objects appear to have color because they absorb a part of the visible spectrum. The remainder passes through, or is reflected, to the observer's eye. The sensation or perception of color, which is defined psychophysically rather than physiologically, is influenced by a number of factors, including:

HUE OR TONE.   This is a function of the wave length. Thus red and green, each of different wave lengths, are different hues.

BRIGHTNESS, which depends upon the intensity of the light. Thus, a single hue, such as green, can have many degrees of brightness. Brightness may be compared to mixtures of black and white to produce gray, in the sense that as one adds black, brightness is lessened. This is because black absorbs all wave lengths and lessens the amount of reflected light. Brilliance is the subjective sensation due to brightness.

SATURATION OR PURITY, which depends upon the mixture with white light. The more white light and, therefore, the more of other colors, the less saturated or pure is a given hue. Colors exhibiting saturation are commonly referred to as pale or pastel.

It has long been known that there are certain primary colors, such that any color of the spectrum can be matched by mixing two primary colors in correct proportions. The primary colors (when dealing with light) are red, green, and blue (or violet). The matching is not quite precise, however, unless a third color is used. For example, if one wished to match a spectral yellow with a mixture of red and green, a precise match is obtained only if some blue is added to the yellow. Methods of color matching are useful in studying defects in color vision, since color blindness can be classified on the basis of defects in primary colors.

There have been, and are, a number of theories of color vision. The one most widely accepted is the three-color theory (Young-Helmholtz Theory), according to which there are three types of retinal receptors (cones), each sensitive to one of the primary colors. It is now known that the absorption spectra for human cones fall into three separate groups (Fig. 12–11), for blue, green, and yellow-red, which correspond to the primary colors. Each cone contains only one of the three pigments.

Color perception may be affected by a number of factors. For example, if a small object of a specific color is placed in the field of vision so that light from it falls on a specific part of the retina, the color perceived may vary according to the part of the retina stimulated. This difference is due in part to the incidence of the light. Light entering the eye through the center of the pupil is more or less parallel to receptors, but light entering at the edge of the pupil strikes receptors at an angle (because the eyeball is curved). The color perceived is different in the two instances.

The important role of the thalamus and the cerebral cortex in color vision is being actively investigated. Interpretation depends in part upon patterns of firing from color-coded receptive fields, upon later coding (signals may be "destroyed" during transmission), and upon the functional attributes of the cortex. For example, although color vision begins with a three-color, three-receptor system, no receptor has a straight line to the brain. Instead, single cells deal simultaneously with information from two sets of cones. Both at the ganglion cell layer, and at subsequent central stations, nerve cells code different colors by integrating excitatory and inhibitory signals from two populations of cones with overlapping spectral sensitivities.

Defective Color Vision. Defective color vision ("color blindness") is a common defect, being found in some degree in about 8 per cent of men and 0.4 per cent of women. It may be acquired, but is otherwise a strongly sex-linked characteristic. Color blindness may be classified according to primary color defect.

TRICHROMATS (persons with three-color vision) include those with normal vision, those with anomalous (weak) red vision (protanomaly), and those with anomalous green vision (deuteranomaly).*

DICHROMATS (persons with two-color vision) include those who cannot perceive red (protanopia); those who have green blindness (deuteranopia), but who can match spectral colors with red and blue, and to whom the luminosity of colors appears normal; and, finally, and quite rarely, those who are blue (violet) blind (tritanopia). The fovea of man appears to be tritanopic, the blue end of the spectrum being absorbed by media and by the yellow pigment of the macula. Diurnal mammals with pure cone retinae have yellow lenses, thus limiting the amount of blue reaching the retina.

MONOCHROMATS (persons with total color blindness) are quite rare. There appear to be two kinds, with and without photophobia (pain on exposure to strong light). The ones with photophobia seem to react as if they had no cones in their retinae.

---

*The words indicating the type of color defect are of Greek origin. *Protos* means first, hence protanomaly (weakness of) and protanopia (loss of or without) are defects in the first of the three primary colors. *Deuteros* means second, hence deuteranomaly and deuteranopia are defects in the second of the primary colors. *Tritos* means third, and tritanopia is a defect in the third primary color.

The above classification is based on subjective defects in perception, which are undoubtedly due to the presence of an abnormal cone pigment or to the absence of a cone pigment.

BINOCULAR VISION.   When one looks at an object, an image is formed in each eye, and impulses go from each eye to both cerebral hemispheres. But only one object is seen. To obtain this result, the points of the image must fall on corresponding parts of the retinae. Thus the temporal half of the left eye and the nasal half of the right eye are corresponding halves. If there is a disturbance of binocular vision, such as may follow paralyses of extrinsic eye muscles, then double vision or *diplopia* may result. This is because image points do not fall upon corresponding parts of the retinae, and two images are seen. Diplopia can be demonstrated by lightly pressing upon the lateral side of one of the eyes while gazing steadily at an object some distance away. The pressure shifts the eye so that images are formed on noncorresponding portions of the retina, and diplopia results. If diplopia is due to a persistent disorder, one lasting for weeks or months or longer, false images usually become suppressed.

CENTRAL CONNECTIONS OF THE RETINA

The two optic nerves converge at the base of the brain to form the optic chiasma. A partial decussation occurs here in a manner indicated in Figure 12–13. Behind the chiasma, the axons continue into the optic tracts, which curve around the outside of the cerebral peduncles and disappear from the surface.

Some of the axons terminate in or near the region of the superior colliculi. Because of these connections, reflex pupillary reactions or body movements in response to light can occur; the pattern of movement and the orientation of objects are important in the reflex skeletal muscle effects. Most of the optic fibers, however, end in the lateral geniculate body of the thalamus and are relayed by way of the internal capsule to the occipital lobes. Here they end around the calcarine fissure in a cortical area numbered 17, the primary receptive area (Fig. 18–4, p. 407). As in the postcentral gyrus, the entering fibers dispose themselves throughout the fourth cell layer (Fig. 17–2, p. 377). They are so concentrated here that they form a white band or stripe, visible to the naked eye. Because of this, the visual cortex is also called the *striate cortex.*

The cells of the lateral geniculate body are probably organized like the ganglion cells, with center-surround fields. The visual cortex, however, is organized differently. Its cells respond to straight edges of light-dark contrast from objects that, for maximum effect, need a specific kind of orientation (edge-on) to the retinal receptive field. One of the major features is that the brain can distinguish between (1) image motion on the retina brought about by object movement and (2) image motion brought about by

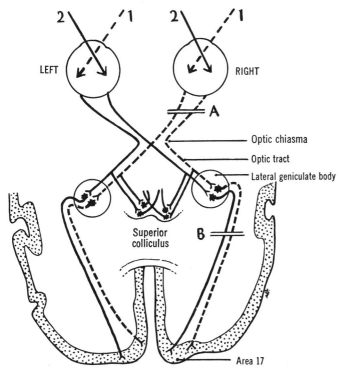

Figure 12–13. The visual pathways. Arrows numbered *1* indicate that light from objects in the right visual fields (when looking straight ahead) reaches the left halves of the retinae. The reverse is true for the opposite visual fields. The collaterals from the visual path (to the superior colliculi for reflexes) are really separate fibers and not branches of true visual fibers. Cutting the optic nerve at *A* causes complete blindness in that eye. A lesion at *B*, however, causes blindness in the left half of each field of vision (arrows numbered *2*).

active eye movements (including saccadic eye movements). Thus, as in other sensory systems, visual information reaching the brain is highly abstract, the result of step-by-step transformation of the input to the retina.

As indicated in Figure 12–13, the fibers from the medial or nasal half of each retina cross, whereas those from the lateral or temporal half do not. This means that objects on the right are visualized by left area 17 and vice versa. This perception is therefore contralateral, as it is in other sensations.

Contralateral vision perception can be demonstrated by a simple experiment. Close the eyes and turn the right eye toward the nose, then press lightly on the temporal side (right side) of the right eyeball. A bright ring or a blue ring with a bright halo is seen in the nasal or left field of the right eye. This shows that stimulation of the right half of the retina produces an effect which appears to come from the opposite or left part of the visual field.

That retinal images are also reversed may be demonstrated in

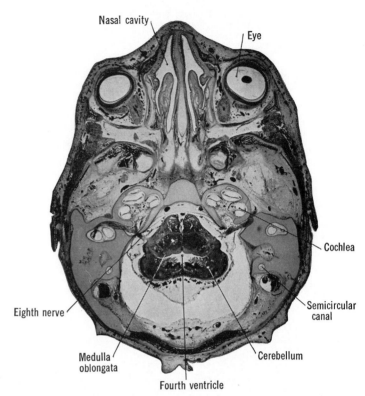

Figure 12-14. Photomicrograph of a horizontal section of the head of a four month human fetus to show the position of the cochlea, which is large in proportion to the head at this age. Note the left eighth nerve dividing into cochlear and vestibular portions, the latter going into the macula utriculi.

a number of ways. The retina is sensitive to any x-rays that may happen to penetrate the eye. Metal letters placed in front of closed eyes and exposed to x-rays are recognized as shadows against a bright background. (The x-rays that reach the retina apparently cause it to fluoresce.) Since x-rays are not refracted or bent during their passage through the eyes, the shadows are not inverted upon the retina. The brain performs its customary reversal during interpretation and the letters appear upside down. If the letters are to appear upright, they must be inverted in front of the eyes. There is not, however, a conscious analysis of retinal inversion. Perception is of objects in visual fields and not of impulses from the retinae. From infancy on, determination of the position of an object by vision is substantiated by impressions produced by that object on other senses, such as touch. Thereafter, impulses from specific retinal areas become visual perceptions for objects in certain portions of the visual field.

The interpretation of these cues from retinal stimulation probably depends to a great extent upon learning. If subjects wear lenses that invert the retinal fields, the images on the retina become upright and the perceived field is inverted. In spite of the resulting confusion, the subjects can, by wearing the lenses for considerable periods of time, adjust themselves fairly well to the situation and perform coordinated movements.

LESIONS OF THE VISUAL SYSTEM

The anatomy of the visual system is such that damage in various portions of the optic pathways causes visual defects with differences which enable one to locate such lesions rather accurately. Destruction of one optic nerve, for instance, will cause complete blindness in that eye. Destruction of the pathway on one side behind the chiasma (Fig. 12–14) will not cause total blindness, but blindness in half of the visual field of each eye, a *hemianopia.* If such a lesion is on the left side, the patient will be unable to see objects on the right side when looking straight ahead.

HEARING

Hearing follows the stimulation of certain specialized epithelial cells by sound waves. These cells are part of a receptor system situated in the *labyrinth,* or inner ear (Fig. 12–15). The labyrinth is a group of small fluid-filled chambers and canals, one of which, the *cochlea,* is concerned with auditory mechanisms. There is an intricate, delicate mechanism by which sound waves enter the external ear and are then funneled into the middle ear, from which three tiny bones transmit the vibrations to the fluid-filled cochlea.

THE EXTERNAL AND MIDDLE EARS

As shown in Figure 12–15, the external ear includes the *auricle,* which is attached to the side of the head, and the *external acoustic meatus* or ear canal. Whether the auricle is of any importance in humans is doubtful. The ear canal transmits the air vibrations to the middle ear. Separating this canal from the middle ear cavity is a thin *tympanic membrane,* or ear drum. To it is attached one of the three ossicles that form a chain across the middle ear cavity. When vibrations of air strike the tympanic membrane, they cause it to move at the same frequency as the impinging waves. These vibrations are transmitted through the ear ossicles in such a manner that the innermost ossicle, the *stapes,* moves inward when the tympanic membrane moves inward. It can be seen from Figures 12–15 and 12–16 that the foot of the stapes impinges upon one of the fluid-filled canals of the cochlea, and its vibrations

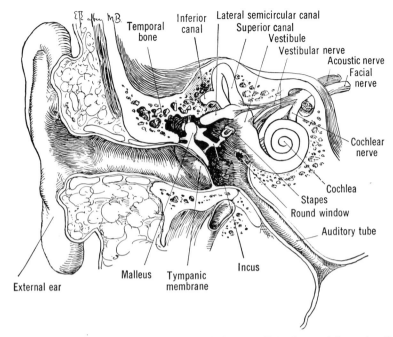

Figure 12-15. Semischematic drawing of the ear. Note the ossicles extending across the middle ear cavity. The greater part of the course of the facial nerve through the ear has been omitted. (Modified from Max Brödel.)

are, therefore, transmitted to the fluid. It can also be seen from these figures that at the other end of the fluid system is an aperture, the *round window,* which is closed off by a thin membrane. Since fluid is incompressible, an increase in pressure at the end where the stapes is located is compensated for by a bulging outward of the membrane in the round window.

Marked changes in external air pressure might seriously affect the tympanic membrane were it not for the fact that the middle ear cavity communicates with the pharynx by means of the *auditory tube* (Fig. 12-15). Pressure on both sides of the membrane may be equalized through this passage way. All are familiar with the "popping" of the ears when ascending or descending considerable distances. This is due to periodic openings of the auditory tube at the point where it reaches the pharynx.

THE INNER EAR AND COCHLEA

The cochlea is a fluid-filled cavity in the temporal bone, being arranged in coils resembling those of a snail shell. Within the cavity is a small fluid-filled duct, the *cochlear duct,* in which are found the specialized epithelial cells of the *spiral organ* (Fig. 12-16). Some of the cells have fine stereocilia at their free ends. Other cells surround and support the hair cells. Fibers of the cochlear division of the eighth nerve end around the bases of the hair cells. The bipolar cell bodies giving origin to these fibers form the *spiral ganglion,* which is located in the bony portion of the cochlea. Their central processes are directed toward the brain stem.

As shown in Figure 12–16, the hair cells rest upon a mem-

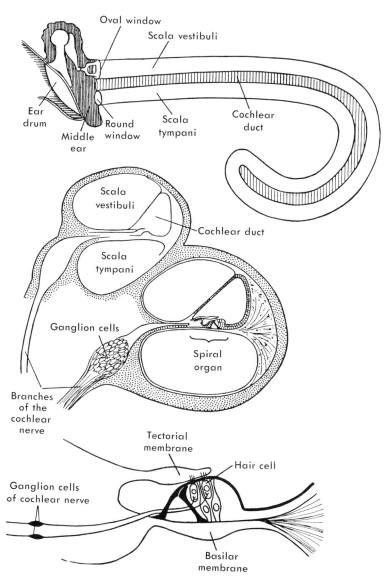

Figure 12–16. Various schema of the inner ear. The top drawing represents the cochlea as if it were uncoiled. Note how the stapes fits into the oval window. The scala vestibuli communicates with the scala tympani which terminates at the round window. Compare with Figure 12–15. The middle drawing represents the cochlea cut at a right angle to or across the first plane, indicating the shape and relationships of the cochlear duct. The peripheral processes of the bipolar ganglion cells extend to the spiral organ. The lower drawing is of the spiral organ. Most of the cells have been omitted, since all are either hair cells or supporting cells.

brane, the *basilar membrane.* This is composed of *auditory strings* that vary in length in different portions of the cochlea. Above the hair cells is a mass of gelatinous material, the *tectorial membrane,* into which some of the stereocilia project. These stereocilia are anchored to a cuticular plate, much as the hair cells of the maculae are (Fig. 12–21, p. 277). There is no kinocilium, but the basal "remnant" of one is present in the cuticular notch.

Cochlear Functions. Broadly speaking, nerve impulses are produced as follows: Vibrations of air strike the tympanic membrane and are transmitted by the ear ossicles to the cochlea, where waves are set up in the fluid and in the basilar membrane. The immediate stimulus of the cochlear hair cells is produced by a relative motion between the cells and their stereocilia. An adequate stimulus is undoubtedly the bending of the stereocilia and thus the deformation of the apical pole of the hair cell. The bending of the stereocilia· can be brought about by at least two mechanisms. In one, the tallest of the hair cells (outer hair cells), whose stereocilia project into the overlying, less freely movable tectorial membrane, are displaced relative to the tectorial membrane. This displacement is directly proportional to a displacement of the basilar membrane. Thus, the outer hair cells are displacement detectors. The short hair cells (inner hair cells) are free standing; their stereocilia do not enter the tectorial membrane. Bending of these stereocilia probably results from viscous forces exerted by the fluid around them. These forces depend upon velocity of fluid flow, which in turn depends upon the rate of displacement of the basilar membrane. Hence, the inner hair cells are velocity detectors. Thus, sound waves bring about fluid waves, and these in turn cause a displacement of the basilar membrane which, directly and indirectly, brings about a mechanical distortion of the hair cells.

Just how the sound waves are ultimately transduced into nerve impulses is uncertain. It may be that the hair cells are like piezoelectric crystals, which upon being deformed, develop an electrical change. Whatever the mechanism, the hair cells are mechanoreceptors, and the deformation stimulates the adjacent nerve endings. The deformation is accompanied by a rapidly developing potential change which can be recorded. This is the *microphonic potential.* The system is extraordinarily sensitive, more than could be expected of a passive system. It behaves much as if the cells were amplifiers.

There is also a resting potential in the cochlea, the spiral organ being negative to the fluid in scala tympani and scala vestibuli. It is not known whether this potential, or the microphonic potential, or both, are directly involved in depolarizing cochlear nerve fibers.

There are efferent nerve endings on the hair cells. These endings have synaptic vesicles, and the functions of the fibers and endings may be to reduce the output of the receptors.

It was mentioned previously that the basilar membrane is composed of auditory strings of varying lengths. There are several theories about the mechanisms by which the basilar membrane and hair cells can discriminate frequencies. According to the *place theory* a pure tone will throw a stretch of the basilar membrane into vibration, with a maximum amplitude of vibration at some point.

One version of this, the Helmholtz resonance theory, is that the auditory strings are of such lengths that for any audible frequency, there is a string or group of strings that will be thrown into vibration, that is, will resonate. Another theory holds that a pure tone produces a standing wave in the basilar membrane, the position of the wave changing according to the frequency of the tone. There is, however, considerable evidence that sound waves produce traveling waves along the membrane. These waves have a flat maximum that shifts in location along the membrane as frequency changes. The theories are not radically different. Whatever the type of vibration, there is a maximum at some point, and nerve fibers from this point will discharge at a higher rate than other nerve fibers from the area of the wave vibration. The basilar membrane in the apical part of the cochlea is wider than elsewhere, and this region responds mainly to low tones.

Central Auditory Connections. When the central fibers of the cochlear division of the eighth nerve reach the brain stem, they end in masses of gray matter, the *cochlear nuclei*. These nuclei are complex structures that provide for reflexes by connections to various cranial nerve nuclei, that are involved in coding functions, and that project to higher centers. The transmission axons form a myelinated tract on each side, the *lateral lemniscus* (Fig. 12–17). There are several synaptic interruptions along this ascending pathway, but eventually the fibers reach the medial geniculate body of the thalamus and are then relayed to the temporal lobe, specifically to the portion of the superior temporal gyrus that forms Area 41 (see Fig. 18–3, p. 407). This and adjacent cortex form the primary receptive area for hearing.

As the lateral lemniscus ascends in the brain stem, one of the major synaptic interruptions mentioned above is in the inferior colliculus. It relays to the medial geniculate body, but it also serves as a major reflex center and in addition sends projections to the cerebellum.

PROPERTIES AND QUALITY OF SOUND

These are pitch, intensity, and timbre, which are mostly psychological factors that cannot be completely correlated with physiological processes.

Pitch. Pitch refers to the level in the musical scale in which a sound may be placed. It is closely related to the frequency or

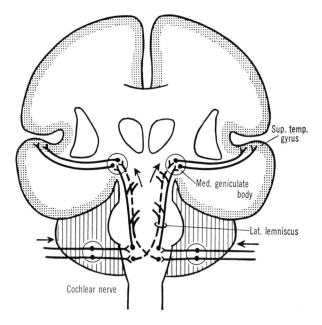

Figure 12–17. Simplified version of the auditory pathways. The cochlear nerves carry impulses from the receptors, the primary neurons being bipolar cells. The brain stem path (lateral lemniscus) is probably a multineuron path, but the relays have been omitted. The branches indicated are those that form reflex connections.

periodicity of the sound wave, but the exact nature of that relationship is still a mystery.

Loudness.   In ordinary usage loudness is synonymous with intensity, but this is not strictly accurate. Intensity is a physical value which refers to the energy of power of the sound waves and is proportional to the amplitude of these waves. Loudness is a subjective sensation. That the two are not the same is shown by the fact that while tones of high pitch are inaudible to man, no matter what their intensity, they may be audible to other animals, such as the dog.

There is in common usage a unit for expressing differences in intensity of two sounds which is based on a logarithmic scale. If one sound has a power ten times greater than another, it is said to be 1 bel greater (log of 10=1). But the bel is too large a unit, and one-tenth of this or 1 decibel (db) is used. Within the auditory range 1 decibel is a change just detectible subjectively. Bels and decibels used without a reference level are meaningless. To say that a sound wave is 1 decibel more than another means nothing, since both may still be inaudible. Accordingly, a standard reference may be used. This is 0.0002 dyne/cm.^{2}, and the threshold of hearing at 1000 cycles is of this order of power. From this point the audible range extends 120 decibels, that is, 12 bels or 10^{12} times. The upper limit represents the loudest sound tolerable to the human ear.

Timbre or Quality.   This is related to wave form and harmonies, and is the property by which two sounds of the same pitch and intensity can be distinguished. As in the case of pitch, the exact relationship is unknown. The tonal quality of a musical instrument cannot be defined in terms of physiological processes.

Audiograms. Normal hearing can be tested in a variety of ways. One method is by means of an audiogram. The range of vibrations or frequencies audible to the human ear is from approximately 20 to 20,000 per second, with considerable individual variation. Furthermore there is a striking difference in sensitivity at different frequencies. When the relation between sensitivity and frequency is plotted, the resulting curve (audiogram) is that shown in Figure 12–18. There are various ways of testing sensitivity against wavelength; all of them show that the human ear is most sensitive at frequencies between 2000 and 4000 cycles per second. At about 2000 cycles, the cochlea is comparable in sensitivity to the retina. By this is meant that under optimum conditions one can detect sounds of such low intensities that the amplitude of vibration at threshold is no more than the longer wave lengths in the visible spectrum.

Audiograms have proven to be extremely useful in clinical testing for hearing losses.

LESIONS OF THE AUDITORY SYSTEM

If a cochlear duct or nerve on one side is destroyed, complete deafness on that side results. But a unilateral lesion within the central nervous system which affects one of the auditory paths does not cause complete deafness, since each lateral lemniscus carries fibers derived from both cochleae, as shown in Figure 12–17. A unilateral lesion, therefore, does not interrupt all impulses derived from the cochlea of the same side.

Diseases of the middle ear may cause middle ear or transmission deafness. Sounds are heard incompletely, if at all, because pathological changes of the ossicles or tympanic membrane interfere with their transmission. If the vibrations are strong enough to set bone in motion, or are started in bone, then they may reach the

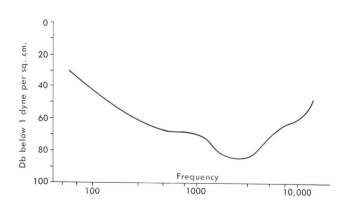

Figure 12–18. Threshold sensitivity of human ear obtained by stimulating the ears at different wave lengths. The ear is most sensitive to frequencies between 2000 and 4000 cycles per second.

cochlea, and perception is ultimately possible. This can be demonstrated by placing the base of a vibrating tuning fork on the skull.
The vibrations are audible, but disappear when the fork is held in
the air beside the ear. Patients with middle ear deafness have
difficulty in ordinary conversation, but may hear well over the
telephone because the sounds are conducted through the bones of
the skull. Hearing aids are, therefore, useful in such cases, but not
when deafness is due to destruction of a cochlea or cochlear
nerve (nerve deafness).

BALANCE OR EQUILIBRIUM

What is ordinarily called the sense of balance or of equilibrium
is functionally integrated with the kinesthetic sense. An important
component of the sense of balance arises from the stimulation of
certain receptors in the labyrinth (these receptors and their
connections are also of major importance in the reflex control
of locomotion and posture). One of the labyrinthine canals, the
cochlea, was discussed in the preceding section of this chapter.
The rest of the labyrinth consists of a small chamber, the *vestibule,*
which communicates with three small *semicircular ducts,* each of
which is in the form of a half-circle (Fig. 12–19) and is contained
within a semicircular canal in the bone. There are two small membranous sacs in the vestibule, the *utricle* and *saccule.* In each of
these is a specialized epithelial layer or *macula,* around the cells
of which fibers of the vestibular portion of the eighth nerve terminate. Also, at one end of each semicircular canal there is a specialized epithelial layer, a *crista,* around whose cells other fibers of
the vestibular nerve terminate. All the nerve fibers are peripheral
processes of bipolar cells in the nearby *vestibular ganglion.* The
central processes enter the brain stem near the junction of the
pons and medulla oblongata.

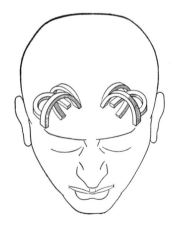

Figure 12–19. A drawing indicating the semi-circular ducts in
relation to each other and to the rest of the head. Compare with
Figure 12–15 in which they are shown with the rest of the ear.
Note that the two lateral ducts are in the same plane, and
therefore form a functional unit with the posterior or inferior
duct of the opposite side. The ducts are much smaller than indicated here.

THE SEMICIRCULAR DUCTS

The semicircular ducts are small membranous tubes filled with a slightly viscous fluid. The structure of each crista is similar to that of the spiral organ. That is, there are hair cells (mechanoreceptors) held together or supported by sustentacular cells, and the stereocilia of the hair cells are embedded in an overlying structure consisting of fibrils embedded in a gelatinous ground substance (see Figs. 12–20, 12–21). Vestibular nerve fibers terminate at the bases of the hair cells. Pressure changes in the fluid of the ducts constitute effective stimuli. The mechanisms are probably membrane deformations, similar to those that occur in the cochlea.

Each of the three ducts on either side of the head occupies a different plane in space (Fig. 12–19), so that when the head is moved or rotated in any direction, the cells in one or more cristae are stimulated because of pressure changes that come about in the following manner: When the head is turned, say to the right (clockwise), the fluid in the horizontal ducts tends to remain stationary because of its inertia. The actual result is that a hydrostatic pressure develops. In clockwise rotation the pressure is exerted against the anterior end of the right horizontal duct, the end which contains the crista.

Similar phenomena are seen when a glass of water is rotated. At first the water remains stationary. Then, as inertia is overcome, the water rotates with the glass. Translated into familiar, everyday experience, similar phenomena are experienced when a car accelerates rapidly. Anyone in the seat tends to remain where he was, so to speak, and the result is the development of pressure against the car seat. But within a short time, particularly if the car reaches a uniform rate of speed, the sensation of pressure stops because inertia has been overcome and the car and person are in effect traveling at the same rate. If, now, the car slows or stops suddenly, anyone in the car tends to keep on going in the same direction, just as one tends to keep going in the same direction when the car goes around a curve. Likewise, when the rotation of the glass of water is suddenly stopped, the water keeps on rotating for a time.

In the case of the ducts, continued clockwise rotation can be carried out if the whole body is rotated. This is most easily done by sitting in a special chair which can be turned (children commonly do this by sitting in a swing which is wound up and then allowed to unwind). When rotation reaches a uniform rate, there is no pressure in the ducts. When rotation stops, the fluid tends to keep on going in the direction of rotation; as a result pressure develops against the crista in the anterior end of the left horizontal duct.

The result of stimulating the cristae, aside from the perception of movement, is commonly some kind of reflex response, usually a characteristic movement of the eyes termed *nystagmus*. Nystagmus may also occur as a result of disease of the vestibular system.

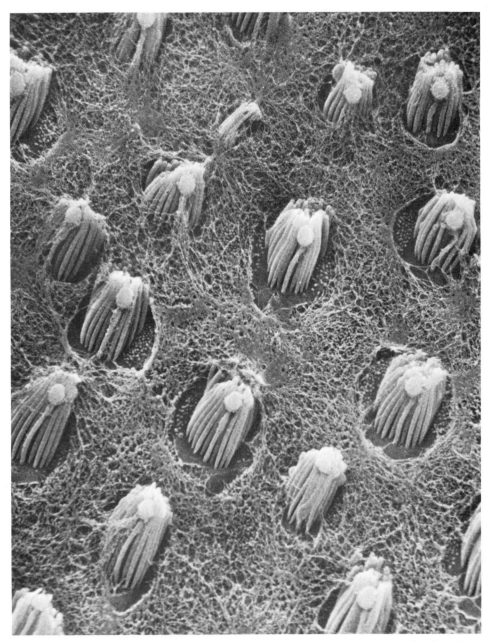

Figure 12-20. Scanning electron micrograph of frog macula sacculi showing directional orientation of ciliary tufts and a matlike base from the otolithic membrane. The unidirectional oriented kinocilium terminates in a large bulb that distinguishes it from the numerous stereocilia (see Figure 12-21). Magnification about 5000x. (From Hillman, D. E., and Lewis, E. R., in Science, *174*:416–419, 1971. By courtesy of the authors and publisher.)

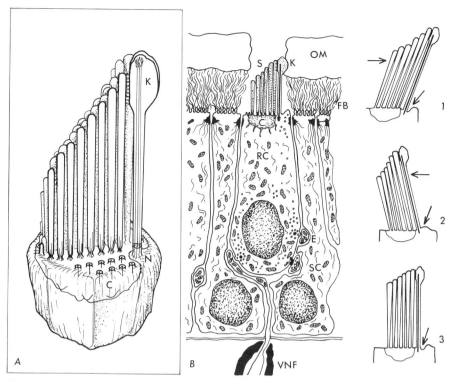

Figure 12–21. A: Diagram to show the vestibular ciliary apparatus at the apical end of a receptor cell in the frog. The stereocilia stand on a cuticular plate (C). The kinocilium (K) is positioned over a notch (N) in the cuticle, where its base is in contact with the cytoplasm. Due to a filamentous attachment of the kinociliary bulb to adjacent stereocilia, the pliable region in the area of the cuticular notch can yield to axial motion of the kinocilium. Two rows of stereocilia are cut at their bases. B: Diagram of a section of saccular epithelium with its receptor cell (RC), ciliary apparatus with kinocilium (K), stereocilia (S), cuticle (C), and otolithic membrane (OM), together with the filamentous base (FB) that supports the otoliths, and the supporting cells (SC). E: efferent ending. VNF: Afferent ending of vestibular nerve fiber, 1, 2, and 3: Diagrams showing the effect of bending the cilia toward and away from the kinocilium. The relatively firm cuticular base and the attachment of the kinocilium to adjacent stereocilia causes the pliable receptor cell membrane in the region of the cuticular notch to be thrust up and down. Axial pull (resulting from an upside-down-position, but not shown here) is also an effective stimulus. (From Hillman, D. E., in Progr. Brain Res., 37:69–75, 1972, and Hillman, D. E., and Lewis, E. R., in Science, 174:416–419, 1971. By courtesy of the authors and publisher.)

In such instances, it may be necessary to test a duct separately, using nystagmus (or its absence) as an end point. This can be done by irrigating the external ear canals with hot or cold water. The temperature changes are sufficient to reach the internal ear and set up convection currents in the fluid in the semicircular duct. These currents create pressures that stimulate, just as if the subject were being rotated. With hot water the currents tend to rise, and with cold water, to fall. Consequently it is necessary to have the subjects so tilt their head that the duct under study is vertical in order to create pressure changes at whatever end of the canal the examiner wishes.

THE UTRICLE AND SACCULE

The maculae of the utricle and saccule resemble the cristae in structure. Each consists of sustentacular cells and hair cells. The stereocilia and associated kinocilium of each hair cell project into an overlying mass *(otolithic membrane)* consisting of fibrils embedded in a gelatinous ground substance and containing small masses of calcium carbonate called *otoliths.* The general arrangement of the ciliary tufts and the mechanical deformation that activates the hair cells are shown in Figures 12–20 and 12–21. Vestibular nerve fibers end around the bases of the hair cells, and the mechanism of stimulation is probably basically similar to that in the cochlea.

The functions of the saccules in man are not known with any certainty. The maculae of the utricles are sensitive to any position that the head occupies in space, whether it is moving or not. The otoliths, because of gravity, probably maintain or increase the mechanical deformation of the hair cells.

CENTRAL VESTIBULAR CONNECTIONS

Impulses over nerve fibers from the maculae and cristae travel centrally to the brain stem and cerebellum. In the brain stem they end in masses of gray matter, the vestibular nuclei, which are specialized portions of the reticular formation. These relay impulses to the spinal cord by way of the vestibulospinal tracts and the medial longitudinal fasciculi (Fig. 12–22). They also relay impulses to various nuclei of cranial nerves, particularly those supplying extrinsic eye muscles, by way of the medial longitudinal fasciculi and also diffuse projections through reticular formation. Connections are also made with visceral centers of the brain stem. Impulses are known to reach the cerebral cortex, but the central pathways are not known with any certainty. There is some evidence that they are topographically the same as the auditory paths and that the primary receptive area is probably the superior temporal gyrus, near or in the auditory area.

FUNCTIONS OF THE VESTIBULAR SYSTEM

This system is important in the control of muscular activity (as a part of the extrapyramidal motor system), for reasons mentioned in Chapter 10 and discussed in more detail in Chapter 14. In spite of the importance of this system in balance or equilibrium

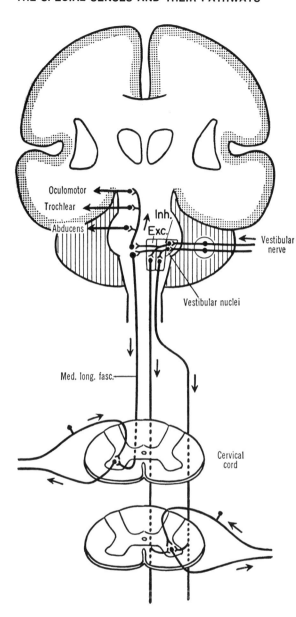

Oculomotor

Trochlear

Abducens

Inh.

Exc.

Vestibular nerve

Vestibular nuclei

Med. long. fasc.

Cervical cord

Figure 12-22. Simplified version of vestibular pathways. The primary neurons are bipolar cells. Direct connections with the cerebellum have been omitted. The vestibular nuclei are represented as projecting to excitatory and inhibitory mechanisms of the brain stem and to various motor nuclei by way of the medial longitudinal fasciculus (both fasciculi are used). The vestibulospinal tract (from the lateral vestibular nucleus) was omitted because it follows much the same course as does the tract from the excitatory center. The ascending path to the cerebral cortex has also been omitted. It is probably similar to that for auditory fibers.

and position sense, reflex functions often overshadow sensory functions. The cristae in semicircular ducts are stimulated mainly by changes in rate of movement, during acceleration or deceleration, and especially in rotational movement. The ducts thus function in kinetic or phasic activity. The maculae utriculi are stimulated mainly when the head is being held in one position, during movement uniform in rate, and during linear acceleration or deceleration. Macular functions are, therefore, mainly static in nature. These distinctions are extremely general. There is actually considerable overlap in functions.

LESIONS OF THE VESTIBULAR SYSTEM

Rapid or prolonged rotations or other types of movement may produce severe side effects, such as vertigo, nausea, and vomiting. These symptoms are the familiar ones of seasickness. Some persoms are so sensitive that these symptoms may follow relatively mild rotations.

Although a number of disorders affect the vestibular system, the symptoms may be difficult to interpret. For example, an inflammatory process in the vestibular system of one side may produce symptoms such as nystagmus, dizziness, or nausea because it irritates or stimulates on that side. But a lesion that destroys the opposite side, by leaving an unopposed or unbalanced normal side, may produce apparently identical symptoms. Consequently, it is necessary to have confirmatory signs referable to other nerves. For example, a destructive lesion of the right vestibular nerve will almost surely destroy the right cochlear nerve. The patient will have, therefore, complete nerve deafness on that side, a symptom that in itself so localizes the lesion that there may be little point in analyzing the vestibular symptoms in detail.

TASTE

The peripheral receptors for this special sense are located in the mucous membrane of the tongue, palate, pharynx, and larynx. Taste, as ordinarily perceived, is a complex sensation, which can be equated with flavor and often includes smell, texture, temperature, and even pain, as well as "true taste." The interference with taste during a cold is the result of a temporary loss of smell. The receptors for taste are found in *taste buds.* These are small cellular areas located in the mucous membrane. They contain specialized cells that are surrounded by nerve endings (Fig. 12–23). These cells

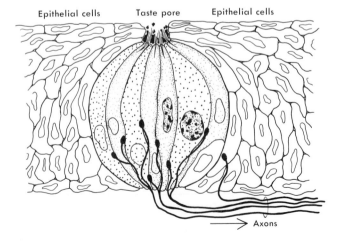

Figure 12–23. Schematic representation of a taste bud showing the two main types of cells. The gustatory cells have hair-like processes at their apex which project into a dense, homogeneous substance in the taste pore. The other main cells are supporting cells; they are somewhat broader and lack processes. Nerve fibers (peripheral processes of unipolar neurons) end in relation to both types of cells. (Based on Murray, R. G., and Murray, A., in Wolstenholme, G. E. W., and Knight, J., editors: Taste and Smell in Vertebrates. London, J. & A. Churchill, 1970.)

Epithelial cells   Taste pore   Epithelial cells

Axons

originate from ordinary epithelium. The buds themselves are constantly renewed and re-innervated. Food substances dissolved in saliva are able in some way to stimulate these cells, and this stimulation in turn initiates impulses in the nerve fibers. Single receptors may be sensitive to one or more of a number of substances characterized as sweet, salt, bitter, and sour, and perhaps others as well. The characterizations are made on the basis of sensations. They can scarcely be separated from behavioral responses, such as the acceptance or rejection of foodstuffs or other substances such as quinine or sugar.

Nerve impulses are transmitted centrally over the facial nerves from the anterior two-thirds of the tongue, by way of the glossopharyngeal nerves from the posterior third of the tongue and part of the pharynx, and over the vagus nerves from the pharynx and larynx. The primary neurons are unipolar cells located in ganglia along the course of these nerves. The central processes of these cells enter the medulla oblongata. Some secondary fibers establish reflex connections, and others ascend to the opposite thalami (commonly stated to be by way of the medial lemnisci, but this is by no means certain), and thence to the postcentral gyri, the primary receptive areas.

SMELL

The olfactory receptors are located in the upper part of the nasal mucous membrane on each side of the nasal cavity. This membrane, which is pigmented in many vertebrates, consists of bipolar nerve cells surrounded and supported by non-nervous cells (Fig. 12–24). The surface of the membrane is covered with a watery fluid. Small particles of gases go into solution in this fluid and are then able to stimulate the bipolar cells by a means as yet uncertain (molecules of different odorants migrate at different rates across the mucous membrane; this is a kind of chromatography that may play an important role). Whatever the means, it is an exceedingly sensitive mechanism by which incredibly small amounts of gaseous substances can be detected. The fact that wood has an odor, for instance, means that oils in the wood are given off in the air and reach the olfactory membrane. The olfactory sense is much more sensitive than that of taste and distinguishes a greater variety of modalities.

The bipolar cells are chemoreceptors with short processes, the olfactory rods. The rods extend to the free surface of the mucous membrane where they end as a brush of filaments. The central processes of the bipolar cells form the filaments of the olfactory nerves (other nerve fibers are also present in the olfactory mucous membrane; presumably some of them exert an efferent control). The olfactory nerve fibers ascend through tiny openings in the base of the skull (Fig. 12–25) and end in masses

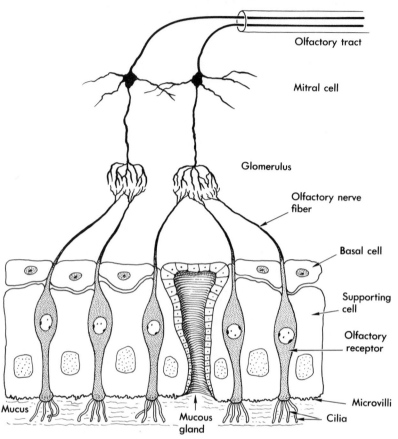

Figure 12-24. Schematic representation of olfactory epithelium and the central projections of the olfactory receptors to the olfactory bulb, where the connections are highly simplified. The orientation is like that of Figure 12–26, with the epithelium downward and the olfactory nerve fibers ascending. (Modified from Moulton, D. G., and Beidler, L. M., in Physiol. Rev., 47:1-52, 1967, and from Schneider, R. A., in New Eng. J. Med., 277:299-303, 1967.)

of gray matter, the olfactory bulbs. Axons from cells in the bulbs travel posteriorly as the olfactory tracts to the primary olfactory cortex in the anterior portion of the piriform area (Fig. 12–26). (In contrast to all other sensory pathways, no thalamic relay intervenes between receptor and primary receptive area.) The subsequent pathways are complex and widespread. Olfaction is an important and sensitive quality in which discrimination is heavily dependent upon synaptic activity in the bulb and piriform cortex. The reflexes that olfaction may initiate are often rapid and forceful, as, for example, violent nausea from a putrid odor. Yet because of many factors in civilized life, such as smoking, contamination of city air, and the like, interferences with and even losses of smell are so common that unless such a loss is restricted to one side of the nose, it cannot be regarded as a definitely important clinical sign.

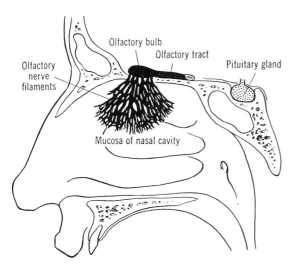

Figure 12–25. Drawing of olfactory structures in the nasal cavity (a sagittal section, exposing the interior of the nose). Numbers of axons interlace as they ascend through the floor of the skull. The olfactory tract is cut anterior to its termination (see Figure 12–26).

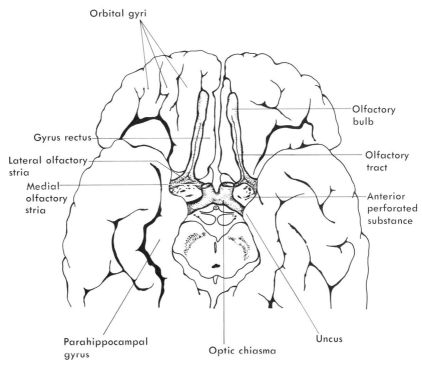

Figure 12–26. The base of the brain (from Figure 7–7, p. 132), anterior portion, to show the division of the olfactory tract into medial and lateral olfactory striae. The lateral stria ends chiefly in the piriform cortex, the medial in the septal area.

SUMMARY

The special senses include vision, hearing, balance, taste, and smell. All of these terms refer to psychological phenomena that can only in part be related to physiological processes.

Vision begins with the excitation of photoreceptor cells by photochemical processes resulting when visual pigments absorb light. The photoreceptor cells are the rods, which serve visual sensitivity, and the cones, which serve visual acuity and color vision. Rhodopsin is the visual pigment in rods. The absorption spectra for three cone pigments corresponds approximately to the three primary colors (blue, green, and yellow-red). The rods and cones are connected to bipolar cells, and these in turn to ganglion cells, while interneurons (horizontal and amacrine cells) establish extensive lateral connections. The retina is organized so that ganglion cells have receptive fields characterized by antagonistic center-periphery zones. The axons of ganglion cells form the optic nerves, which intermingle at the chiasma in such a way that impulses resulting from light entering the eye from one side of the body finally reach the opposite primary area (Area 17), located on either side of the calcarine fissure of the occipital lobe.

Hearing begins with the transduction of sound waves into nerve impulses. This occurs as the sound waves impinge upon the fluid-filled spaces of the inner ear, and produce fluid waves and displacement of the basilar membrane so that the stereocilia of the hair cells of the spiral organ are deformed. The deformation activates cochlear nerve fibers, and nerve impulses are then transmitted bilaterally over a complex central pathway to the primary receptive areas in the superior temporal gyrus (Area 41 and adjacent cortex). The human ear is sensitive to vibrations of about 20 to 20,000 cycles per second, and maximally sensitive at between 2000 and 4000 cycles. The important qualities of sound are pitch, loudness, and timbre or quality; these are mostly perceptual phenomena.

The cristae of the semicircular canals and the maculae utriculi and sacculi are important components of kinesthetic mechanisms and of the reflex control of movement and posture. In all of these structures, the mechanoreceptors are hair cells with stereocilia and kinocilia. Deformation of these cells activates vestibular nerve fibers. The semicircular canals are important in angular acceleration and deceleration. The utricle and saccule are stimulated during maintained position and during linear acceleration and deceleration. The nerve impulses that travel centrally over vestibular nerve fibers establish major reflex connections, and also reach the primary receptive areas, which are probably in the superior temporal gyri.

Solutions of food substances stimulate receptors in taste buds of the tongue, palate, pharynx, and larynx. The nerve impulses are transmitted centrally over the facial, glossopharyngeal, and vagus nerves to the brain stem. From here they eventually reach the primary receptive areas, the postcentral gyri.

Smell depends upon the stimulation of bipolar cells in the olfactory mucous membrane by substances dissolved in the overlying watery fluid. The central processes of these bipolar cells form the olfactory nerves, which end in the olfactory bulbs. From here the impulses travel by the olfactory tracts to the primary receptive area, the piriform cortex.

NAMES IN NEUROLOGY

HERMANN LUDWIG FERDINAND HELMHOLTZ (1821–1894)

Helmholtz was a German physician, physiologist, and physicist and one of the giants in scientific attainment. He was a man of widespread interests who, at various times, occupied chairs of physiology, anatomy, pathology, and physics. He applied the law of conservation of energy to all living material. He showed that muscles were the main source of animal heat. During the years 1850–1852, he measured the velocity of the nerve impulse. In 1851 he invented the ophthalmoscope and, with the aid of other instruments of his own devising, measured ocular constants and explained the mechanism of accommodation. During the years 1856–1867, he wrote his *Handbook of Physiological Optics,* which is a scientific classic. In spite of all this work, he found time to publish on acoustic mechanisms, including the functions of the tympanic membrane and the ear ossicles. From him we have our most widely accepted theory of cochlear functions. From 1887 on he made outstanding contributions in the fields of dynamics, hydrodynamics, thermodynamics, and electrodynamics.

JAN EVANGELISTA PURKYNĚ (Johannes Purkinje) (1787–1869)

The Czech biologist Purkyně was an outstanding investigator who made major contributions to our knowledge of nerve cells, the heart and its nerve supply, and embryology. Born in Bohemia, he studied philosophy and medicine in Prague from 1813 to 1818. Five years later he was appointed to the chair of physiology and pathology at the University of Breslau (now Wroclaw). After 27 years, he returned to Prague as professor of physiology and remained there for the rest of his life. He was the first to use a microtome in the preparation of microscopic slides and also developed many other aids for microtechnique. He studied nerve cells, glands, the heart, and other organs. The characteristic large neurons of the cerebellum and the conducting fibers of the heart bear his name, as does the shift from the scotopic to the photopic curve. He did not confine his interests to anatomy, but studied fingerprints, noted that deaf mutes could in some instances hear through the bones of the skull, and investigated the effects of opium, belladonna, and other drugs. Moreover, he played a major role in the formation of the cell theory; in 1837, two years before the formulation of the cell theory by Schleiden and Schwann, he pointed out the similarity of animal and vegetable cells.

THOMAS YOUNG (1733–1829)

Young, a Quaker physician in England was widely acknowledged as one of the most intellectually brilliant men of the eighteenth century. After qualifying in medicine—following social and academic tours of London, Edinburgh, Göttingen, Dresden, and Cambridge—he set up practice in London. Popular as a practicing physician, he nevertheless devoted himself to mastering his many interests. He made important original contributions in three major fields: physiological optics, the theory of light, and the deciphering of the Egyptian hieroglyphics. He studied accommodation, gave the first description of astigmatism, and stated that color vision was possible because of retinal structures sensitive to red, green, and violet. He also studied blood flow and stated the laws governing it. He introduced concepts of energy and work done and defined the nodulus of elasticity, "Young's modulus." Because of his many interests, his ideas were not always fully developed, and many others enjoyed the credit of his discoveries. (Herivel, H.: Thomas Young [1773–1829], Endeavour, 32:15–18, 1973.)

REFERENCES

These first two references are modern classics, Polyak on the structure and neurological connections of the human retina, and Walls on the comparative anatomy and functions of the eye.

Polyak, S. L.: The Retina. Chicago, University of Chicago Press, 1941.
Walls, G. L.: The Vertebrate Eye. Bloomfield Hills, Mich., Cranbrook Institute of Science, 1942.

The following are valuable source books:

von Békésy, G.: Experiments on Hearing (transl. and edited by Wever, E. G.). New York, McGraw-Hill Book Company, Inc., 1960.
Dallos, P.: The Auditory Periphery. New York, Academic Press, 1973.
Dartnall, H. J. A. (editor): Photochemistry of Vision. In Handbook of Sensory Physiology, vol. VII/1. Berlin, Springer-Verlag, 1972.
Fuortes, M. G. F. (editor): Physiology of Photoreceptor Organs. In Handbook of Sensory Physiology, vol. VII/2. Berlin, Springer-Verlag, 1972.
Rodieck, R. W.: The Vertebrate Retina. San Francisco, W. H. Freeman and Company, 1973.
Straatsma, B. R., et al., (editors): The Retina, Berkeley, University of California Press, 1969.

The following are papers and reviews on specific subjects.

Boycott, B. B., and Dowling, J. E.: Organization of the primate retina: light microscopy. Royal Soc. Lond., Philos. Trans., B., 255:109–184, 1969.
Davis, H.: Biophysics and physiology of the inner ear. Physiol. Rev., 37:1–49, 1957.
Daw, N. W.: Neurophysiology of color vision. Physiol. Rev., 53:571-611, 1973.
Dowling, J. E., and Boycott, B. B.: Organization of the primate retina: electron microscopy. Proc. Royal Soc., B., 166:80-111, 1966.
Klinke, R., and Galley, N.: Efferent innervation of vestibular and auditory receptors. Physiol. Rev., 54:316-357, 1974.
Moulton, D. G., and Beidler, L. M.: Structure and function in the peripheral olfactory system. Physiol. Rev., 47:1-52, 1967.
Pfaffman, C.: Taste, its sensory and motivating properties. Amer. Sci., 52:187-206, 1964.
Rushton, W. A. H.: Pigments and signals in colour vision. J. Physiol., 220:1-31P, 1972.
Shepherd, G. M.: Synaptic organization of the mammalian olfactory bulb. Physiol. Rev., 52:864-917, 1972.
Wightman, F. L., and Green, D. M.: The perception of pitch. Amer. Scientist, 62:208-215, 1974.

Chapter 13

THE ORGANIZATION
OF THE SPINAL CORD
AND ITS NERVES

The presentation of central nervous system structure and function has been made, up to now, from what might be termed a longitudinal point of view, considering motor and sensory functions in toto. This and the following chapters consider local and regional functions, with emphasis on segmental and suprasegmental mechanisms.

THE SPINAL CORD

The spinal cord is similar in structure and function in all vertebrates. It is segmental in arrangement, and it carries out sensory, integrative, and motor functions. These may be categorized as reflex activity, reciprocal activity, monitoring and modulation, and transmission.

White Matter. The white matter differs but little in its fundamental arrangement throughout the spinal cord (Fig. 13–1). It is contained within three funiculi on each side, as indicated in Figure 13–2. These funiculi vary in shape and size at different levels, because of variations in the shape of the gray matter and because of additions of ascending and terminations of descending fibers. The funiculi are morphological divisions that contain tracts, which are the functional units of the white matter (Fig. 13–2). However, tracts cannot be distinguished from each other in normal material. The lateral corticospinal tracts, for example, can be morphologically demonstrated only by their absence, as shown in Fig. 10–11 (p. 213). The fibers of the lateral spinothalamic tract are

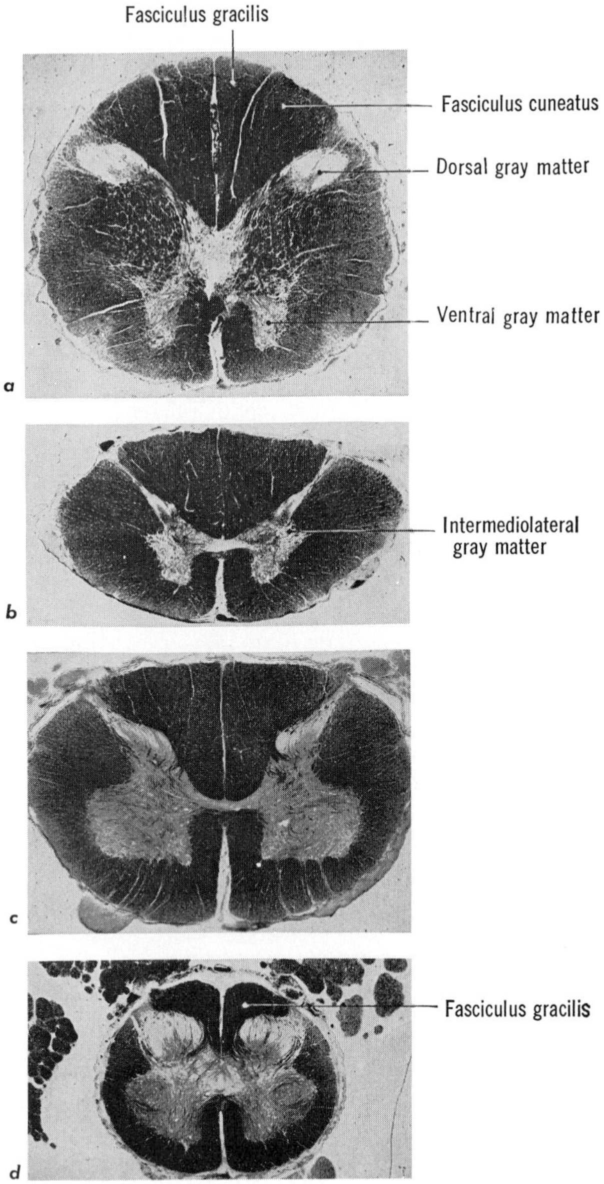

Fasciculus gracilis

Fasciculus cuneatus

Dorsal gray matter

Ventral gray matter

a

Figure 13-1. Photomicrographs of cross sections of a human spinal cord. a, Upper cervical; b, thoracic; c, lumbar; d, sacral. The dorsal gray matter labeled in a is the substantia gelatinosa. Note that the gray matter varies in shape and volume. The structures around the spinal cord in d are spinal roots of the cauda equina. Tracts cannot be distinguished in the normal material. Compare with Figures 10–11 and 11–11, pp. 213 and 241.

Intermediolateral gray matter

b

c

Fasciculus gracilis

d

intermingled with spinocerebellar fibers (Fig. 13–2). Thus the lateral and anterior funiculi contain ascending and descending tracts that are anatomically congruent.

A large part of the white matter is composed of spinospinal or propriospinal fibers, that is, fibers that begin and end within the spinal cord, thereby linking various levels and providing for coordinated activity. These spinospinal fibers range from short ones that interconnect levels within a given region (such as from one cervical segment to another), to long ones that pass from one region to another (for example, from cervical to lumbar).

The anterior and lateral funiculi contain most of the ascending and descending tracts (in some species, corticospinal fibers descend in the posterior funiculi). The posterior funiculi are of special interest because they are traditionally assigned to sensory-discriminative functions. Yet, as discussed previously, this concept is being called into question.

Excluding those fibers that ascend only part way in the posterior funiculi (e.g., those from neuromuscular spindles), the posterior funiculus is composed chiefly of fibers from rapidly adapting mechanoreceptors (in the cervical region it also carries some second-order fibers whose functional significance is not yet known). Complete posterior funiculus section at any level, even in humans, causes surprisingly little sensory deficit; patients can still carry out discriminations of weight, texture, two points, and position. The characteristic defects in motor behavior were pointed out previously (p. 232). It should be noted that many of the disorders that affect the posterior funiculi rarely limit themselves to these funiculi and, moreover, commonly involve the adjacent spinocervicothalamic tract. Finally, it should be pointed out that the posterior funiculi are organized somatotopically, e.g., according to precise peripheral fields with no overlap, in contrast to the dermatomal organization of the spinal nerves.

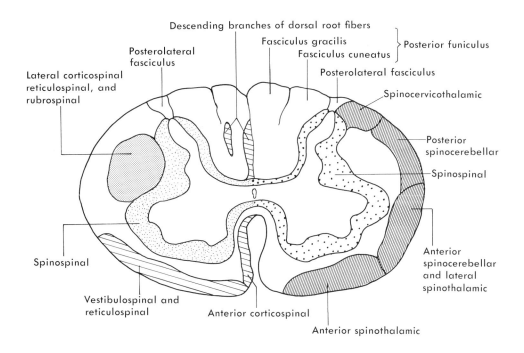

DESCENDING TRACTS   ASCENDING TRACTS

Figure 13–2.   The main tracts of the spinal cord. Ascending tracts are shown on the right side and descending tracts on the left.

Gray Matter. Gray matter has a fundamental arrangement that is modified locally, as indicated in Figure 13–1. This is the result of differences in numbers and types of its contained neurons. Thus the gray matter of the cervical and lumbosacral regions is more abundant because these regions supply the limbs. That of the thoracic and upper lumbar segments of the spinal cord is less in amount because it supplies only the trunk. It is characterized, however, by a lateral projection of its intermediate portion which contains the autonomic neurons whose axons leave the spinal cord as preganglionic sympathetic fibers (p. 338).

The cells of the gray matter are arranged in 9 layers (Fig. 13–3), (10 if the central gray matter is included), most of which extend from one end of the spinal cord to the other. From dorsal to ventral, the first 6 layers comprise the dorsal gray matter (the 6th layer is present only in the cervical and lumbosacral enlargements). The cells of these layers are predominantly interneurons and transmission neurons, as described in Chapter 11. The approximate correlation of numbered layers to classical names is as follows: Layers 2 and 3 comprise the *substantia gelatinosa,* which is capped by layer 1; these three and layer 4 form the head of the dorsal gray matter. Layers 4 and 5, which form the neck of

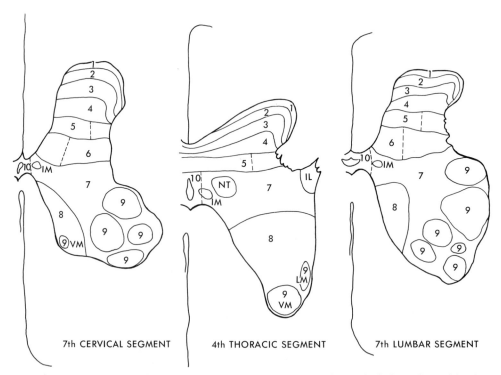

7th CERVICAL SEGMENT   4th THORACIC SEGMENT   7th LUMBAR SEGMENT

Figure 13–3. Diagrams of the layers of gray matter in cervical, thoracic, and lumbar levels of the spinal cord of the cat. IM, intermediomedial portion of 7th layer; NT, nucleus thoracicus; IL, intermediolateral nucleus (origin of preganglionic sympathetic fibers). The various subdivisions of layer 9 represent nuclei for various groups of muscles. (Based on Rexed, B., in J. Comp. Neurol., *96:*415, 1952, and *100:*297, 1954.

the dorsal gray, comprise the *nucleus proprius* (layer 6, which forms the base of the dorsal gray, is sometimes included). Layers 7 to 9 occupy intermediate to ventral positions: layer 7 contains autonomic cells, layer 8 has many commissural neurons, and layer 9 contains interneurons, e.g., Renshaw cells, cells of origin of *gamma efferents,* and large *alpha* motor cells that are arranged into nuclei for the supply of muscle groups.

The anterior spinocerebellar tract originates from cells in the lateral portions of layers 5 to 7, and the posterior spinocerebellar tract originates from the *nucleus thoracicus* in the medial part of layer 7.

The foregoing account is based on the spinal cord of the cat; there is reason to believe that a similar arrangement holds for primate spinal cords. It should be emphasized, however, that there are no sharp lines between the layers; rather, they overlap considerably. Moreover, there are significant differences in the findings and conclusions of various investigators regarding the composition and function of the several layers, and relatively few of the constituent cells have been adequately characterized anatomically and physiologically.

FUNCTIONS OF THE SPINAL CORD

The functions of the spinal cord have been studied by a variety of experimental approaches, and by analyses of clinical disorders. Among the various experimental approaches are those that attempt to assess intrinsic functions by isolating the spinal cord from higher level control, thereby producing what is termed a "spinal animal." In such an animal, certain reflex patterns may be elicited in a relatively unmodified form. How closely these patterns resemble those of the normal animals depends upon the species under study. If, for example, the spinal cord of a frog is severed, spinal cord functions are depressed immediately after the section, but within a few minutes it is possible to demonstrate reflex withdrawal to painful stimuli, reflex squatting and swimming movements, and a variety of reactions similar to those seen in normal frogs. The spinal cord of the frog is therefore capable of much autonomous activity. Little of this activity, however, is spontaneous; that is, it does not take place without adequate external stimuli.

In higher animals, such as the cat or dog, the period of depression (spinal shock) may last several hours or days. Subsequently, certain patterns of reflex behavior can be demonstrated. Although spinal cats and dogs cannot stand, or can stand for short periods of time only, if they are properly supported and adequate stimulation is supplied, alternating flexion and extension movements that resemble running patterns may be elicited. The reflexes forming these patterns are combinations of the fundamental types discussed previously (p. 115). There it was pointed out that the monosynaptic two-neuron or stretch reflex is a highly restricted or *local reflex* of both phasic and static types. The phasic type, that is, the knee jerk, can be elicited in spinal cats and dogs, but the degree to which the static type is present is variable. Those animals that exhibit some degree of reflex extensor activity also show periods of reflex standing, whereas in others the knee jerk may be the only type of extensor response that can be demonstrated.

Studies of spinal animals show that the multisynaptic (polysynaptic) reflexes, together with monosynaptic reflexes, are organized into patterns that can be categorized as withdrawal, crossed extension, thrust, and long spinal. Some of these are most easily elicited by painful stimuli. For example, a painful stimulus to the foot may be followed by *withdrawal* of that limb. At the same time, interneurons project to various levels of the opposite side of the gray matter and provide for extensor activity (*crossed extensor* or *segmental static reflex*). This total reaction is a mechanism for providing support when a limb is lifted from the ground. It is obviously an important component of posture and locomotion as well as of responses to nociceptive stimulation. Some components of locomotion may be characterized as *thrust,* and more complex reactions and mechanisms require coordination of all limbs by *long spinal reflexes.* Certain general principles regarding more complicated patterns can be pointed out.

Reflexes exhibit *local sign* and *specificity.* For example, scratching movements may follow light scratching of the skin of the flank, but not of the foot. A painful stimulus to the skin of the flank is followed, not by scratching, but by withdrawal.

Reflexes exhibit *rhythm,* which appears to be an intrinsic property of the spinal cord. For example, one may scratch the skin of the flank of a spinal dog at a certain frequency, say several times a second. Yet the scratching movements that the animal carries out reflexly are not necessarily the same number of times per second. They may be much slower, and independent of stimulus frequency to the extent that the rate of scratching remains the same even when the stimulus frequency is varied. Likewise, for certain species, it is likely that a basic rhythmic discharge from gray matter is responsible for the locomotor pattern of activity. Afferent stimuli, then, although extremely important in locomotion, modify the basic rhythm rather than determine it.

Reflexes may be *allied.* For example, the scratch response consists of several simpler types of reflexes which are coordinated into a fairly complicated pattern.

Not infrequently, the cutaneous stimulation is subthreshold, that is, ineffective. In such cases a similar subthreshold stimulus applied nearby at the same time (simultaneous combination) or applied to the same region immediately after the first (successive combination) will summate with the first and produce a response. *Summation of subthreshold stimuli* is commonly seen in connection with many reflexes.

Some reflexes are *antagonistic,* as in the case of extensor and flexor components of locomotion, in the sense that they initiate movement in opposing directions. When they are coordinated into locomotor patterns involving forelimbs and hindlimbs, they form what are called *intersegmental reflexes* (long spinal). Intersegmental relationships are further illustrated by the changes subsequent to spinal transection in a decerebrate animal (p. 310). If the transection is made in the thoracic region, stretch reflexes in the forelimbs become exaggerated, indicating that the caudal portion of the spinal cord had been carrying out an inhibitory function.

It is apparent that the spinal cord in cats and dogs does not function as well as that of the frog when separated from the rest of the nervous system. The higher the animal in the vertebrate scale, the more dependent on higher centers and the less autonomy there is of the spinal cord. This can be shown by references to spinal shock in humans, a condition that also demonstrates the role of the spinal cord in autonomic activities.

Spinal Shock in Humans. When the spinal cord is completely severed above the fourth cervical segment, death rapidly follows because of the interference with respiration (p. 316).

Transection at lower levels is compatible with life. The initial effect is a complete cessation of spinal cord functions below the lesion. This *spinal shock* is much more pronounced in humans than in lower vertebrates; it is characterized by complete flaccid paralysis, absence of reflexes and sensation below the level of the lesion, and marked disturbances of bladder and rectal functions. The reasons for spinal shock are not fully understood. One of the main factors is sudden section of descending tracts, because if a transection develops slowly over days or weeks, shock may not appear. In experimental animals it can be shown that if the isolated cord is severed again, the cord distal to the second transection does not develop signs of shock. Evidently, then, fibers descending from higher levels are implicated initially, but not in the second transection.

There are certain fundamental reactions to any pathological changes in the nervous system, their specificity depending on whether there is a destruction of nervous tissue or an irritation (stimulation), (1) If part of the nervous system has been destroyed, two fundamental reactions occur: (a) functions performed by the affected area are lost, and (b) abnormal phenomena appear because of the hyperactivity of areas normally held in check by, inhibited by, or opposing the affected part. In an upper motor neuron lesion, for instance, the paralysis is a loss of function; the spasticity and hyperactive reflexes are abnormal phenomena. (2) If a disorder irritates part of the nervous system by a stimulating action, the fundamental reaction is an exaggeration of the normal functions of the affected area. In poliomyelitis, for instance, there may be irritation of motor neurons, and muscle spasm results. Any or all of the fundamental reactions may occur in a neurological disorder. Furthermore, some lesions are initially irritative and later destructive; in such cases the type of fundamental reaction may change during the course of the disorder. Both types of reaction occur in spinal shock.

Following cord transection, there are generally the following stages: spinal shock, minimal reflex activity, flexor spasms, and alternating flexor and extensor spasms. In most instances of uncomplicated long-surviving cases of complete cord transection, extensor activity below the level of transection becomes dominant.

Flaccid paralysis, with complete loss of all reflexes, persists during spinal shock. The paralyzed bladder contains stagnant urine, a potential source of infection, and care must be taken to prevent infections from involving the urinary system.

As spinal shock subsides, the isolated part of the spinal cord becomes more or less automatic in function. Muscles are not severed from motor neurons except at the level of the transection itself and reflex arcs are, therefore, intact. But all descending motor tracts are severed and reflex arcs are, therefore, modifiable by local influences (cutaneous stimulation, muscle stretch, or *gamma* efferents). All ascending tracts are cut and sensation is completely lost below the level of the lesion.

The first signs of reflex activity appear in the distal parts of the limbs, one to six weeks after transection. These consist of mild reflex contractions of flexor muscles following cutaneous stimulation.

Flexor activity becomes more marked until flexor spasm or *mass flexion* is seen. In its best developed form this consists of withdrawal of the limbs, with flexion at hip, knee, and ankle, and strong Babinski responses, these occurring in response to cutaneous stimulation. Tendon reflexes become very active, and at a variable time after transection can be elicited in extensor muscles, for example, a phasic type of knee jerk.

Commonly, extensor spasm (straightening of lower limbs) begins to appear and eventually becomes predominant (*mass extension*). Extensor activity is best elicited by stretch of muscles. In a few instances, extension may be so pronounced that patients, on being placed in a standing position, may continue to stand reflexly, even though no voluntary control exists.

Autonomic functions are lost during the period of spinal shock. With recovery, evidences of sympathetic activity reappear. The cutaneous vessels constrict, and sweating may be reflexly induced. Thus a mass flexion is accompanied by sweating in the affected areas. The upper limit of the area of sweating indicates the approximate level of the cord lesion. This illustrates the localized distribution of the autonomic outflow.

With recovery from spinal shock, the bladder may function almost automatically and become a "cord bladder", tending to fill and empty spontaneously. The bladder normally functions as follows: Urine formed by the kidneys flows down the ureters into the urinary bladder. The walls of the bladder are composed of smooth muscle, which continues along the urethra. Under normal conditions the smooth muscle of the bladder wall is contracted to a certain degree. These contractions are mediated by the parasympathetic system. When the amount of urine in the bladder increases enough to raise the intravesical pressure, several things may happen. Afferent impulses due to the increase in pressure are interpreted as a vague sensation of bladder fullness. If voiding is initiated, the smooth muscle of the bladder contracts. At the same time, the urethral musculature contracts, the part of the urethra immediately below the bladder becomes shorter, and the opening between the bladder and the urethra widens. The external abdominal muscles likewise contract, thereby increasing intra-abdominal pressure and aiding in the evacuation of the bladder. Here, then, is a situation in which smooth muscle supplied by the parasympathetic system is partially under voluntary control and is coordinated in its activity with skeletal muscles. If the bladder is not emptied, the afferent impulses inhibit the parasympathetic cells in the sacral cord. The smooth muscle relaxes and the pressure drops until afferent impulses cease and the muscle resumes its tonicity. As more urine enters, the same processes may be repeated. But there is a limit to the relaxation of the bladder. When a certain pressure is reached, the sensation of fullness becomes acutely and increasingly uncomfortable.

Early in spinal shock the bladder is paralyzed; it fills with urine that cannot be voided except by artifical means. But as the shock disappears, the reflex arc begins to function. Eventually, the para-sympathetic cells in the sacral cord begin to function and may be excited by afferent impulses resulting from a rise in intravesical pressure. When the bladder begins to contract reflexly, an auto-matic or "cord bladder" is established.

Other types of visceral activities are affected by cord transec-tions. In spinal man, during the period of shock, the nervous mechanism controlling evacuation of the rectum is almost com-pletely depressed. With gradual recovery from the shock, local reflexes appear whose stimulus seems to be distention of the rectum, the response of which consists in rectal contraction and relaxation of the sphincters at the anal orifice.

Likewise, sexual functions are interfered with. Psychic stimuli are generally unable to influence sexual activity. But there appears to be an area in the lumbosacral cord capable of initiating inte-grated sexual activity, not only after direct stimulation of the external genitalia, but frequently after any type of cutaneous stimulation.

SPINAL NERVES

All outward expressions of behavior are mediated through effectors and no matter what they are, the final or ultimate path from the central nervous system is the motor neuron of the brain stem and spinal cord, the final common path. This path (*alpha motor neurons*) is distributed to skeletal muscles that developed in the embryo segment corresponding to the cord segment of the ventral root. However, in the limbs, there is no true segmental distribution to muscles (p. 172).

The fibers of the dorsal roots that supply skin are segmentally distributed, even in the limbs. The area of skin supplied by each dorsal root is termed a dermatome (p. 168). The size of this area, as determined physiologically (and clinically), is variable and depends upon the effectiveness of transmission in the gray matter. The excitability of transmission over a root is enhanced by terminals from adjacent roots. Hence, if the dorsal roots adjacent to an intact root are cut, the dermatome of that root becomes smaller as determined by sensitivity to stimulation. If more adjacent roots are cut, the dermatome becomes still smaller. Conversely, the size of a dermatome may be expanded enormously by giving subconvulsive doses of strychnine sulfate.

The fact that afferent fibers are collected into dorsal roots is utilized clinically in spinal anesthesia. The introduction (in the sitting position) of a local anesthetic, such as *procaine,* into the subarachnoid space is followed by analgesia of first the sacral areas, then the lumbar, and so forth, depending on the amount of anesthetic injected and the height to which it is allowed to rise. Such anesthetics affect nonmyelinated and small myelinated fibers first. Consequently, the sense of pain disappears first, and that of pressure last. During an operation, therefore, pain may be absent, but pressure sense may still be present.

Nerve Components.   The fibers contained within a nerve may be classified according to the structures they supply. This has considerably simplified and clarified our concepts of cranial nerves (p. 306). In spinal nerves, four types or components of fibers are present. These are arranged in a manner relating to the position of the embryonic sulcus limitans. It will be recalled that within the neural tube those neuroblasts lying ventral to the sulcus limitans (that is, in the basal plate), become efferent. The dorsally placed afferent fibers, on the other hand, enter the alar plate and synapse with the cells developing there. The same relationship is present in the adult.

Ventral roots contain large myelinated fibers (*alpha*) supplying skeletal muscle and small myelinated fibers (*gamma*) to spindle muscle fibers. These are efferent fibers to somatic structures, hence are called somatic efferent fibers, and their cells of origin are in the most ventral part of the gray matter (layer 9). Many ventral roots also contain small myelinated fibers destined for visceral structures. These *general visceral efferent* fibers, whose cells of origin are in layer 7, are preganglionic axons of the autonomic system. The term "general" is used in contrast to special visceral efferent fibers present in certain cranial nerves (Table 14–1, p. 307).

Dorsal roots contain *general somatic afferent* and *general visceral afferent* fibers, which supply somatic (skin, muscles, and so forth) and visceral structures, respectively.

Spinal nerves, since they are formed by dorsal and ventral roots, contain all four components. This is true of major peripheral nerves, but branches of these vary in composition. Thus a nerve to skin lacks somatic efferent fibers.

In the upper levels of the cervical spinal cord, large motor neurons are found in intermediate as well as in ventral gray matter. The axons of cells in the intermediate gray leave, not by way of spinal roots, but instead emerge laterally and form the spinal portion of the accessory nerve, which ascends through the foramen magnum and joins the medullary portion. These axons comprise a functional component that belongs with the brain stem.

PERIPHERAL NERVES

Nearly all major peripheral nerves include fibers from several spinal nerves (p. 168). For example, the femoral nerve in the thigh is derived from the second, third, and fourth lumbar spinal nerves and supplies the skin over the anterior surface of the thigh and the extensor muscles of the leg. The obturator nerve is also derived from the second, third, and fourth lumbar nerves, but it supplies a different skin area and the abductor muscles of the thigh. Thus these lumbar nerves are distributed by way of different peripheral nerves. Furthermore, the fourth lumbar nerve contributes to the sciatic nerve.

When a spinal nerve is severed, therefore, the effects are found in parts of several peripheral nerve areas. A lesion of the second lumbar spinal nerve, for instance, is followed by involvement of part of the femoral and part of the obturator nerve supply. A lesion of a peripheral nerve, however, involves parts of several spinal nerves. These facts are of clinical importance, in determining the location of a lesion causing muscle paralyses or sensory losses, or both.

If a peripheral nerve is completely severed, the muscles supplied by the nerve undergo a sudden, complete, flaccid paralysis. Reflexes as well as sensation are lost. The anesthesia covers an area less than the anatomical distribution because of the overlap from neighboring peripheral nerves. Without proper care the muscles may atrophy before regeneration can occur and atrophy will inevitably follow if there is no regeneration.

As nerve fibers begin to regenerate, spontaneous pains may occur in the area of distribution of the nerve. This results from an irritation at the growing ends, and the pain is of a projection type. When connections are re-established, the muscles slowly regain their tone, atrophic changes lessen, and the field of sensory impairment gradually narrows and disappears. Sensations of pain and temperature return first, partly because small fibers grow faster, and partly because nonmyelinated fibers from neighboring normal areas grow into the denervated skin. The regeneration of the larger peripheral nerves may take a year or two.

A description of a radial nerve injury suffices to illustrate. This nerve supplies the extensors of the forearm, wrist, and proximal phalanges, so that these muscles become paralyzed and a "wrist drop" results. The fingers tend to bend because the flexor muscles are unopposed. Sensory losses are slight because there is a considerable overlap; only a small area on the back of the hand between the thumb and first finger becomes anesthetic. If the cut ends are united, regeneration may occur in a year or less.

SUMMARY

The spinal cord retains, to a certain extent, the segmental character of the neural tube. The gray matter has a basic arrangement which is modified by local changes in character and number of contained neurons, which are arranged in 9 layers that extend from one end of the cord to the other. The white matter is arranged in funiculi which are also modified locally. Tracts, such as the lateral spinothalamic, are not anatomically demonstrable in normal material.

In the spinal cord the basic reflexes are coordinated in local and general movement patterns. These, such as stepping or walking, are spinal mechanisms, but cannot function autonomously. Certain higher centers must be present before the spinal cord can function normally.

Transection of the cord in humans is followed by spinal shock, with complete flaccid paralysis and loss of sensations. Autonomic functions, such as sweating and evacuation of the urinary bladder, are restricted to local reflexes operating over cord levels.

Spinal nerves contain general somatic afferent and general visceral afferent components, which enter dorsal roots; and somatic efferent and general visceral efferent fibers derived from motor neurons by way of ventral roots. The major peripheral nerves likewise contain these components.

Lesions of spinal and peripheral nerves differ in their effects because (1) a spinal nerve reaches its area of supply through several different peripheral nerves and composes only part of each, and (2) a major peripheral nerve contains parts of several spinal nerves.

REFERENCES

See also the references on pages 219 and 244.

Eccles, J. C., and Schade, J. P., (editors): Organization of the Spinal Cord; Physiology of Spinal Neurons (vols. 11 and 12, Progress in Brain Research). Amsterdam, Elsevier Publishing Company, 1964.

Kirk, E. J., and Denny-Brown, D.: Functional variation in dermatomes in the macaque monkey following dorsal root lesions. J. Comp. Neurol., *139*:307–320, 1970. An important paper on the size of dermatomes and their relation to central excitability.

Kuhn, R. A.: Functional capacity of the isolated human spinal cord. Brain, *73*:1–51, 1950. A very thorough study, especially valuable because patients were observed for long periods of time, and cord transections were verified at surgery.

Pubols, B. H., Jr. and Pubols, L. M.: Forelimb, hindlimb, and tail dermatomes in the spider monkey (*Ateles*). Brain Behav. Evol., *2*:132–159, 1969. Somatotopic representation in the lemniscal system.

Riss, W.: Introduction to a general theory of spinal organization. Brain Behav. Evol., *2*:51–82, 1969. The role of interneurons in reflexes produced by cutaneous and proprioceptive stimulation.

Wall, P.: The sensory and motor role of impulses traveling in the dorsal columns toward cerebral cortex. Brain, *93*:505–524, 1970. A paper dealing with concepts of major importance.

Chapter **14**

THE ORGANIZATION OF
THE BRAIN STEM
AND ITS NERVES

The brain stem is comprised, from rostral to caudal, of the diencephalon, mesencephalon, pons, and medulla oblongata. It contains, in addition to the tracts that ascend and descend to it and through it, collections of nerve cells that (1) comprise major integrating centers for sensory and motor functions; (2) form the nuclei of most of the cranial nerves (all of the cranial nerves, except the first, are attached to the brain stem); (3) form centers concerned with a variety of visceral, endocrinological, behavioral, and other functions; (4) are associated with most of the special senses; (5) control muscular activity in the head and part of the neck; (6) supply structures derived from the pharyngeal arches; and (7) are connected with the cerebellum.

Although the diencephalon is regarded as a part of the brain stem, its major components, the thalami and hypothalamus, are usually discussed in conjunction with cerebral structures and the autonomic nervous system (p. 333).

FUNCTIONAL MORPHOLOGY OF
THE BRAIN STEM

The major features of the gross morphology of the brain stem were discussed in Chapter 7. The purpose of the following discussion is to outline some of the internal anatomical arrangements and regional functions before turning to more detailed considerations of common brain stem functions.

THE MEDULLA OBLONGATA

The medulla oblongata is the caudal portion of the brain stem. The ninth to twelfth cranial nerves are attached to it, it contains the upper portion of the central canal, and it serves as the floor of the lower half of the fourth ventricle. The change from the spinal cord to the medulla oblongata at the level of the foramen magnum is more evident microscopically than grossly. The lower limit of the pyramidal decussation marks the transition. Above this level, the *nucleus gracilis* and the *nucleus cuneatus* are evident, as are the *medial lemnisci,* which become increasingly prominent (Fig. 14–1). The bilaterally placed *olivary nuclei,* characterized by their crumpled shape, begin at the approximate level at which the

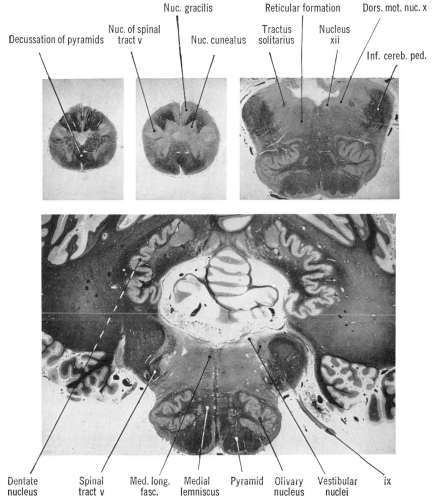

Figure 14-1. Transverse sections of medulla oblongata and cerebellum. Weigert stain.

medial lemnisci appear; they extend upward to the pons. The olivary nuclei, which are a major source of climbing fibers to the cerebellum (by way of the inferior cerebellar peduncles), are important components of cerebellar functions. They have a large input from mechanoreceptors, are under the influence of the sensorimotor cortex by way of indirect descending paths, and receive projections from the red nuclei and the visual and auditory systems.

The *motor nuclei of the hypoglossal nerves* lie in the dorsal part of the medulla oblongata, in the floor of the fourth ventricle (Fig. 14–1), and on each side of the median plane. Lateral to each hypoglossal nucleus is the *dorsal motor nucleus of the vagus.*

Dorsally situated on each side in the medulla oblongata is a small bundle of myelinated fibers, the *tractus solitarius.* The *spinal tract of the trigeminal nerve* forms the dorsolateral surface of the lower part of the medulla; more rostrally it lies deep to the inferior cerebellar peduncle.

Much of the central portion of the medulla oblongata consists of the reticular formation; it is a mixture of white and gray matter which contains many types of neurons (Fig. 7–18, p. 141, and Fig. 14–1. Some of the functions of the reticular formation are discussed later (p. 318). Throughout the medulla, cells subserving different functions may lie side by side. For example, the vagus, glossopharyngeal, and accessory nerves supply striated muscles by axons derived from large neurons in the medulla oblongata and upper cervical cord. These neurons form an inconspicuous nucleus (*nucleus ambiguus*) in the reticular formation. Other cells in the same general region are involved in cardiovascular and respiratory mechanisms (p. 314).

THE PONS

The pons consists of a large, rounded ventral portion and a dorsal portion that is chiefly a rostral continuation of the reticular formation of the medulla oblongata. The trigeminal nerve is attached to the lateral aspect of the pons; the sixth, seventh, and eighth cranial nerves are attached at the junction of the pons and the medulla.

The ventral portion of the pons contains masses of cells, the *pontine nuclei,* whose axons project laterally and form the middle cerebellar peduncles. These nuclei are separated by bundles of corticospinal and corticobulbar fibers which descend through the pons. The dorsal portion of the pons is separated from the ventral by the medial lemnisci, which, as they enter the pons, become oriented transversely instead of dorsoventrally (Fig. 14–2). With this rearrangement, the *medial longitudinal fasciculi* remain in their dorsal location, on each side of the median plane. These fasciculi, which can be readily followed into the midbrain, also descend into the cervical portion of the spinal cord. They are important association bundles that carry ascending and descending

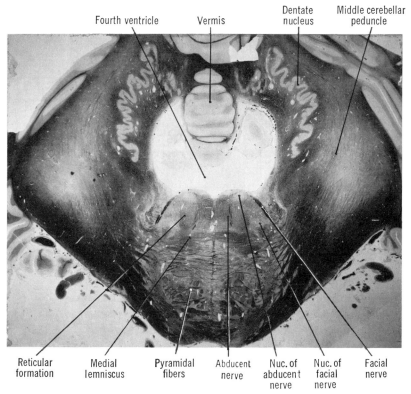

Fourth ventricle Vermis Dentate nucleus Middle cerebellar peduncle

Reticular formation | Medial lemniscus | Pyramidal fibers | Abducent nerve | Nuc. of abducent nerve | Nuc. of facial nerve | Facial nerve

Figure 14–2. Transverse section of the pons and cerebellum. Pyramidal fibers form small bundles in the ventral part of the pons. Weigert stain.

fibers that link various motor nuclei. In their course through the medulla, they are immediately dorsal to the medial lemnisci (Fig. 14–1).

The dorsal portion of the pons contains nuclei related to the trigeminal, abducent, and facial nerves. At the junction of the pons and medulla, the cochlear nerve ends in the *ventral* and *dorsal cochlear nuclei,* which are placed on the ventrolateral and posterior aspects of the inferior cerebellar peduncles, respectively. The vestibular nerve enters medial to the peduncle and ends in four nuclei (*medial, lateral, superior,* and *inferior vestibular nuclei*). The reticular formation of the pons contains important visceral and motor centers, which are discussed later, and also portions of the biogenic amine system (e.g., see locus ceruleus, pp. 306 and 319).

THE MIDBRAIN

The midbrain, which is joined to the base of the brain and is thereby continuous rostrally with the diencephalon, is distinguished by the two massive *cerebral peduncles* which form its anterior portion and which lie in front of the cerebral aqueduct (Fig. 14–3). Each peduncle consists of a dorsally placed *tegmentum* and a ventrally placed *crus cerebri*. They are separated by the *substantia nigra* whose dorsal portion consists of a compact zone of melanin-containing cells. These cells are a part of the dopaminergic system (p. 319) and project to the striatum.

Each crus cerebri, which consists chiefly of pyramidal fibers, is continuous above with the internal capsule as the latter emerges from the base of the brain. Below, the crura break up into bundles that descend through the pons. The area between the two crura is termed the *interpeduncular fossa.* A number of small vessels enter the fossa and supply the midbrain, and because of the perforations caused by their entrance, the surface of the fossa is termed the *posterior perforated substance.*

The tegmentum contains: (1) the *nuclei* of the *oculomotor* and *trochlear nerves*; (2) the rostral portions of the medial longitudinal fasciculi; (3) a number of other important nuclei, some of which comprise portions of the *limbic midbrain area*; and (4) the *red nuclei.* The two superior cerebellar peduncles ascend through the tegmentum, crossing as they do so.

The limbic midbrain area consists of neurons that form the ventral portion of the central gray matter and the medial portion of each tegmentum. The cells form a part of the dopaminergic system, they have powerful inputs from more caudal levels and

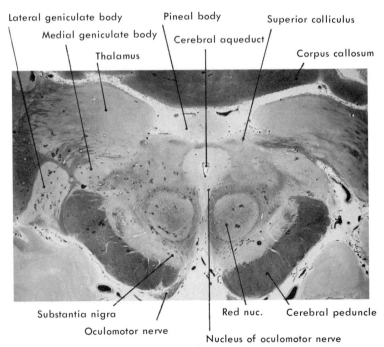

Figure 14–3. Transverse section of the midbrain. Weigert stain.

from the hippocampus, and they project to nuclei in and near the septum. Functional considerations are discussed on p. 321.

The red nuclei are important elements of the extrapyramidal system; their chief input is from the dentate nuclei of the cerebellum. Each red nucleus usually contains large neurons that project to various nuclei on the opposite side of the brain stem and to the opposite side of the spinal cord (*rubrospinal tract*). Each one also contains many small neurons whose axons remain uncrossed, projecting to reticular and inferior olivary nuclei.

The portion of the midbrain behind the cerebral aqueduct is the *tectum* or *roof*, which is a plate of nervous tissue with four rounded elevations, the two *superior* and two *inferior colliculi.* The colliculi have important intrinsic functions. For example, the two superior colliculi are important visual centers. Their cells, which are organized into layers, receive fibers from the retina (each colliculus is activated by light from the opposite visual fields) and from areas of the cerebral cortex. They also have a somatic input from ascending paths and an auditory input from the inferior colliculi and auditory cortex. The collicular cells project (1) to the oculomotor, trochlear, and abducent nuclei; (2) to other motor nuclei by way of *tectobulbar* and *tectospinal tracts*; and (3) to the cerebellum. Many of the cells in the superior colliculi fire only in response to movement in the visual fields. Moreover, it appears that the cells in the deeper layers of the superior colliculi are organized to integrate information about the location and direction of auditory and visual movement, and thereby to help the eyes in detecting and following moving objects. The superior colliculi are also important integrating centers for certain kinds of voluntary eye movements (e.g., upward gaze, saccadic movements, p. 209). Finally, the superior colliculi are important reflex centers. Examples of reflexes are blinking in response to an object that appears suddenly in the visual field (the object does not necessarily have to be seen) and generalized startle reactions to such a stimulus. Pupillary constriction in response to light (p. 338) is also a visual reflex, but the integrating component is a function of the *pretectal region,* which is gray matter that lies between the colliculi and the thalami.

The two inferior colliculi are important elements of the auditory system. They receive ascending auditory fibers, as well as fibers from somatic pathways, and they project to the brain stem, spinal cord, cerebellum, superior colliculi, and medial geniculate body. The inferior colliculi are important reflex and integrating centers. Examples of reflexes are a turning of the eyes, head, or body, or a general startle reaction, in response to a sudden noise.

PINEAL BODY

The *pineal body,* or *epiphysis* (Fig. 14–3) lies at the posterior end of the third ventricle, at the junction of midbrain and diencephalon, where it is topographically associated with the roof of the midbrain. The role of the pineal body in neuroendocrinological mechanisms is discussed on p. 352.

FOURTH VENTRICLE AND CEREBRAL AQUEDUCT

The fourth ventricle is broad in its midportion, but it narrows below as it continues into the central canal, and above, where it is continuous with the cerebral aqueduct. Its floor is formed by the medulla oblongata and pons, and is divided into right and left halves by a longitudinal *median sulcus.* Each half is further divided into medial and lateral areas by the *sulcus limitans.* The floor is marked by various elevations that correspond to underlying tracts and cranial nerve nuclei. At the upper end of the sulcus limitans there is a small, pigmented area, the *locus ceruleus.* The locus ceruleus is the caudal end of a highly vascular column of melanin-containing cells that synthesize norepinephrine (p. 319).

In the caudal part of the fourth ventricle, at each lateral edge, is a slight eminence termed the *area postrema.* This area contains neuroglial cells, nerve cells, and many blood vessels (the endothelial cells of the capillaries lack tight functions, hence a blood-brain barrier is absent); the nerve cells are connected with the nucleus of the tractus solitarius, are thought to be chemoreceptors of some kind, and appear to be involved in the mechanisms of vomiting.

As indicated previously, the cerebral aqueduct marks the division between the cerebral peduncles and the roof of the midbrain. The oculomotor and trochlear nuclei lie immediately in front of the aqueduct. The cells in the gray matter around it (*periaqueductal gray*) are important components of visceral and limbic mechanisms.

CRANIAL NERVE COMPONENTS

The major differences between cranial and spinal nerves were discussed in Chapter 2, in which the concept of functional components was presented. There and in other chapters it was pointed out that in the developing spinal cord the basal plate was related to motor functions and the alar plate to sensory functions. This topographical arrangement is present in adults. The development of the brain stem, however, is such that the alar plate moves laterally as the roof of the fourth ventricle widens, and the basal plate becomes medial in position. Hence, in adults, the motor nuclei form medially placed cellular columns and the sensory nuclei form lateral columns. The four functional components that are present in spinal nerves can be found in certain cranial nerves, and their cells of origin and termination form the columns mentioned above. Table 14–1 tabulates the cranial nerve components, and Figure 14–4 illustrates their fundamental arrangements in the brain stem and indicates certain additional components that are not present in spinal nerves. Although no component forms a complete longitudinal column, the cells of a specific component at any one level occupy the same topographical position as the cells of that component at another level. For example, the motor cells that supply the tongue and the extrinsic muscles of the eye form nuclei that lie in the floor of the fourth ventricle or aqueduct, adjacent to the median plane.

What are the reasons for the additional components present

Table 14-1. Components of cranial nerves

Cranial Nerve	Component	Function
Olfactory	Special visceral afferent (Sometimes classified as special somatic afferent)	Smell
Optic	Special somatic afferent	Vision
Oculomotor*	Somatic efferent	Movements of eyeball
	General somatic afferent	Proprioception from extrinsic eye muscles
	General visceral efferent (parasympathetic)	Accommodation and pupillary constriction
Trochlear*	Somatic efferent	Movements of eyeball
	General somatic afferent	Proprioception from extrinsic eye muscle
Trigeminal	Special visceral efferent	Movements of mastication
	General somatic afferent	General sensations from face and head
Abducent*	Somatic efferent	Movement of eyeball
	General somatic afferent	Proprioception from extrinsic eye muscle
Facial	Special visceral efferent	Facial expressions
	General visceral efferent (parasympathetic)	Salivation and lacrimation
	Special visceral afferent	Taste
Vestibulocochlear (or eighth nerve)	Special somatic afferent	Hearing and equilibrium
Glossopharyngeal	Special visceral efferent	Pharyngeal movements
	General visceral efferent (parasympathetic)	Salivation
	Special visceral afferent	Taste
	General visceral afferent	Visceral reflexes; sensation in tongue and pharynx
	General somatic afferent	Sensation from external ear
Vagus	Special visceral efferent	Pharyngeal and laryngeal movements
	General visceral efferent (parasympathetic)	Movements and secretion of thoracic and abdominal viscera
	Special visceral afferent	Taste
	General visceral afferent	Visceral reflexes; sensation in tongue and pharynx
	General somatic afferent	Sensation from external ear and scalp
Accessory	Special visceral efferent	Movements of pharynx, larynx, head, and shoulders
	General visceral efferent (parasympathetic)	Same as vagus
Hypoglossal	Somatic efferent	Movements of tongue

*The general somatic afferent fibers in these nerves probably enter trigeminal branches through extracranial anastomoses and have their cell bodies in the trigeminal ganglion or mesencephalic nucleus.

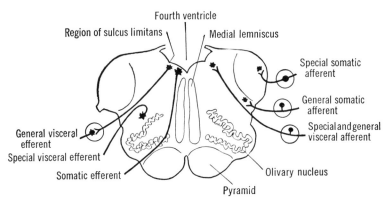

Figure 14-4. Schematic representation of cranial nerve components and their cells of origin and termination in the medulla oblongata. Afferent fibers are shown on the right, and efferent on the left.

in cranial nerves and for their arrangement? The reasons for the most part have been demonstrated by studies of amphibian forms; the arrangement seems fundamentally similar in humans.

Obviously, some of the additional components relate to the special senses. The classification of taste and smell as *special visceral afferent,* and vision, hearing, and balance as *special somatic afferent,* is arbitrary. The term *special visceral efferent* refers to the motor supply of muscles that develop from the pharyngeal arches. The muscles of mastication arise from the first pharyngeal arches and are supplied by the motor nuclei of the trigeminal nerves. The facial muscles arise from the second arches and are supplied by the facial nerves. The muscles of the pharynx and larynx arise from the third, fourth, and fifth arches and are supplied by the glossopharyngeal, vagus, and medullary portions of the accessory nerves; all of the nerve fibers concerned arise from cells in the columns formed by the nuclei ambigui. The spinal parts of the accessory nerves supply those parts of the sterno-cleidomastoid and trapezius muscles which appear to be derived from the pharyngeal arches.

It must be emphasized again that the classification into functional components has obvious limitations but is useful in tracing relationships and in developing functional correlations.

TRIGEMINAL SENSORY COMPLEX

The major general sensory supply of the head and neck is by the trigeminal nerves and the upper cervical dorsal roots. There is a minor contribution by the glossopharyngeal nerve to the supply of the external ear and a contribution by the vagus nerve to the supply of the external ear and adjacent scalp. The cutaneous fibers of these two nerves enter the central trigeminal connections.

The trigeminal nerve has three major peripheral divisions, the ophthalmic, maxillary, and mandibular nerves. The area of skin supplied by these nerves can be regarded as a dermatome. The contiguous dorsal roots that overlap this dermatome are the second to fourth cervical. The central processes of the cells in the trigeminal ganglion enter the pons where some end in the main sensory nucleus. The remainder turn downward and form the spinal tract of the trigeminal nerve, some fibers extending as far caudally as the second or third cervical segment. The fibers end in the nucleus of the spinal tract of the trigeminal nerve, which is continuous caudally with the substantia gelatinosa. The spinal nucleus is probably organized like spinal sensory gray matter, containing interneurons that act upon transmission cells. Some cervical dorsal root fibers ascend in the spinal tract, and some of the cells in the spinal nucleus relay impulses from these cervical fibers.

Within the spinal tract, the fibers descending from the ophthalmic division are most ventral in position, those of the maxillary division are intermediate, and those of the mandibular division are dorsal. Differing results of sectioning the tract for the relief of pain are related in part to the location and extent of the surgical section. However, just as in the case of spinal dermatomes, the central interaction and summation of impulses must be taken into account.

The distribution and overlap of the trigeminal nerve and the upper cervical dorsal roots are much greater than is generally supposed. When the spinal tract of the trigeminal nerve is sectioned, the loss of sensation is greatest in the areas of skin with the most overlap. The loss of pain is most noticeable in these same areas. The explanation is that a cell transmitting from these areas does not fire unless impulses converge on it from at least two different nerves. Hence, just as in the case of spinal dermatomes, loss of one input reduces central excitability and input from skin that is still innervated by overlap is ineffective. Strychnine temporarily restores sensation. Likewise, if the upper cervical dorsal roots are cut, the area of cutaneous distribution of the trigeminal nerve, as determined by sensory testing, expands temporarily but enormously when strychnine is administered.

MOTOR FUNCTIONS OF THE BRAIN STEM

The motor organization of the brain stem appears to be similar in most vertebrates, although individual parts and regions may vary greatly in importance and functional specialization. In the lower vertebrates, the brain stem may be the chief area that controls muscular activity. In the higher vertebrates, the stem is an integral part of a system that involves the cerebral cortex, basal ganglia, and cerebellum (Chapter 10).

The cells in the brain stem that are concerned in the control of muscular activity are scattered throughout the reticular formation. Some of the cells, located chiefly in the medulla oblongata, comprise an inhibitory mechanism. The specific cells and nuclei concerned are not completely known. They project to motor nuclei in the brain stem, and to the spinal cord as *reticulospinal tracts.* They exert a powerful depressing influence through connections with anterior horn cells, *gamma* efferent neurons, and interneurons in the intermediate layers.

Other cells in the reticular formation of the medulla oblongata and pons comprise an excitatory mechanism by way of reticulospinal fibers that descend to the spinal cord. In addition, the lateral vestibular nucleus (one of the nuclei in which the vestibular nerve ends) forms a part of the excitatory mechanism, through its projection, the *vestibulospinal tract.*

The concept of inhibitory and excitatory centers that act upon the neurons supplying skeletal muscle is a simplistic, but nevertheless useful, one. It seems likely that the cerebral cortex, basal ganglia, and cerebellum exert many of their peripheral effects by activating, modulating, or inhibiting the brain stem mechanisms.

A number of brain stem functions concerned with posture and movement are carried out reflexly, and some can be demonstrated in isolated form. For example, nystagmus (p. 275) can be brought about by rotating a sitting subject (or by appropriately warming or cooling the ear canals). The rotation stimulates semicircular canals according to the manner discussed previously (p. 275). When rotation begins, the eyes exhibit a form of rhythmic oscillation called nystagmus, which is a series of relatively slow tracking movements, each followed by a rapid (saccadic) movement to a new position. When the rotation reaches a steady state, the nystagmus stops. But when rotation stops, the nystagmus reappears and persists for fifteen to twenty seconds or more. This is a reflex result of postrotational pressure in the semicircular canals. Other types of brain stem reflexes can also be demonstrated in normal subjects. Examples are the jaw jerk (reflex contraction of jaw-closing muscles in response to sudden stretch); the corneal reflex (blinking when a cornea is touched); blinking in response to objects appearing suddenly in the visual fields; and sudden muscular responses to noise.

Integrative brain stem mechanisms, however, are more difficult to demonstrate. One method has been to study animals in which the brain stem is isolated from higher centers. It was pointed out previously (p. 291) that, after spinal cord transection in higher animals, the reflex extensor activity decreases. A different result is obtained, however, if the brain stem is transected at the level of the midbrain, thereby producing a *decerebrate animal.* In such an animal, the brain stem is superimposed on the spinal cord and can influence or modify its functions. Most of the cranial nerves and many of the cerebellar connections are still intact. A decerebrate cat exhibits strong, maintained contractions in extensor muscles, so much so that, if placed upright with the proper support, the limbs can support the body weight. The animal cannot, however, carry out any voluntary locomotor activity. If pushed over, it falls and cannot right itself. It must be fed and, since temperature control is lacking, it must be kept warm. Blood pressure is reflexly maintained, and respiration is slow and deep.

A concept that is rather generally held postulates that the brain stem excitatory and inhibitory mechanisms exhibit autonomous activity when isolated from descending control, and that the excitatory mechanisms involving postural muscles predominate. In other words, the cells in the excitatory centers discharge repetitively to the spinal cord, whereas the cells in the center that inhibits extensor activity are silent and are activated only when impulses from the appropriate sources reach them. In a decerebrate animal, then, impulses continually reach the motor cells supplying antigravity muscles, either stimulating them or so facilitating them as to make them more susceptible to afferent impulses from muscles. Impulses also reach the motor cells giving rise to *gamma* efferents, causing their discharge rate to increase, and thereby increasing the sensitivity of the spindles. The *gamma* system appears to be more easily influenced by impulses from the brain stem than are the large motor cells. Finally, the interneurons involved in reflexes are also influenced by descending impulses.

Decerebrate rigidity can be extinguished or greatly diminished by cutting dorsal roots or the descending motor tracts. Inhibition of muscular activity can also be carried out in a coordinated manner by the spinal cord. If, after decerebration, the spinal cord is transected in the thoracic region, the stretch reflexes and the rigidity of the forelimb become even more marked. Evidently the lumbar portion of the cord inhibits motor cells of the cervical region.

Decerebrate rigidity is seldom seen in humans. When it does occur, it resembles in many respects that which is seen in lower animals. Less severe motor disorders are common, however, and certain aspects are similar to decerebrate rigidity. For example, it was pointed out (p. 214) that in an upper motor neuron lesion, exaggerated deep reflexes and spasticity are characteristic findings. If the causative lesion is in the internal capsule, the result is akin to decerebration in that some of the connections between higher centers and the brain stem are cut so that the excitatory mechanisms become autonomous and the inhibitory ones relatively inactive. The spasticity that is seen is therefore similar to rigidity. Spasticity will also result from a spinal cord lesion when such a lesion destroys the inhibitory paths in the lateral funiculi, leaving only the excitatory ones intact.

The predominance of extensor tone in a decerebrate cat makes normal walking impossible, although phasic types of reflexes and a pattern of locomotion can sometimes be demonstrated, provided that the animal is suspended so as to eliminate the reflex effects of weight acting upon postural muscles. These phasic reflexes, however, are more easily demonstrated if the basal ganglia are present (see later discussion). In a true decerebrate animal, the coordinated reflexes that are readily obtained are static in nature.

STATIC COORDINATED REFLEX ACTIVITY

Local. If a limb of a decerebrate animal touches the ground, it stiffens enough to offer support. The intrinsic mechanisms are stretch reflexes operating locally, initiated by stretch of antigravity muscles and pressure upon the foot. The local reaction may be illustrated in a somewhat different manner. If the animal is supported off the ground and the foot is touched, or slightly pressed, the limb extends. The extension continues as the finger is slowly drawn away, the foot appearing to follow the finger like a magnet. This is the *positive supporting reaction.*

Segmental and Intersegmental. The classic example of the segmental reaction is the crossed extensor reflex. This is obtained in a spinal as well as in a decerebrate cat (p. 292). It may be accompanied by extension of the opposite forelimb, so that there is an intersegmental reaction forming a pattern resembling a phase in locomotion.

General. This includes the reactions to changes in position of the head and neck. These are (1) the tonic neck reflexes, and (2) tonic labyrinthine reflexes.

Tonic neck reflexes are best demonstrated after the labyrinths have been destroyed. If the head is turned to one side, the limbs on that side increase in extensor tone, thus providing a mechanism for supporting the body on the side toward which the cat is looking. The reaction depends upon proprioceptive impulses from the neck muscles on being stretched and from the joints between the cervical vertebrae. Long propriospinal fibers conduct the impulses to the ipsilateral motor neurons.

Tonic labyrinthine reflexes are best shown after the cervical dorsal roots are cut so as to eliminate tonic neck reflexes. Changes in the position of the head are again followed by maintained reactions. If the cat is placed on its back with the head somewhat elevated, a maximal tone appears in the limbs, which become fully extended. In intermediate head positions, the tone is less than maximal. In this particular plane the maculae utriculi are maximally stimulated by gravity. Impulses reach the vestibular areas and thence the motor neurons of the spinal cord. Although these are static and not acceleratory phenomena, there is considerable evidence that the semicircular canals subserve some functions in this instance. If the maculae are destroyed, tonic labyrinthine reflexes may yet be demonstrated. This leads to the concept that acceleratory reactions are predominantly but not entirely vested in the canals and that static reactions are predominantly but not exclusively vested in maculae utriculi. Since extensor tone is maintained as long as the head occupies a position under these conditions, Magnus (p. 326) termed these responses *attitudinal reflexes.* Under most circumstances the tonic neck and labyrinthine reflexes operate together, producing coordinated reactions.

PHASIC COORDINATED REFLEX ACTIVITY

As mentioned above, phasic reflexes are not easily demonstrable in a decerebrate animal. If, instead of transecting the midbrain of an experimental animal, the upper brain stem and basal ganglia are spared (by appropriate section through the thalami, producing what is known as a *thalamic* or *midbrain animal*), dynamic or phasic coordinated reflexes can be more readily demonstrated. These are displayed in the ability of the cat to right itself, or to return to a standing position after changes in position, and to carry out a fairly well-coordinated type of locomotion. In a normal animal, these reactions can be analyzed by excluding first one and then another of the various sensory and reflex fields. It must be emphasized that in the absence of cerebral cortex they depend upon the basal ganglia and the cerebellum, acting upon the lower brain stem mechanisms. The dynamic reactions are also known as *righting reflexes,* of which there are five types, as follows.

Labyrinthine-Righting Reflexes. If an animal is blindfolded and placed in any position off the ground, the head returns to the normal horizontal position. The midbrain and the labyrinths appear to be essential for this reaction.

Body-Righting Reflexes Acting on the Head. The labyrinths must be destroyed. If the blindfolded animal is then placed on its side, the head assumes a normal position. But this can be prevented if a board is placed on the upper surface of the body with enough pressure to equalize the pressure of the body weight exerted on that surface lying on the ground. The reflex depends then upon unequal stimulation of pressure receptors in the body.

Neck-Righting Reflexes. If the neck has once been turned in response to labyrinthine-or body-righting reflexes, proprioceptive receptors in the neck muscles are stimulated. This is followed by a reflex rotation that brings the body into line with the head and neck.

Body-Righting Reflexes Acting on the Body. In order to demonstrate these fully, the labyrinths must be destroyed and the animal blindfolded. If the forelimbs and shoulder are placed lateral to the ground, the hindlimbs tend to rotate to the horizontal position. This reaction can be prevented by equalizing the pressure with a board, as before.

Optic-Righting Reflexes. In the tests listed above, animals are blindfolded to exclude optic-righting reflexes. These are important in the normal animal, but, since they depend upon the cerebral cortex, they are absent in a midbrain animal. If the labyrinths are removed and cervical dorsal roots sectioned in an otherwise normal animal, righting reflexes can be demonstrated when the eyes are open, but not if the animal is blindfolded.

Primates differ from quadrupeds in that a midbrain primate, even though exhibiting righting reflexes, cannot stand. The loss of cerebral cortex is much more important than it is in lower vertebrates.

AUTONOMIC FUNCTIONS OF THE BRAIN STEM

Many of the cells in the reticular formation are concerned with autonomic activities. The cells are smaller than somatic motor neurons, but like them, are scattered throughout the pons and medulla, so that cells subserving somatic functions and those serving autonomic functions may lie side by side. Some of the autonomic cells are involved in relatively simple reflex mechanisms. For instance, certain cells scattered in the upper medulla and lower pons near the tractus solitarius form the *salivatory nuclei.* Their axons form preganglionic parasympathetic fibers that reach cranial parasympathetic ganglia by way of the facial and glossopharyngeal nerves; the postganglionic fibers supply salivary glands and control secretory processes in these glands. The cells of the salivatory nuclei may be reflexly activated by impulses resulting from taste or smell, or psychically by impulses from the cerebral cortex. The psychic influence is usually inhibitory, as, for example, dryness of the mouth in many emotional states. The salivatory system was extensively used by Pavlov (p. 326) in his studies of conditioned responses.

The purpose of the following discussion is to present certain examples of important intrinsic autonomic functions of the brain stem which are coordinated with somatic mechanisms. A broader coverage of central and peripheral autonomic mechanisms is provided in Chapter 15.

CONTROL OF RESPIRATION

Although the muscles of respiration are skeletal in type, the respiratory process itself is reflexly controlled. No one can voluntarily stop breathing to the point of asphyxiation. The following brief account of respiratory mechanisms is based mainly upon studies carried out in the cat, but there is reason to suppose that similar mechanisms are present in humans.

Scattered throughout the reticular formation, dorsal to the olivary nuclei, are small neurons that project to those motor neurons in the cervical part of the spinal cord which give rise to the phrenic nerves that supply the diaphragm. The reticular neurons also project to those cells in the thoracic part of the spinal cord which supply the intercostal and abdominal musculature.

If groups of the reticular neurons are stimulated with electric currents, two different effects can be demonstrated, depending upon the placement of the electrodes. More caudally placed stimuli produce inspiratory movements that are maintained for the duration of the stimulus. The neurons that are stimulated form *inspiratory centers,* one in each half of the medulla (Fig. 14–5). More cephalically placed stimuli in the medulla cause expiratory movements, and the cells mediating this activity form *expiratory centers,* which project to the same regions of the spinal cord.

The inspiratory centers appear to be dominant (perhaps reflecting the fact that in quiet breathing, expiration is chiefly a function of the intrinsic elasticity of the lungs). If the respiratory centers are isolated from all afferent impulses, the inspiratory

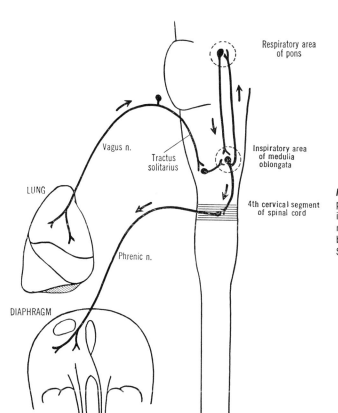

Respiratory area of pons

Vagus n.

Tractus solitarius

Inspiratory area of medulla oblongata

LUNG

4th cervical segment of spinal cord

Phrenic n.

DIAPHRAGM

Figure 14–5. Schematic, simplified diagram of the pathways in a respiratory reflex. The terminals in the lung are stimulated by expansion during inspiration. See text for description.

centers discharge continuously, and the animal dies in a state of prolonged inspiration. Normal respiration is reflexly controlled by modifying the intrinsic activity of these centers.

Within the lungs there are interoceptive receptors that are sensitive to the stretch resulting from the expansion of the lungs during respiration. The nerve impulses that result traverse the vagi, enter each tractus solitarius of the medulla oblongata, and are relayed to the respiratory centers. When the impulses reach a certain frequency, they inhibit the inspiratory center. Inspiration, therefore, lessens and stops; expiration supervenes. The stimulation of lung receptors naturally decreases in intensity. Below a certain frequency the inhibition of inspiratory centers lessens and they again resume activity.

If the vagi are cut, respiration slows and deepens, but does not stop. It stops only when the brain stem is transected immediately above the medullary centers. In each side of the pons there is a respiratory center that receives fibers from the medullary centers and in turn projects to them. These pontine centers, upon receipt of impulses at or above a certain frequency, discharge to and inhibit the inspiratory centers. Expiration thus intervenes. Hence, either vagal impulses or pontine centers can produce fairly normal respiration, but, if both are absent, the animal dies in prolonged inspiration.

That the cervical cord is unable to maintain respiration automatically is shown as follows: If the cord is severed just below the fourth or fifth cervical segment, respiration continues because the control of the diaphragm is intact. But if the transection is above this level, the fibers descending from the medulla oblongata are severed. Death rapidly follows because of the asphyxia resulting from failure of respiration. This explains why transections of the cord high in the cervical levels are rapidly fatal in humans. It also explains why medullary lesions may be fatal if they involve much of the reticular formation.

The respiratory centers receive impulses from higher centers, so that their activity may be considerably modified, either voluntarily or during emotional stress, but in neither case can reflex functions be completely suppressed.

The respiratory centers are directly sensitive to gaseous tensions in the blood flowing through them. Thus, an increase in carbon dioxide in the lungs is followed by an increase of carbon dioxide in the blood and then by an increase in the rate and depth of respiration which serves to blow off the excess carbon dioxide.

At the bifurcation of each common carotid artery is a small tissue mass, the *carotid body*, which contains receptors that are likewise sensitive to changes in gaseous tensions of the blood flowing by them. The impulses traverse the glossopharyngeal nerves to the respiratory centers and result in reflex mechanisms similar to those cited in the preceding paragraph.

Respiration thus illustrates a marvelous coordination of complex somatic and visceral functions. An example of an equally important coordinated activity is given below in a discussion of the digestive system.

CONTROL OF MOVEMENTS IN THE DIGESTIVE SYSTEM

When food enters the mouth and is tasted and smelled, or even before it enters the mouth, saliva reflexly flows into the oral cavity. Its contained enzymes begin the digestion of certain constituents of the food.

Swallowing initiates other types of reflexes. The first part of swallowing is the thrusting of food into the oral pharynx by the tongue. The impact of the food upon the walls of the pharynx stimulates receptors in the walls. The nerve impulses reach the medulla oblongata over the vagus and glossopharyngeal nerves, and are distributed to special visceral efferent cells in the motor nuclei of these nerves. There is then set into play a complex series of involuntary muscular actions. The palate and upper part of the pharynx constrict so as to prevent food from entering the nasal cavity. The upper part of the larynx constricts so as to shut off passage to the lungs. The muscles around the bolus of food contract, while those immediately ahead of it relax so as to receive it. The wave of contraction, preceded by a wave of relaxation, proceeds from the pharynx into the esophagus and thence to the stomach. The timing of this mechanism is even more intricate when one realizes that initially the activity involves striated muscle, but that in the middle of the esophagus the musculature becomes smooth. Hence the impulses shift from the special visceral efferents of these nerves to the general visceral efferents of the vagus nerves (from the dorsal motor nuclei). Furthermore, sympathetic fibers are involved, because inhibition of the muscles, as evidenced by the wave of relaxation, is a function (at least in part) of the sympathetic system. Impulses descend from the medulla oblongata to the thoracic cord, then out to the sympathetic ganglia and eventually to the esophagus. This type of activity, in which there is a wave of relaxation preceding a wave of contraction, is known as *peristalsis,* and is one of the fundamental types of coordinated activity of the digestive system, especially in the gastrointestinal canal. Here, at junctional areas (e. g., gastroesophageal, pyloroduodenal, ileocecal), sphincter activity is coordinated with peristaltic activity. The sphincters must open at appropriate times, and the contraction and relaxation of the smooth muscle of the sphincters is under both neural and humoral control.

Gastrointestinal movements may be reversed in vomiting. This is accompanied by simultaneous contraction of the external abdominal muscles and descent of the diaphragm, thereby increasing the intra-abdominal pressure and forcing intestinal contents orally. Whether or not vomiting results from activity of a special center is unknown, although cells in the area postrema are thought to be involved. Vomiting may be reflexly induced by impulses resulting from irritation of gastric mucosa, from putrid odors, and so forth. There is a drug, *apomorphine,* which induces vomiting by acting directly on certain brain stem cells (e.g., cells in the area postrema are known to be sensitive to apomorphine). Increased intracranial pressure may stimulate these cells, so that otherwise unexplained violent vomiting is an important sign of increased intracranial pressure.

THE RETICULAR ACTIVATING SYSTEM, THE BIOGENIC AMINE SYSTEM, AND STATES OF CONSCIOUSNESS

RETICULAR ACTIVATING SYSTEM

The term *reticular formation* refers to an anatomical arrangement of cells and fibers which forms the central portion or core of the brain stem, which receives diffuse, multisynaptic inputs from the spinal cord, and which projects diffusely to the spinal cord and to more rostral structures. The term *reticular activating system* refers to a physiological system. Stimulation of various areas of the midbrain portion of the reticular formation leads, in unanesthetized animals, to an arousal reaction—that is, a sleeping animal awakens. The arousal reaction is accompanied by a desynchronization of the electroencephalogram (p. 379). Thus, it appears that the reticular activating system plays an important role in conscious states and attention. There has developed substantial evidence that the reticular activating system is a function of the reticular formation, and that its effects upon the cerebral cortex depend also upon certain thalamic nuclei (non-specific thalamic nuclei) that relay to the thalamus. Moreover, it seems likely that the reticular activating system projects to the limbic system and that it plays a role in behavioral mechanisms (see p. 236 for a discussion of pain mechanisms).

It has long been supposed that general anesthetics are effective because they depress the reticular activating system, and thereby secondarily depress the cerebral cortex. (Some anesthetics, however, continue to depress the cortex in decerebrate animals.)

What has been lacking is a correlation between the reticular activating system and localizable groups of neurons. It now appears that activating mechanisms and maintenance of consciousness may be a function, at least in part, of brain stem neurons that synthesize monoamines and that neurons synthesizing acetycholine may also play an important role.

MONOAMINERGIC AND CHOLINERGIC SYSTEMS

The monoamines (also called biogenic amines) include the catecholamines, norepinephrine and dopamine, and the indole amine, serotonin. They have already been discussed in Chapters 4 and 5. They are uniquely important because of their role in animal and human behavior, and because many (perhaps most) of the central nervous system cells that synthesize the monoamines have been identified. The cellular localization of the amines followed upon the development of histochemical fluorescence methods. When these amines are exposed in tissue sections to formaldehyde under appropriately humid conditions, they condense to form intensely fluorescent isoquinoles. The color of the fluorescence differs according to the wavelength of the fluorescence. Thus, serotonin appears bright yellow, and the catecholamines bright green. The method permits the localization of the cell bodies and their axons; the findings have been confirmed by experiments employing surgical or biochemical lesions, and also by study of clinical disorders (e.g., parkinsonism, p. 387).

There are three major groups of monoamine-synthesizing neurons. We have gained our knowledge of them chiefly through experiments on rats; there is substantial evidence, however, that the arrangements in humans are similar.

Norepinephrine.   Groups of neurons that synthesize norepinephrine are found throughout the lateral portions of the reticular formation of the brain stem (Fig. 14–6), especially in the locus ceruleus. The axons of the norepinephrine-synthesizing cells have a widespread distribution to the spinal cord, cerebellum (here they appear to inhibit Purkinje cells), and forebrain (Fig. 14–7). A major rostral pathway is by way of the medial forebrain bundle (Fig. 17–12, p. 391), and the heaviest projections are to the hypothalamus and limbic system. Terminals are also present in the neocortex.

Dopamine.   The neurons that synthesize dopamine form three well-defined groups (Figs. 14–7, 14–8). Two are present in the midbrain. One is in the compact zone of the substantia nigra and projects to the striatum and amygdaloid body; the other is in the limbic midbrain area and projects to nuclei in the septum and anterior perforated substance. A third group of dopamine-synthesizing cells is located in the arcuate nuclei of the hypothalamus (p. 333); their axons project to the median eminence (p. 351). Other dopamine projections may also be present in the brain (e. g., to the neocortex), but as yet are not definitely known.

Serotonin.   The serotonin-synthesizing neurons are located in and near the median plane of the brain stem in what are termed

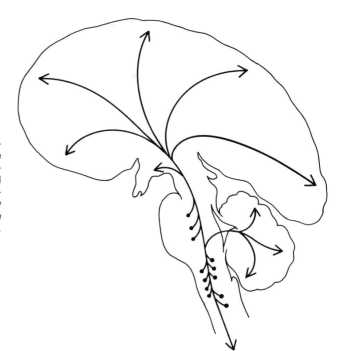

Figure 14–6. Schematic representation of the location in the brain stem of neurons that synthesize norepinephrine. Lateral view. Note the widespread distribution of axons (indicated by arrows) to the spinal cord, the cerebellum, and the forebrain.

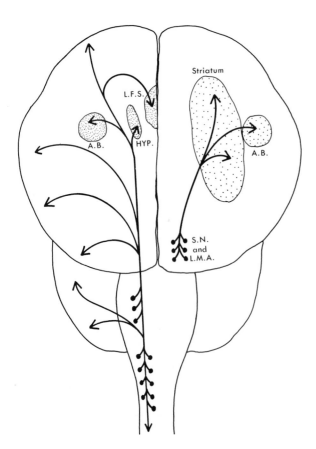

Figure 14–7. Schematic representation of a posterior view of the location in the brain stem of cells that synthesize norepinephrine (left side) and dopamine (right side). The norepinephrine cells are distributed to the spinal cord, cerebellum, and forebrain (as shown also in Figure 14–6); the forebrain distribution is to the amygdaloid body (A.B.), the hypothalamus (HYP.), and the limbic forebrain system (L.F.S.). The dopamine cells shown in this view occur in the substantia nigra (S.N.) and limbic midbrain area (L.M.A.). Their axons are distributed chiefly to the striatum and amygdaloid body (A.B.). Dopamine cells in the hypothalamus are shown in Figure 14–8.

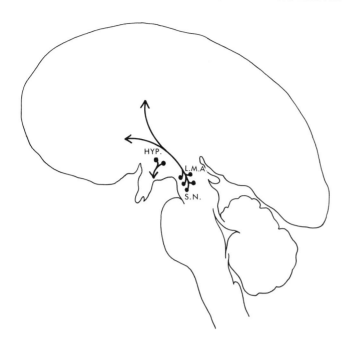

Figure 14–8. Schematic representation of a lateral view of the location of dopamine-synthesizing cells in the midbrain (see Figure 14–7) and in the hypothalamus (HYP.). S.N. indicates substantia nigra, and L.M.A., limbic midbrain area.

the *raphe nuclei.* Their axons are distributed to essentially the same regions as the norepinephrine cells.

Functions. The three biochemical systems have extraordinary significance for behavior, states of consciousness, and mental disorders. Moreover, they function in an integrated manner in a variety of somatic and autonomic mechanisms. However, the cells are not uniform in function. That is to say, some norepinephrine-synthesizing cells, even in the same nuclear configuration, carry out certain functions, whereas other such cells may have different functions. Many of the functions of these three biochemical systems remain to be determined. Nevertheless, the following generalizations can be made.

All of the biochemical systems are important to states of consciousness.

The nigrostriatal dopaminergic pathway is involved in the control of muscular activity by the basal ganglia (Chapter 17).

The norepinephrine projections to the hypothalamus, and the dopamine neurons within the hypothalamus, are involved in neuroendocrinological mechanisms.

Projections from the rostral portion of the brain stem (probably norepinephrine-synthesizing cells in the midbrain) project to the thalamus and neocortex and probably represent the reticular activating system.

The important role of the biochemical pathways in behavior was introduced in the discussion of pain (p. 240), and is emphasized by the fact that depletion of the biogenic amines can precipitate profound depression. Selective biochemical destruction of the central catecholamine cells and fibers (by injection of 6-hydroxydopamine in the central nervous system of experimental animals) leads to significant behavioral changes. Bilateral destruction of the locus ceruleus may be followed by impaired learning. The activation of certain catecholamine cells appears to be essential for intracranial self-stimulation (electrical stimulation through implanted electrodes); the cells that are most essential are in the midbrain limbic area, the nigrostriatal system (thus, dopamine plays a role in behavior as well as in motor control), and the locus ceruleus.

The continuing elucidation of the biochemical pathways has helped to clarify the actions of psychopharmacological drugs (drugs that act on the central nervous system and that influence or modify behavior, perception, affect, and state of consciousness). Among such drugs, few have been as important as the major tranquilizers or *neuroleptics*. *Reserpine* is one such drug (p. 110); it brings about a depletion of biogenic amines. The antipsychotic actions of various major tranquilizers can be classified according to their ability to blockade the dopamine or norepinephrine receptors, and it seems clear that dopamine receptor-blockade is essential for effective antipsychotic action. Large numbers of *phenothiazine* drugs have been used in the treatment of psychoses, and many have severe extrapyramidal side effects because of their interference with the dopaminergic nigrostriatal pathway (p. 387).

A number of drugs are used as antidepressants. *Monoamine oxidase inhibitors* are an important class of antidepressant drugs. *Amphetamine* and some related compounds have long been used as psychological stimulants and hallucinogenic agents. Amphetamine has several major effects upon monoamine storage and release, and is also a monoamine oxidase inhibitor. In large doses, it can produce a psychosis that is clinically indistinguishable from an acute paranoid schizophrenia. It can exacerbate the symptoms of schizophrenic patients, even when only small doses are used.

There are many hallucinogenic drugs, and some of them (e.g., *lysergic acid diethylamide*, LSD) appear to act upon the monoaminergic systems.

Acetylcholine. This important transmitter is known to be synthesized by motor neurons (p. 104). Based upon histochemical localization of acetylcholinesterase, it also seems likely that cholinergic neurons have a wide distribution in the brain stem and forebrain (especially in the tegmentum and basal ganglia), although identification and location are less precise than in the case of the monoaminergic neurons.

STATES OF CONSCIOUSNESS

The conscious state can scarcely be defined in neurophysiological terms. It is psychological as well as physiological and cannot be ascribed to a specific "center" in the central nervous system. There are, however, pathological changes in the state of consciousness that are of clinical importance, and which follow brain stem damage. It has long been known, for example, that injury to the upper brain stem, especially its central portion, can produce an enduring loss of consciousness termed *coma*. Moreover, there are lesser degrees of change that may follow damage to the same regions, and a variety of drugs can induce similar changes. The purpose of the following discussion, however, is to call attention to sleep, which is a circadian alteration in state of consciousness, one that is dependent in part upon brain stem mechanisms.

Sleep is an example of a circadian rhythm that occurs in reptiles, birds, and mammals, and which involves the monoaminergic systems of the brain stem. (It does not necessarily occur at night; many animals are nocturnal and sleep during the day.) In mammals, sleep follows a characteristic pattern known as the basic sleep cycle, which can be classified according to the presence of rapid eye movements (*REM sleep*), and to the absence of such movements, (*NREM sleep*). In human NREM sleep, the brain is relatively quiet and muscles show electrical and reflex activity. In REM sleep, the brain is extremely active and rapid eye movements occur, but skeletal muscles are inhibited and areflexic. Usually there is a regular alternation between NREM sleep and REM sleep. Each alternation (basic sleep cycle) lasts from 70 to 120 minutes (average about 90), and is usually repeated four to six times during the night. The cyclic pattern is established before birth, and infants show a much higher percentage of REM sleep than do adults.

The onset of sleep is normally of the NREM type; it is arbitrarily divided into four stages, as follows: (1) Drowsiness, with a relatively low voltage electroencephalograph (EEG, p. 381); (2) increasing drowsiness. With the beginning of deep sleep, sleep "spindles" appear in the EEG; (3) and (4) deep sleep, with high voltage, slow waves in the EEG. Some dreaming may occur during NREM sleep.

NREM deep sleep then gives way to REM sleep, which lasts about 20 or 30 minutes. Rapid eye movements are present and the muscles of the middle ear may be active, but tone is lost in most other muscles. Dreams are a characteristic feature, the EEG is fast and asynchronous, autonomic activity is noticeably increased (the brain is awake and the muscles are paralyzed), and large spike discharges occur in the pons, lateral geniculate body, and visual cortex. When REM sleep ends, another cycle begins. During the night, the length of REM sleep usually increases, and the depth of sleep may not be as great (perhaps only stages 3 or 2 are reached in NREM sleep).

Experimental work indicates that sleep is an active process that is dependent upon neurons in the hypothalamus and basal forebrain the activity of which is strongly controlled and modulated by elements of the monoaminergic and cholinergic systems. In addition, the medial and spinal vestibular nuclei appear to be essential in the production of rapid eye movements, and the inhibitory neurons of the reticular formation are responsible for the general loss of muscle tone.

Serotonin-synthesizing cells seem to be necessary for the induction of NREM sleep, especially its slow wave stages, although the mechanisms by which this is brought about remain unknown. Destruction of raphe nuclei results in an *insomnia* that is proportional to the extent of destruction. Serotonin also seems to be necessary, in some unknown way, for the onset of REM sleep, although the actual production of this stage of sleep is controlled by the norepinephrine-synthesizing cells. (Cholinergic neurons may also be involved.) It is known that cells of the locus ceruleus fire slowly during drowsiness and deep sleep, but in rapid bursts during REM sleep, and that REM sleep disappears if they are destroyed.

Aside from the fact that sleep undoubtedly permits some restoration of the brain, the functions of sleep are still a mystery. Sleep deprivation results in few organic changes; the effects are mostly psychological. The nature and purpose of REM sleep have attracted much attention. An interesting and likely hypothesis has been presented that REM sleep is a mechanism that aids in establishing the neuromuscular coordination necessary for voluntary conjugate eye movements, and ensuring, throughout life, a periodic reinforcing before awakening. This hypothesis helps to explain the prominence of REM sleep in infants, in whom precise coordination has to be developed, and the decreasing prominence of REM sleep throughout adult life.

Disorders of sleep are common and often serious, and range, for example, from insomnia to *narcolepsy*. Narcolepsy is a sleep attack that is characterized by a sudden change from wakefulness directly to REM sleep.

SUMMARY

The spinal cord becomes the medulla oblongata at the foramen magnum. Above this level the major tracts are topographically rearranged and nuclei of cranial nerves appear. Functional components found in spinal nerves are also present in certain cranial nerves. In addition, there are others: special visceral efferent supplying pharyngeal arch muscles; special visceral afferent (taste and smell); and special somatic afferent (hearing, balance, and vision).

The medulla oblongata is in part a rostral continuation of the spinal cord. Associated with the ninth to twelfth cranial nerves, it contains an important core of reticular formation, it is the site of much of the trigeminal sensory complex, and it is distinguished by the olivary nuclei, which have major projections to the cerebellum by way of the inferior cerebellar peduncles.

The posterior portion of the pons, with its reticular formation, is a rostral continuation of the medulla oblongata. The anterior portion is prominent, owing to the pyramidal fibers descending through it, and the presence of pontine nuclei, from which axons extend to form the middle cerebellar peduncles.

The midbrain consists of the cerebral peduncles in front and the roof behind. The peduncles each consist of tegmentum, substantia nigra, and crus cerebri, and the superior cerebellar peduncles cross as they ascend through them. The medial portions of the tegmenta, together with the ventral portion of the peri-aqueductal gray, form the midbrain limbic area. The red nuclei, which are located in the tegmentum, project to the brain stem and spinal cord, and are involved in the control of movement. The roof contains the superior and inferior colliculi, which are concerned with visual and auditory mechanisms, respectively. The superior colliculi are involved in the location and tracking of movement.

The trigeminal sensory complex is responsible for the general sensory components from the head and neck. The fibers enter the brain stem over the fifth, ninth, and tenth cranial nerves and form the spinal tract; the fibers end in the main sensory and spinal nuclei. The spinal nucleus is continuous caudally with the substantia gelatinosa. The cutaneous distribution of the trigeminal nerve forms a dermatome; its contiguous dorsal roots are the second to fourth cervical. Central summation is involved, just as in the spinal cord.

The reticular formation, including the vestibular nuclei, contains motor neurons, some of which are excitatory in function and others inhibitory. A decerebrate animal is one in which the brain stem is sectioned between the basal ganglia and the reticular formation. The excitatory mechanisms become active, the inhibitory mechanisms relatively silent, and the result is an increased, exaggerated postural activity termed decerebrate rigidity. The reticular formation mechanisms are modified by impulses from the labyrinths, the paleocerebellum, the midbrain, and the cerebral hemispheres, so that a variety of static reflexes can be demonstrated. Coordinated phasic mechanisms can take place if the midbrain and basal ganglia connections are intact.

Many cells in the reticular formation of the brain stem subserve visceral functions. The most important of these are the control of blood pressure, cardiac activity, respiration, and alimentary movements. Still other reticular cells are concerned with many aspects of consciousness, attention, and behavior. There are three groups of such cells that are now known to synthesize norepinephrine, dopamine, and serotonin; cholinergic cells are also present in the brain stem and forebrain. The norepinephrine cells, which are located laterally in the brain stem, including the locus ceruleus, project to the spinal cord, cerebellum, and forebrain. The serotonin cells, located in raphe nuclei, project to the same regions. The dopamine cells, located chiefly in the midbrain, project to the striatum and limbic system. Others, in the hypothalamus, project to the median eminence.

Depletion of the biogenic amines can lead to profound depression, and drugs that stimulate the system can bring about acute psychotic states. The antipsychotic drugs, e.g., the phenothiazines, act by dopamine-receptor blockade.

The reticular activating system is important in states of consciousness having circadian changes which include sleep. Normal sleep, which is dependent (at least in part) upon the combined functions of the serotonin, norepinephrine, and cholinergic systems, follows a characteristic pattern, the basic sleep cycle. There are four to six such cycles per night, each consisting of a regular alternation between NREM sleep (quiet brain and potentially excitable muscles) and REM sleep (active brain, rapid eye movements, dreams, and atonic muscles).

NAMES IN NEUROLOGY

RUDOLPH MAGNUS (1873–1927)

Born in Germany, Magnus studied medicine mainly at Heidelberg, where he carried out research on the cardiovascular, renal, and intestinal systems. He also studied pituitary functions during a stay in Edinburgh. In 1908, shortly after a winter spent at Liverpool with Sherrington working on reflexes, he was appointed professor of pharmacology at Utrecht. There he began his classic experiments on the reflexes of balance and on the whole question of body posture, as well as studies on choline and the effects of drugs on the nervous system. His experiments proved to be the foundation for modern studies of posture, locomotion, and vestibular functions.

IVAN PETROVICH PAVLOV (1849–1936)

Born in central Russia, Pavlov studied medicine in St. Petersburg (now Leningrad). After receiving his M.D. there, he spent two years in Germany, studying the circulatory system in Leipzig, and gastrointestinal secretion in Breslau. In 1891, he became director of the physiology department in the Institute for Experimental Medicine in St. Petersburg. Working with animals, he devised an operative procedure for gastric and pancreatic fistulas which left the nerve supply intact. In animals, if the esophagus is severed, gastric reactions with and without food can be studied. Pavlov later devised a fistula for salivary ducts and over many years carried out his famous experiments on conditioned responses and higher levels of nervous function. In 1904 he was awarded the Nobel Prize, as much for his important contributions for physiology as for his studies of conditioned reflexes.

REFERENCES

See also the references cited on pages 159 and 418.

The following two references are classical reviews of pioneering studies of brain stem mechanisms in motor control.

Magoun, H. W.: Caudal and cephalic influences of the brain stem reticular formation. Physiol. Rev., *30*:459–474, 1950.

Magoun, H. W., and Rhines, R.: Spasticity: The Stretch Reflex and Extrapyramidal Systems. Springfield, Ill., Charles C Thomas, 1947.

These following references are excellent source books.

Granit, R.: The Basis of Motor Control. New York, Academic Press, 1970.

Kales, A. (editor): Sleep. Physiology and Pathology. Philadelphia, J. B. Lippincott Company, 1969.

Leavitt, F.: Drugs and Behavior. Philadelphia, W. B. Saunders Company, 1974.

Longo, V. C.: Neuropharmacology and Behavior. San Francisco, W. H. Freeman and Company, 1972.

The following are important reviews and analyses of important topics and issues.

Armstrong, D. M.: Functional significance of the connections of the inferior olive. Physiol. Rev., *54*:358-417, 1974.

Berger, R. J.: Oculomotor control: a possible function of REM sleep. Psychol. Rev., *76*:144-164, 1969.

German, D. C. and Bowden, D. M.: Catecholamine systems as the neural substrate for intracranial self-stimulation: A hypothesis. Brain Res., *73*:381-419, 1974.

Gordon, B.: The superior colliculus of the brain. Sci. Amer., *227*:72-82, 1972.

Jouvet, M.: Neurophysiology of the state of sleep. Physiol. Rev., *47*:117-177, 1967. The role of monoamines and acetylcholine-containing neurons in the regulation of the sleep-waking cycle. Ergebr. Physiol., *64*:166–307, 1972.

Massion, J.: The mammalian red nucleus. Physiol. Rev., *47*:383-436, 1967.

Moruzzi, G.: The sleep-waking cycle. Ergebr. Physiol., *64*:1-165, 1972.

Schildkraut, J. J.: Neuropharmacology of the affective disorders. Ann. Rev. Pharmacol., *13*:427-454, 1973.

Snyder, S. H., Banerjee, S. P., Yamamura, H. I. and Greenberg, D.: Drugs, neurotransmitters, and schizophrenia. Science, *184*:1243-1253, 1974.

Walshe, F. M. R.: The neurophysiological approach to the problem of consciousness. pp. 181–189, in M. Critchley, J. O'Leary, and B. Jennett (editors). Scientific Foundations of Neurology. Philadelphia, F. A. Davis Company, 1972.

Zarcone, V.: Narcolepsy. New Engl. J. Med., *288*:1156–1166, 1973.

The following are key scientific papers.

Denny-Brown, D., and Yanagisawa, N.: The function of the descending root of the fifth nerve. Brain, *96*:783-814, 1973.

Miller, R. A., and Strominger, N. L.: Efferent connections of the red nucleus in the brain stem and spinal cord of the rhesus monkey. J. comp. Neurol., *152*:327-346, 1973.

Nauta, W. J. H.: Hippocampal projections and related neural pathways to the mid-brain in the cat. Brain, *81*:319-340, 1958.

Nieuwenhuys, R.: Topological analysis of the brain stem: a general introduction. J. comp. Neurol., *156*:255-276, 1974.

Nobin, A., and Björklund, A.: Topography of the monoamine neuron systems in the human brain as revealed in fetuses. Acta physiol., scand., Suppl. 388, 1973.

Olson, L., Boreus, L. O., and Seiger, Å.: Histochemical demonstration and mapping of 5-hydroxytryptamine– and catecholamine– containing neuron systems in the human fetal brain. Z. Anat. Entw. Gesch., *139*:259-282, 1973.

Ungerstedt, U.: Stereotaxic mapping of the monoamine pathways in the rat brain. Acta Physiol., scand., Suppl. 367, 1971.

Chapter 15

AUTONOMIC AND NEUROENDOCRINE FUNCTIONS

The nervous system has three major effector systems. One system is that which supplies skeletal muscle. The other two are the autonomic nervous system and the neuroendocrinological system. These two are key elements in the mechanisms whereby the body keeps its internal environment (*milieu intérieur* of Bernard) constant. That is, they help to maintain temperature, fluid balance, ionic composition of the blood, and other internal processes. The maintenance of the internal environment is termed *homeostasis*.

AUTONOMIC NERVOUS SYSTEM

The autonomic nervous system supplies the viscera and is sometimes called the visceral nervous system. The term viscera is a general one, and is difficult to define precisely. Anatomically, the term refers to the organs that contain cardiac muscle fibers, smooth muscle, and glands. The term autonomic also carries an implication that this part of the nervous system deals with processes not under voluntary control. The distinction, however, is more apparent than real. Many muscles (e. g., the diaphragm) are not subject to complete voluntary control. Organs containing smooth muscle may be as much under voluntary influence or control as many so-called voluntary muscles. Moreover, certain organs, such as the pharynx and esophagus, contain striated muscle but are classified as viscera. Skin, which is usually not classified as a viscus, contains many glands and smooth muscle fibers. Blood vessels often have smooth muscle fibers.

In its narrow sense, then, the term viscera refers to the heart, and to the organs and tissues containing smooth muscle and glands, which are controlled or regulated by the autonomic nervous system. (The autonomic control of endocrine glands is considered under neuroendocrine mechanisms.) In the broader sense, the term visceral activity is more useful. However ill-defined it may be or how unaware of it one may be, visceral activity is a complex pattern involving sensory and motor nerve fibers, many parts of the central nervous system, and various neuroendocrinological mechanisms. The regulation of body temperature is an excellent example of such a complex pattern of activity.

Cold-blooded vertebrates, such as fishes, amphibians, and reptiles, have body temperatures that vary with the ambient temperature. Warm-blooded animals, such as birds and mammals, keep their body temperatures constant within certain limits and are therefore to some extent independent of their thermal environment. Heat production and heat loss are relatively balanced. The heat that is produced by metabolic activity is lost chiefly through radiation from the blood vessels that lie near the surface of the body. A certain amount of heat is also lost with the evaporation of sweat, through the air and water vapor exhaled from the lungs, and with the excreta. If more blood flows through the surface vessels per unit of time, and especially if more vessels are made available for blood to flow through, more heat will be lost by radiation. The autonomic nervous system can regulate the caliber of the blood vessels by, for example, activating the smooth muscle of the vessels with a resultant narrowing of the diameter of the vessels. It can also control special vessels that act as shunts. If these shunts are closed, blood is diverted to the surface vessels.

This overall control of blood flow may be initiated in a number of ways. For example, skin exposed to cold air becomes blanched or pale, owing to a reflex constriction of the vessels in it, coupled with an opening of the vascular shunts. This reflex action involves a pathway of the type shown in Figure 15–1. The cold air stimulates thermoreceptors. The resulting nerve impulses reach the spinal cord or brain stem where they activate motor cells of the autonomic nervous system. These cells send fibers to peripheral ganglia, the cells of which send postganglionic fibers that activate the smooth muscle of the surface vessels, thereby constricting them and narrowing their lumen. At the same time, some fibers activate the smooth muscle of the shunts so that these vessels open and divert blood away from the surface vessels. The resultant decrease in heat radiation helps to maintain the internal body temperature, although the skin may be cold, both subjectively and objectively.

The foregoing brief description illustrates a complete reflex mechanism, the output of which is by way of the autonomic

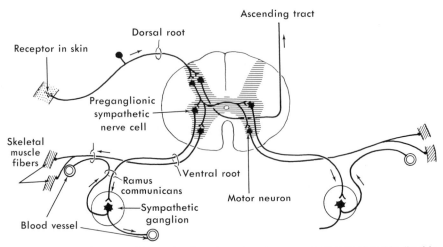

Figure 15–1. Diagram illustrating how impulses from a receptor in the skin (in this case a temperature receptor) reach motor neurons supplying skeletal muscles and also neurons in the intermediate gray matter. By way of these connections the impulses reach smooth muscle in blood vessels of the trunk and limbs. The impulses may also reach the brain.

nervous system. It illustrates that this output consists, in its simplest form, of a pathway of two succeeding nerve cells. The first cell is located in the brain or spinal cord, the second in a ganglion outside of the brain and spinal cord (both are classified as general visceral efferent components). The axons of the first cells are termed *preganglionic fibers.* The axons of the ganglion cells, which form the neuro-effector junctions, are termed *postganglionic fibers.*

The locations, arrangements, and connections of the two nerve cell pathways form the basis of an anatomical classification or subdivision of the autonomic nervous system into *sympathetic* and *parasympathetic systems* (Fig. 15–2). Anatomically and functionally, however, the autonomic nervous system is much broader than the simplistic classification given above would indicate. The motor fibers comprising this system are closely associated with sensory fibers in all of their functions and are an integral part of the entire nervous system, being activated by nerve impulses arising reflexly at local levels or from higher centers of the brain.

In carrying out its general functions, the autonomic nervous system is concerned with a number of specific regulatory functions, such as body temperature, blood pressure, respiration, digestion, intermediate metabolism of foods, and excretion. It enables the body to handle emergencies or sudden environmental changes and is thus an important feature of the mechanisms by which a person reacts to stress. Finally, the autonomic nervous system is an integral feature of behavioral and emotional actions and responses. It must be emphasized that in all of these activities, sensory fibers and sensory mechanisms are indispensable fea-

tures. Most viscera have sensory fibers arising from them, some
concerned with pain but many concerned with reflex mechanisms.
These fibers (general visceral afferent) reach the brain and spinal
cord by traveling in autonomic and peripheral nerves, often
side-by-side with autonomic fibers.

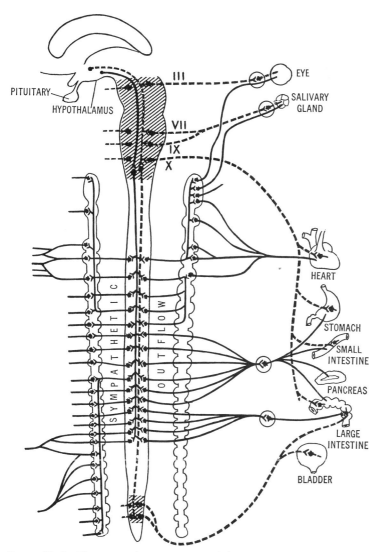

Figure 15-2. The general arrangement of the autonomic nervous system. The projections from the hypothalamus to the pituitary gland have
been omitted, while those to lower centers are shown in solid lines (sympathetic) and broken lines (parasympathetic). The portions of the brain
stem and sacral cord from which the parasympathetic preganglionic
fibers leave are indicated by oblique lines, and the sympathetic outflow
from the thoracic and upper lumbar cord is labeled. Autonomic fibers to
organs of the head and trunk are shown on the right side, while those on
the left side represent the sympathetic outflow to blood vessels, sweat
glands, and smooth muscle fibers attached to hairs.

For purposes of simplicity, the autonomic nervous system is presented as if it were a series of physiological and anatomical levels that differ in function in that the higher the level, the more widespread and general its function; the lower the level, the more restricted and specific its functions. The lowest level consists of the two nerve cell pathway mentioned above, the autonomic nervous system of classical description.

The various levels begin with the cerebral hemispheres, in which certain parts of the cerebral cortex and some subcortical structures are involved in autonomic functions. These portions of the hemispheres send fibers to lower levels, especially to the hypothalamus, which has vascular and nervous connections with the hypophysis, and which also sends nerve fibers to brain stem centers. These in turn send nerve fibers to parasympathetic and sympathetic neurons in the brain stem and spinal cord. The axons of these cells leave the central nervous system as preganglionic fibers and synapse in sympathetic or parasympathetic ganglia. The postganglionic fibers supply the appropriate effectors.

CEREBRAL HEMISPHERES

There is no region of the cerebral cortex that is specifically and solely involved in autonomic activity. Rather, when the neocortex controls, regulates, or activates a visceral function, it does so during the course of some other activity. For example, cortical activity leading to muscular contraction also brings about an increase in blood flow in the contracting muscles. Other examples of the role of the cerebral cortex could be provided; all of them are mediated by cortical projections to the diencephalon and brain stem. The parts of the cerebral hemisphere that figure most prominently in autonomic functions include much of the cortex of the frontal lobes together with the limbic system (see Chapter 17). It is the powerful connections between the limbic system and the hypothalamus and midbrain that are chiefly responsible for making possible the autonomic functions of the cerebral hemispheres.

Autonomic functions are important elements in many behavioral mechanisms, and the cerebral cortex can be viewed as the "high level mediator," probably suppressing or inhibiting many outward expressions of behavior (sham rage can be elicited in animals with much of the cortex removed). The interrelationships of autonomic functions and behavior are illustrated by the fact that there is no autonomic activity that cannot be modified, or even completely disorganized, by emotional upsets. Beginning with what is usually considered relatively "normal," one can cite blushing. This is a sudden dilatation of blood vessels, usually but not always limited to those of the face, in response to an emotional situation or the memory of one. Fright, anger, or apprehension may completely upset digestive processes and, at the same time, may cause blood pressure to rise and the heart rate to increase. Students are well acquainted with such phenomena before examinations; speakers may know them as stage fright.

HYPOTHALAMUS

The hypothalamus is located at the base of the brain where it forms the floor and the lower portions of the walls of the third ventricle (Figs. 7–14 and 7–15, pp. 139 and 140). Although it comprises but a small part of the brain, the hypothalamus is structurally complicated; it consists of a number of different nuclei with widespread connections, and it is traversed by major fiber-bundles (e. g., fornix and medial forebrain bundle).

Anteriorly, the hypothalamus begins at the lamina terminalis and the optic chiasma. Just posterior to the chiasma is the *infundibulum,* to which the hypophysis is attached and which contains the portal system of vessels that relate the hypothalamus to the hypophysis (p. 349). Behind, the infundibulum is continuous with a slightly bulging region in the floor of the third ventricle termed the *tuber cinereum.* The floor then increases in thickness at the transition to the mesencephalon. Here, in front of the interpeduncular fossa, are the two *mamillary bodies,* one on each side of the median plane. The optic tracts extend posteriorly from the chiasma, one on each lateral aspect of the hypothalamus.

Internally, the hypothalamus contains the lower part of the third ventricle. On each lateral wall of the third ventricle, the *hypothalamic sulcus* demarcates the thalamus and hypothalamus. Anteriorly on each side the fornix forms a curved elevation in front of the interventricular foramen. Below, the third ventricle exhibits two recesses. One, the *optic recess,* extends downward in front of the optic chiasma. The other, the *infundibular recess,* extends downward into the infundibulum.

The close relationship of the hypothalamus with the hypophysis is a reflection of the double embryological origin of the hypophysis (p. 348); the adenohypophysis develops from oral ectoderm and the neurohypophysis develops from the hypothalamus.

Nuclei.   Most of the hypothalamic nuclei have been described and named, but there is still no complete agreement about their organization and connections. The following grouping, which is in common use, is based upon the fact that the hypothalamus on each side of the third ventricle is traversed by the fornix as it courses toward its termination in the mamillary body, thereby dividing each half of the hypothalamus into a medial and a lateral zone.

The medial zone includes an anterior or suprachiasmatic group (*preoptic, supraoptic,* and *paraventricular nuclei*), a tuberal group in the tuber cinereum (*ventromedial, dorsomedial,* and *infundibular* or *arcuate nuclei*), and a posterior or mamillary group (*mamillary* and *posterior hypothalamic nuclei*). The medial zone also includes the gray matter immediately adjacent to the ventricle (*periventricular gray*).

The lateral zone, which is traversed by the medial forebrain bundle, includes the *lateral hypothalamic* and the *lateral tuberal nuclei.*

Connections.   In carrying out its functions, the hypothalamus receives information relating to environmental situations and changes, both external and internal. Information is derived from various factors to which many hypothalamic neurons are directly sensitive, such as the levels of circulating hormones and the temperature and osmotic pressure of the blood. Information is also derived through neural connections, e. g., by way of the following: direct and indirect connections from the cerebral cortex; a major input from the limbic system by way of the fornix (p. 393), impulses from the retina; olfactory impulses by way of the piriform cortex; afferents from the thalamus; direct and indirect input from various sensory pathways; and a powerful input from the biogenic amine systems of the brain stem (p. 319).

The major efferent projections are as follows: (1) *Hypothalamico-hypophysial tract* (p. 351); (2) *Mamillothalamic fasciculus,* a prominent bundle that ascends from the mamillary body to the anterior nucleus of the thalamus; (3) *Mamillotegmental fasciculus,* comprised of fibers that curve backward and downward to the tegmentum; (4) *Periventricular fibers,* which descend in the periaqueductal gray throughout the brain stem, ending mostly in relation to autonomic centers.

Functions.   The hypothalamus is that part of the corticodiencephalic mechanism which activates, controls, and integrates peripheral autonomic mechanisms, endocrine activities, and many somatic activities, and which participates in many of the outward expressions of emotion and behavior. For example, it is known to effect a general regulation of water balance, body temperature, food intake, and the development of secondary sex characteristics, to mention but a few. These actions are important elements of homeostatic mechanisms, and many are also elements of the outward expressions of emotion and behavior. The hypothalamus mediates its functions through neural projections to the brain stem and limbic system, and by way of the hypophysis (neuroendocrinological functions are discussed on p. 347).

An example of hypothalamic function can be provided by a brief account of its role in temperature regulation. Earlier in this chapter, it was pointed out that changes in external temperature stimulate thermoreceptors in the skin. The resulting nerve impulses reach the spinal cord and brain stem, where they initiate local reflexes. They also ascend to the hypothalamus where they activate nuclei that initiate a range of activities designed to conserve heat. In addition, certain cells in the hypothalamus are directly sensitive to changes in temperature of the blood that flows through the area in which the cells are located. The overall result is that if the external temperature drops, some hypothalamic nuclei initiate or regulate the activities that are necessary to prevent heat loss. The converse occurs if the external temperature rises. Under more extreme conditions of cold, metabolic processes are initiated that increase the production of heat (hypothalamic activation of the hypophysial cells that produce the thyroid activating hormone). The thyroid gland regulates the general metabolic level, and when rapid increase in heat production is necessary, can bring about the characteristic contractions of skeletal muscle called shivering. In other words, the hypothalamus acts as a thermostat. Under normal conditions these various mechanisms, under the control of the hypothalamus, brain stem, and spinal cord, maintain body temperature near or at 37° C (98.6° F).

This balanced maintenance of body temperature may be altered in a variety of ways, as when one has a fever, a common sign of a bacterial infection. Bacterial toxins alter the sensitivity of the hypothalamic cells so that they operate as if the thermostat were set at a higher level. For the body temperature to rise to this new level, the processes of heat retention are started. Cutaneous vessels constrict and shunt vessels open, thus reducing the loss of heat by radiation. This may be accompanied by a subjective sense of coldness. Shivering may occur, thereby increasing heat production. The chills that sometimes signify the onset of fever consist of shivering, plus the sensation of cold. Body temperature rises because more heat is produced than is lost. When the new level is reached, compensatory processes occur. More heat is lost, as evidenced by flushing (dilatation of cutaneous vessels). However, the fever does not drop until the infection is over and hypothalamic cells begin to return to normal.

BRAIN STEM

Certain groups of neurons termed "vital centers" are located in the reticular formation of the pons and medulla oblongata. The chief ones are the *respiratory* (p. 314), *vasomotor,* and *cardiac centers.* Still other centers are concerned with swallowing, intestinal movements (p. 317), and the control of micturition; smaller groups of cells are concerned with a variety of still more specific functions (e. g., salivation, control of pupillary diameter, etc.). The various centers receive impulses from higher levels, especially from the hypothalamus, from the spinal cord, and from afferents to the brain stem. Their constituent neurons send their axons to the cells that give rise to the parasympathetic and sympathetic outflows, and to the motor neurons supplying skeletal muscles that happen to be involved.

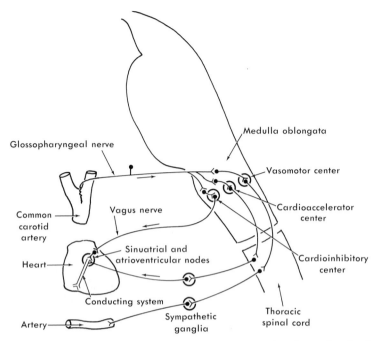

Figure 15–3. Diagram indicating some of the neural pathways involved in reflex control of blood pressure.

Functions. The centers are functionally restricted in the sense that the respiratory centers have no specific vasomotor or cardiac functions, although they may affect the activity of the vasomotor and cardiac centers. But the hypothalamus, which sends fibers to all of these centers, may control or activate them simultaneously as when respiration and blood pressure increase during exercise (or emotional states). An example of the importance of the brain stem centers in homeostatic mechanisms is given in the following description of the reflex control of blood pressure (Fig. 15–3). (A similar example is contained in the description of the reflex control of respiration, p. 314.)

There must be a pressure gradient in order for blood to circulate. This can be measured in terms of the ability of the blood to raise a column of mercury above atmospheric pressure. A device used to measure blood pressure is a *sphygmomanometer.* A hollow cloth cuff is wrapped around the arm and pumped full of air until the flow of arterial blood is stopped. This cuff is connected to a tube filled with mercury, and air pressure in it is thereby exerted against the mercury column. The latter, therefore, rises as the air pressure increases. The height which the mercury column reaches when blood flow is stopped normally averages about 120 mm at rest. This, then, is the highest pressure in the bloodstream. Since it is related to the contraction of the heart, or *systole,* it is termed systolic pressure. Between contractions, that is, during relaxation of the heart (termed *diastole*), the pressure drops to a minimum pressure that averages about 80 mm of mercury. In referring to blood pressure one should always include the two figures, systolic and diastolic; in the example cited the values would be written as 120/80. The 40 mm difference is the pulse pressure and represents the efficiency of the heart in raising pressure above the minimum level and pumping the blood around the body.

Reflex mechanisms help to maintain blood pressure at these average levels. In the bifurcation of each common carotid artery in the neck and also in the wall of the arch of the aorta in the chest, there are mechanoreceptors that are sensitive to changes in blood pressure. Those in the carotid arteries comprise what is termed the *carotid sinus.* The endings in both vessels are stimulated by the distention caused by an increase in blood pressure. The resulting nerve impulses reach the medulla oblongata by way of the vagus and glossopharyngeal nerves (general visceral afferent fibers) and end in the cardiac and vasomotor centers. Some of the neurons in these centers project to the dorsal motor nuclei of the vagus nerves; axons from these nuclei (preganglionic parasympathetic fibers) reach the heart, which they inhibit, thereby slowing its rate of contraction. At the same time, other nerve impulses from the centers descend to the spinal cord. Here they act upon cells of origin of those preganglionic sympathetic fibers that control the diameter of the peripheral arterioles in such a way as to bring about a peripheral vasodilation. The resistance of these vessels to the flow of blood decreases and blood pressure drops. This may be likened to widening the nozzle of a garden hose, as a result of which the force of the stream of water decreases. With the decrease in blood pressure, fewer nerve impulses reach the brain stem centers and the process lessens or reverses. The blood pressure then rises as the peripheral arterioles constrict and the heart rate increases. Under resting conditions, then, there is continually a slight rise, fall, then rise, and so on. The net result is a finely balanced and integrated activity whereby blood pressure is reflexly maintained at an average level.

Other mechanoreceptors and their connections, especially those in the right atrium of the heart, also play major roles in the reflex regulation of cardiac activity. Moreover, it should be emphasized that humoral factors are important in the reflex control of blood pressure, especially during depletion of blood and tissue fluid volume (see p. 354 for a discussion of the renin-angiotensin system).

It is to be noted that in a spinal animal (one in which the junction of the spinal cord and medulla oblongata is severed), neither blood pressure nor respiration can be reflexly maintained. Artificial respiration is necessary to maintain life.

Many other autonomic reflexes occur at brain stem levels.

Some, such as reflex salivation, were discussed in Chapter 14. Other examples include the *light reflex.* If a light is flashed in an eye, both pupils narrow and restrict the amount of light which can enter. The impulses initiated by the light traverse those fibers of the optic nerve which go to the pretectal region. After several synaptic connections, impulses leave by way of the oculomotor nerves (preganglionic parasympathetic fibers) and reach the constrictor muscle of each iris. A widening of the pupils, on the other hand, may result either from sympathetic stimulation of the dilator muscle of the iris, or inhibition of the parasympathetic fibers supplying the constrictor muscles.

SYMPATHETIC AND PARASYMPATHETIC OUTFLOWS AND GANGLIA

The sympathetic and parasympathetic cells in the brain stem and spinal cord comprise still lower and more specific levels of autonomic function. The peripheral ganglion cells to which they project form the lowest and most specific level of autonomic function.

As mentioned previously, the sympathetic and parasympathetic outflows involve two successive neurons. The first cell is in the central nervous system and its axon is preganglionic. The next cell is in a peripheral ganglion and its postganglionic axon supplies an effector. The general arrangement of these outflows, their connections with higher centers, and the structures they supply, are shown in Figure 15–2. Most organs are supplied by both systems, although there are major exceptions. Nearly all peripheral blood vessels, for example, are supplied by the sympathetic system alone. When an organ has a double autonomic nerve supply, the two systems tend to have opposite functions. Thus, the parasympathetic system slows the heart rate and the sympathetic increases it.

Sympathetic System.   This is also called the *thoracolumbar system.* The nerve cells that give rise to the preganglionic fibers form a narrow column (intermediolateral cell column of layer 7) which extends throughout each side of the thoracic and upper lumbar parts of the spinal cord (hence the term thoracolumbar). The axons leave by way of the ventral roots of the corresponding spinal nerves. It is characteristic of preganglionic fibers, at least in higher vertebrates, that they are small myelinated fibers, whereas postganglionic fibers are nonmyelinated. The preganglionic fibers then synapse in peripheral autonomic ganglia, which they reach by way of rami communicantes (Fig. 15–4).

SYMPATHETIC TRUNKS.   These are ganglionated trunks, one on each side of the vertebral column, which extend from the base of the skull to the coccyx. The cervical part of each trunk consists of three or four interconnected ganglia. The uppermost ganglion

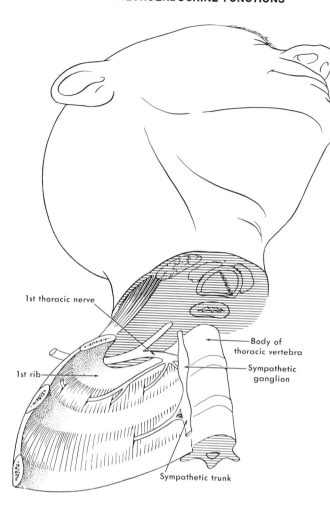

Figure 15-4. A portion of the right sympathetic trunk giving rami communicantes to the first and second thoracic nerves; note relationship to vertebra. (Based on Gardner, E., Gray, D., and O'Rahilly, R.: Anatomy. 4th ed. Philadelphia, W. B. Saunders Company, 1975.)

1st thoracic nerve

Body of thoracic vertebra

Sympathetic ganglion

1st rib

Sympathetic trunk

gives a large branch or branches (postganglionic fibers) that accompany arteries to the face and cranial cavity. The thoracic parts of the trunks commonly have 11 or 12 separate ganglia each. The lumbar parts of the trunks are seldom symmetrical, and the lumbar ganglia are irregular in size, position, and number (3 to 5). The pelvic parts of the sympathetic trunks lie on the sacrum; each usually has 3 or 4 ganglia. The trunks end by joining to form an enlargement, the *ganglion impar,* in front of the coccyx.

The postganglionic fibers that arise in the ganglia of the sympathetic trunks either go directly to adjacent viscera and blood vessels, or they return to spinal nerves by way of rami communicantes and are distributed by way of peripheral nerves (Figs. 15-4, 15-5). They supply secretory fibers to sweat glands, motor fibers to smooth muscle fibers attached to hairs, and vasomotor fibers to blood vessels. The postganglionic fibers that leave the superior cervical ganglia and accompany blood vessels supply the

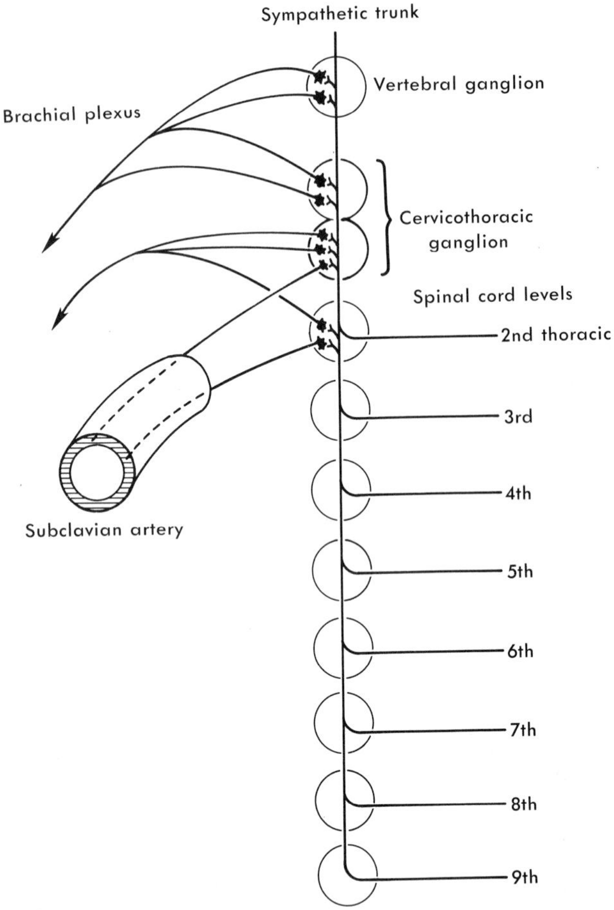

Figure 15-5. Schematic representation of the sympathetic distribution to the upper limb showing that (1) preganglionic fibers arise from several levels of the spinal cord, (2) synapses occur in specific ganglia of the sympathetic trunk and (3) most postganglionic fibers are distributed by way of the nerves of the brachial plexus, but some accompany blood vessels.

salivary and other glands (e. g., pineal body), smooth muscle of the eye, and extracranial and intracranial blood vessels.

Many preganglionic fibers that enter the sympathetic trunks in the thorax and abdomen pass through and emerge as *splanchnic nerves.* These end in various *prevertebral plexuses,* which contain a number of autonomic ganglia. The postganglionic fibers arising from these ganglia go directly to adjacent viscera and blood vessels. However, some preganglionic fibers continue on to the medullae of the suprarenal glands where they form neuro-effector junctions with the glandular cells.

Some of the preganglionic fibers in spinal nerves synapse in *accesory (intermediate) ganglia* without reaching sympathetic trunks (Fig. 15–6). These ganglia are small collections of ganglion cells scattered along spinal nerves and rami communicantes, especially in the cervical, lower thoracic, and upper lumbar regions. Most of these cells send their axons into the spinal nerves with which they are associated. These ganglion cells would not be affected by the usual surgical procedure designed to cut autonomic fibers. Hence, they are a source of residual autonomic function after sympathectomies.

Finally, it should be emphasized that sensory fibers arising from viscera are contained within the various autonomic nerves. Depending upon their functions, they may reach the brain stem by way of the vagus nerves; or they may traverse the sympathetic trunks, reach spinal nerves by way of rami communicantes, and enter the spinal cord by way of dorsal roots.

Parasympathetic System. This is also called the *cranio-sacral system.* The motor cells whose axons form the pregangli-onic fibers are found in the nuclei of origin of certain cranial nerves (oculomotor, facial, glossopharyngeal, vagus, and acces-sory), and also in the sacral part of the spinal cord (hence the term craniosacral).

The preganglionic fibers that leave by way of the oculomotor, facial, and glossopharyngeal nerves synapse in the cranial para-sympathetic ganglia. Table 15–1 lists these ganglia and the struc-tures they supply with postganglionic fibers. The preganglionic fibers in the vagus nerves are joined by those from the accessory nerve and are distributed to viscera in the thorax and abdomen. The ganglia are in or near these viscera.

The sacral preganglionic fibers arise from a column of cells on each side of the middle segments of the sacral cord. The fibers leave by way of the corresponding ventral roots, pass through the sympathetic trunks, and emerge as *pelvic splanchnic nerves,* which are distributed to the pelvic and genital organs and to the distal part of the large intestine (the proximal part is supplied by the vagus nerves).

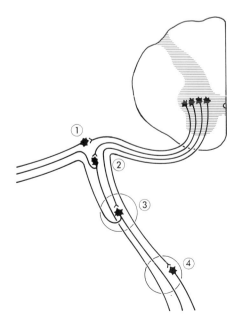

Figure 15–6. Schematic representation of the locations of sympathetic ganglion cells. Ganglion cells may form accessory ganglia in (1) spinal nerves (or in ventral rami), or in (2) rami communi-cantes. Ganglion cells are also present in (3) ganglia of sympathetic trunk, and in (4) preverte-bral ganglia, such as the celiac. (Based on Gardner, E., Gray, D., and O'Rahilly, R.: Anatomy. 4th ed., Philadelphia, W. B. Saunders Company, 1975.)

Table 15-1. Cranial Parasympathetic Ganglia.

Ganglion*	Location	Origin of parasympathetic fibers that synapse in the ganglia	Origin of sympathetic fibers that pass through the ganglia	Chief distribution
Ciliary	Lateral to optic nerve in the orbit	From 3rd cranial nerve (oculomotor)	From superior cervical ganglion by way of internal carotid plexus	Eye (ciliary muscle, sphincter pupillae, dilator pupillae)
Pterygopalatine	In pterygopalatine fossa	From 7th cranial nerve (facial)	From superior cervical ganglion by way of internal carotid plexus	Lacrimal gland and glands in oral, nasal, and palatine mucosa
Otic	Below foramen ovale	From 9th cranial nerve (glossopharyngeal)	From superior cervical ganglion by way of plexus on middle meningeal artery	Parotid gland
Submandibular	On hyoglossus muscle	From 7th cranial nerve (facial)	From superior cervical ganglion by way of plexus on facial artery	Submandibular and sublingual glands

*The parasympathetic ganglia of the vagi and the pelvic splanchnic nerves are located in or near the walls of the organs they supply.

The parasympathetic ganglion cells in the walls of the thoracic, abdominal, and pelvic organs rarely form recognizable ganglia, but instead are usually scattered in the walls. In the alimentary canal, however, these cells occur between the muscle layers in arrangements complicated enough to warrant the term plexuses. Moreoever, there is evidence of intrinsic functions that may be independent of the external nerve supply, and which may be a factor in pacemaker activity (p. 95). In addition, it seems likely that the postganglionic sympathetic fibers entering the plexuses may end on the intrinsic parasympathetic ganglion cells. If so, the sympathetic fibers inhibit intestinal motility by inhibiting the excitatory parasympathetic ganglion cells.

Ganglionic Structure. The sympathetic ganglia are complicated in structure and are incompletely understood. Their neurons are multipolar and each is apparently synaptically connected with many preganglionic fibers. Conversely, a single preganglionic fiber may synapse with many ganglion cells. Moreover, the ganglia often contain chromaffin cells (p. 353) that appear to act as interneurons. These cells show intense fluorescence, they synthesize catecholamines (probably dopamine), and their axons synapse with ganglion cells. They probably regulate transmission through these cells, perhaps by inhibiting them.

The cranial parasympathetic ganglia likewise have a complicated structure that is incompletely understood. In some vertebrates, especially birds, the ciliary ganglia of young animals have large electrical synapses with tight junctions between preganglionic fibers and ganglion cells. In general, each cranial parasympathetic ganglion has a sympathetic root (postganglionic fibers originating in the superior cervical ganglion and passing through the ganglion; Table 15–1), a sensory root (sensory fibers passing through to a cranial nerve and thus to the brain), and a parasympathetic root (preganglionic fibers from the appropriate cranial nerve and synapsing in the ganglion). Each preganglionic fiber synapses with fewer ganglion cells than is the case with sympathetic ganglia.

Functions. With regard to local autonomic reflexes in the spinal cord, these are clearly demonstrable when the spinal cord is severed (the transection must be at the lower cervical segments or lower if respiration is to survive and life to be maintained). A study of such injuries in man as well as in lower animals has given some insight into the autonomic functions of the spinal cord. As has been mentioned before, they are characterized by their restricted nature and are integrated only to a limited degree.

The peripheral autonomic ganglia are restricted in outflow and function. Each ganglion is the final level of autonomic control of a specific structure or region.

PHARMACOLOGY OF THE AUTONOMIC NERVOUS SYSTEM

The anatomical classification that divides the autonomic nervous system into sympathetic and parasympathetic parts is unsatisfactory in certain respects. It implies a rigid or sharp distinction between these divisions that functionally does not always exist. Also, some organs and tissues are supplied by sympathetic fibers that function like parasympathetic fibers, whereas others may be supplied by but one set of fibers. There is in common use another classification that is based upon the types of postganglionic transmitters and upon reactions to certain drugs (see Chapter 5). In this classification, postganglionic fibers are termed *cholinergic* if they release acetylcholine at their terminals and *adrenergic* if they release norepinephrine (noradrenaline).

Much of our knowledge of the autonomic nervous system has been obtained through the experimental use of a variety of important drugs, many of which bring about profound physiological, behavioral, and emotional changes because of their effects on metabolism and synaptic transmission (p. 110). A number of these drugs can be classified according to their autonomic effects. These effects may be chiefly parasympathetic or chiefly sympathetic in nature, or they may interfere with ganglionic transmission.

Drugs that stimulate or inhibit autonomic effectors in the same manner as parasympathetic postganglionic stimulation are known as *parasympathomimetic* drugs. They include acetylcholine and some of its derivatives, alkaloids such as *pilocarpine* and *muscarine* (p. 106), and a variety of anticholinesterases such as *eserine.* Many are produced synthetically, and many may have central actions also.

Sympathomimetic drugs stimulate or inhibit effectors in the same way as sympathetic postganglionic stimulation. These drugs often have profound effects on the central nervous system also. Some of them are the biogenic amines (p. 319). Non-catecholamine sympathomimetic drugs include *amphetamine, cocaine,* and *ephedrine.* They act by bringing about the rapid release of stored noradrenaline in a physiologically active form. Because this release occurs in the central nervous system also, the accentuation of norepinephrine functions brings about profound behavioral and mood changes (Chapter 14). Amphetamine (p. 322) is a notable example of a drug that seriously affects the central nervous system by means of the mechanism just outlined.

Other non-catecholamines that are sympathomimetic include the monoamine oxidase inhibitors. These are a heterogeneous group of drugs that block the actions of monoamine oxidase, causing an increased concentration of the biogenic amines and an enhancement of sympathetic and serotonin activity.

Finally, there are drugs that produce synaptic and effector blockade. They may block transmission in autonomic ganglia; examples include certain quaternary ammonium compounds, as well as anesthetics such as ether, and drugs such as nicotine in high concentration. Peripherally, some drugs compete with acetylcholine at the receptor site, that is, they have an antimuscarin effect. Examples are atropine and scopolamine. A number of drugs block activity at sympathetic postganglionic endings. Some prevent the release of transmitter; an example is *guanethidine,* a powerful anti–high-blood-pressure agent. Others block the effects of noradrenaline directly at either the *alpha-* or *beta*-receptor sites. Examples of an *alpha*-receptor blocking drug are the ergot *alkaloids* (which have other actions also) and *thymoxamine.* Beta-receptor blocking agents include *propranolol.*

COMPARISON OF SYMPATHETIC AND PARASYMPATHETIC FUNCTIONS

The various responses of organs to autonomic impulses are summarized in Table 15–2. These responses are important components of homeostatic mechanisms, as well as of the outward expressions of emotions and behaviors. In carrying out these functions, the sympathetic and parasympathetic systems exhibit distinctive functional attributes.

The sympathetic system tends to respond as a whole, espe-

Table 15–2. Usual Responses of Organs to Autonomic Impulses.

Organ	Cholinergic	Adrenergic
Eye	Stimulates ciliary muscle and sphincter pupillae – pupillary constriction to light and during accommodation	Pupillary dilatation – stimulates dilator pupillae and possibly radial fibers of ciliary muscle
Lung and trachea	Stimulates secretory cells and smooth muscle – serous and mucous secretions, narrowing of bronchioles	Inhibits smooth muscle – relaxation of bronchioles
Lacrimal, nasal, palatine, and salivary glands	Stimulates secretory cells – serous (watery) secretions	Either no important effect, or else a thick, mucous secretion
Gastrointestinal system	Stimulates secretory cells and smooth muscle – digestive secretions, peristalsis, evacuation. Inhibits sphincters	Inhibits peristalsis – stimulates sphincters
Liver and pancreas	Stimulates pancreatic cells, including beta islet cells	Probably no important effect on liver; stimulates alpha cells of pancreatic islets
Suprarenal medulla	Secretion of epinephrine and norepinephrine	
Urinary bladder	Stimulates smooth muscle (detrusor) – emptying of bladder	Questionable effect on emptying. May activate internal sphincter during ejaculation
Uterus	Uncertain and variable	Uncertain and variable
Genitalia	Erection	Ejaculation
Sweat glands	Secretion	No significant effect except in palms
Arrectores pilorum	No effect	Erection of hair – stimulation of smooth muscle
Heart		
S-A node	Decrease in heart rate	Increase in heart rate
Atria	Decrease in contractility	Increase in contractility
A-V node	Decrease in conduction	Increase in conduction
Ventricles	– – –	Increase in contractility
Blood vessels		
Coronary	?	Constriction (α receptor); dilatation (β receptor)
Skin	?	Constriction
Muscle	?	Constriction (α receptor); dilatation (β receptor)
Viscera	?	Constriction; dilatation in liver.

cially during emergencies or sudden environmental changes. The sympathetic system is therefore an important part of the mechanisms by which one responds to stress. Among the situations that cause stress are pain, rage, fright, exercise, cold, the use of many drugs, and asphyxia. All of these may evoke similar patterns of response. For example, a situation that results in rage or fear may also result in a rapid increase in blood pressure, pulse rate, cardiac output, sweating, and blood sugar; all are changes designed for "fight or flight." These acute responses to stress result from sympathetic discharge initiated by cortical and hypothalamic activity. They are generalized and widespread because of the organization of the system (for example, one preganglionic fiber synapses with many ganglion cells), and also because the medullary cells of the suprarenal glands are stimulated and epinephrine is released into the blood stream. Epinephrine may maintain or enhance many sympathetic activities.

In addition to the acute responses to stress, there may be more slowly developing changes in metabolic activities and defense mechanisms. These are brought about by the activation of the hypothalamic-pituitary system, leading to an increased secretion by the pituitary or adrenocorticotrophic hormone. This acts on the cortex of the suprarenal glands, leading to a greater output of the cortical steroid hormones, with changes in metabolic activities and cellular composition of the blood.

The parasympathetic system is concerned with the initiation and maintenance of a number of specific functions, such as digestion, intermediate metabolism of foods, and excretion. These actions are usually initiated in response to specific stimuli; hence the necessity for more specific anatomical arrangements and reflex pathways. Widespread connections such as are characteristic of the sympathetic system would interfere with, or make impossible, the specific parasympathetic functions. Widespread, generalized parasympathetic actions can occur, but they are often abnormal responses to unusual situations, such as bladder and bowel evacuation during unusual stress.

PATHOPHYSIOLOGY

The purpose of the following discussion is to provide a few examples of some peripheral autonomic disorders. The autonomic nervous system is frequently involved in surgical procedures. With the exception of vagotomy in the treatment of gastric ulcer, most surgery of the autonomic nervous system involves sympathetic denervation of a limb with a vascular disease, in order to improve the circulation of that limb. Other procedures include the denervation of the carotid sinus for the relief of fainting and other symptoms of a suddenly falling blood pressure, due to a sensitive sinus. Finally, there are procedures aimed at relieving pain, for example: sympathetic denervation of a limb for phantom-limb pain (p. 239), causalgia, and other painful disorders. The rationale of treating pain by surgery on the autonomic nervous system is often not clear, nor are the procedures always successful. Sometimes they are effective simply because sensory fibers traveling in or through an autonomic nerve or ganglion are severed.

Degeneration and Regeneration. When peripheral autonomic fibers, whether pre- or postganglionic are cut, they degenerate. However, provided that their cells of origin remain intact, regeneration often takes place and function is restored. One of the significant effects of denervation is *denervation sensitivity.* The effector (especially smooth muscle) becomes sensitive to circulating or directly applied transmitters and drugs. For example, certain vascular disorders in which vasoconstriction causes pale, cold, aching fingers and hands may be temporarily relieved by sympathectomy. Unfortunately, these vessels may become so sensitive to circulating adrenaline that they again constrict, sometimes to a greater degree than before.

It is of interest that transplanted hearts are completely denervated. The conducting system of the transplanted heart, however, maintains relatively normal rhythmic activity. There is some evidence that in experimental animals transplanted hearts may be re-innervated, but as yet there is no good evidence that this occurs in humans.

NEUROENDOCRINOLOGY

Neuroendocrinology encompasses those mechanisms that comprise the third effector system of the nervous system. These mechanisms include the autonomic outflow to certain endocrine glands. The effectors are cells that convert neural signals into hormonal outputs (*neuroendocrinological transducer cells*). There are a number of such types of cells (Table 15–3), both within and

Table 15–3. Examples of Neuroendocrine Transducer Cells.

Cell Type	Examples of Input Signals	Hormonal Output Signal
Hypothalamic cells that synthesize releasing factors	Dopamine and other monoamines	Releasing factors → adenohypophysial hormones
Cells of the hypothalamic paraventricular and supraoptic nuclei	Possibly acetylcholine or norepinephrine	Antidiuretic hormone (vasopressin) — oxytocin
Suprarenal medulla (chromaffin cells)	Acetylcholine (preganglionic sympathetic neurons)	Epinephrine and norepinephrine
Cells of pineal body	Norepinephrine (postganglionic sympathetic neurons)	Gonad-inhibiting substance (melatonin?)
Juxtaglomerular cells of the kidney	Norepinephrine (postganglionic sympathetic neurons)	Renin → angiotensin II
β-cells of pancreatic islets	Acetylcholine (postganglionic parasympathetic neurons)	Insulin
α-cells of pancreatic islets	Norepinephrine (postganglionic sympathetic neurons)	Glucagon

(Modified from Wurtman, R. J.: Fed. Proc., *32*:1769, 1973.)

outside the central nervous system, and more will undoubtedly be discovered. All have certain common characteristics. Nerve endings are present in their immediate vicinity, they respond to humoral as well as to neural signals (but the neural input must be intact for humoral inputs to be effective), and the humoral sensitivity may take the form of feedback control (e.g., inhibition by the circulating target organ hormones).

Most of the neurotransducer cells involve the catecholamines or serotonin in their functions. These monoamines serve either as hormones or as input signals that activate or modulate hormonal secretion.

HYPOTHALAMIC-HYPOPHYSIAL SYSTEM

Two groups of transducing cells occur in the hypothalamus, as indicated in Table 15–3; both groups involve the hypophysis. The hypophysis lies in the hypophysial fossa of the sphenoid bone, immediately below the brain, to which it is connected by a stem or stalk (Fig. 15–7). The gland has a double embryological origin, developing partly from the oral ectoderm (pharyngeal region) of the embryo and partly from the hypothalamus.

Adenohypophysis. The part of the hypophysis that arises from the oral ectoderm is termed the *adenohypophysis*. This is fur-

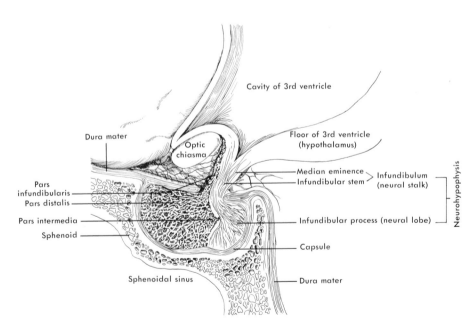

Figure 15–7. Diagram of a median section through the floor of the third ventricle and through the hypophysis. (Based on Guillemin, R., and Burgus, R., in Sci. Amer., 227: 24–33, 1972, by permission of the authors and publisher. Copyright 1972 by Scientific American, Inc. All rights reserved.)

Table 15–4. The hormones of the hypophysis. The target organs are the chief ones, but not necessarily the only ones.

Adenohypophysis		
Hormone	Secreting cell	Target organs
Growth hormones (somatotropic hormone, STH)	Acidophilic cells of pars distalis	Chondroblasts of growth cartilages
Lactogenic hormone, LTH (prolactin)	Acidophilic cells of pars distalis	Milk producing cells of mammary gland. Progesterone secreting cells of corpus luteum of ovary
Gonadotrophic hormones (GTH)	Basophilic cells of pars distalis	
Follicle stimulating hormone (FSH)		Females: growth and maturation of ovarian follicles Males: spermatogenesis in seminiferous tubules of testis
Luteinizing hormones (LH)		Females: follicle rupture and formation of corpus luteum Males: stimulation of interstitial cells of testis (production of testosterone)
Thyrotrophic hormone (TSH)	Basophilic cells of pars distalis	Thyroid cells: synthesis, storage, and release of thyroxine
Adrenocorticotrophic hormone (ACTH)	Chromophobe cells of pars distalis	Suprarenal cortex: release of glucocorticoids
Melanocyte stimulating hormone (MSH)	Probably cells of pars intermedia (perhaps chromophobe cells)	Melanocytes: production of melanin
Neurohypophysis		
Antidiuretic hormone, ADH (vasopressin)	Paraventricular and supraoptic hypothalamic nuclei	Tubules of kidney; smooth muscle of arterioles
Oxytocin	Paraventricular and supraoptic hypothalamic nuclei	Smooth muscle of uterus; myoepithelial cells of mammary gland

ther subdivided into the *pars distalis, pars intermedia,* and *pars infundibularis* (Fig. 15–7), which contain different kinds of epithelial cells. These cells produce various hormones, and a specific cell type is related to each hormone (Table 15–4). The adenohypophysis is also characterized by a special blood supply that forms a portal system (Fig. 15–8). Briefly stated, certain arteries enter the median eminence where they form *sinusoidal capillaries.* These vessels then collect into *portal vessels* that enter the adenohypophysis and form a second set of sinusoidal capillaries, which are the direct supply of the adjacent epithelial cells. These vessels in turn drain into adjacent veins.

The release of adenohypophysial hormones into the general circulation is effected by certain brain hormones. These are termed *releasing factors;* they are polypeptides that are synthesized in the hypothalamus. At least nine have been identified, although for

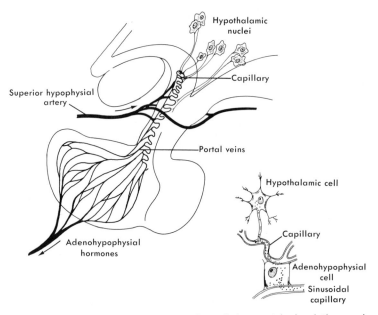

Figure 15-8. Schematic representation of the portal circulation and sinusoids of the adenohypophysis. The figure at the lower right illustrates a portal vessel, which is transporting a releasing factor, interposed between a hypothalamic neuron (neuroendocrine transducing cell) and an adenohypophysial cell which is discharging hormone into a sinusoidal capillary. (Based on Guillemin, R., and Burgus, R., in Sci. Amer., *227*: 24–33, 1972, by permission of the authors and publisher. Copyright 1972 by Scientific American, Inc. All rights reserved.)

most of them the synthesizing cells have not been identified. The releasing factors are delivered to the median eminence where they enter the portal vessels and reach the adenohypophysis. The mechanism of delivery has not been completely established. There is abundant evidence that one mechanism is axonal transport from the synthesizing cells to the median eminence. An additional postulated mechanism is release into the cerebrospinal fluid and subsequent uptake by the ependymal cells of the median eminence.

It is of interest that some of the brain hormones inhibit rather than release the adenohypophysial hormones. *Somatostatin* is a brain hormone that acutely and reversibly inhibits the secretion of growth hormone. Moreover, it inhibits the secretion of glucagon, probably through a direct action on the *alpha* cells of the pancreatic islets.

The biogenic amine system of the brain stem appears to be involved in the control of synthesis of the releasing factors, and is thereby a factor in the circadian rhythm of hormonal output. The growth-releasing factor (synthesized in the arcuate nuclei) acts chiefly during deep sleep; hence the output of growth hormone and its blood levels are highest during slumber. Other input signals that serve as negative feedback mechanisms in the discharge of releasing factors are circulating hormones (especially the ovarian hormones). The hypothalamic neurons that synthesize the releasing factors are sensitive to and inhibited by the circulating hormones.

Neurohypophysis. The portion of the pituitary which develops from the diencephalon is termed the neurohypophysis (Fig. 15–7). Its chief cellular elements, the *pituicytes,* are neuroglial cells. It is connected to the hypothalamus by the *infundibulum* (also known as the *neural stalk*). The infundibulum has two parts, the *median eminence* above and the *infundibular stem* below. The infundibular recess usually extends into the stem. The stem gives way to the *neural lobe* proper (*infundibular* or *neural process*), which receives nerve fibers from hypothalamic nuclei.

Certain hypothalamic nuclei, chiefly the supraoptic and the paraventricular, form the hypothalamicohypophysial tract (also known as the supra-opticohypophysial tract), which projects to the neural lobe (Fig. 15–9). Two hormones are synthesized by the neurons of these nuclei, and travel by axonal transport (probably in precursor form) to the neural lobe where they are stored until discharged into the circulation. The two hormones are the *antidiuretic hormone* (ADH; also known as *vasopressin*) and *oxytocin.* (The antidiuretic hormone is synthesized chiefly in the supraoptic nuclei, and oxytocin chiefly in the paraventricular nuclei).

The antidiuretic hormone produces a rise in blood pressure through activation of vascular smooth muscle only when given in high doses. Its chief action is to work on the tubules of the kidney in such a way as to decrease urine production. It thus constitutes an important means of conserving body water. It is of interest that the cells of the supraoptic nucleus are directly sensitive to the ionic concentration and osmotic pressure of the blood. Changes in these features undoubtedly alter the activity of the nucleus. If the nucleus or its projections are destroyed, a disorder known as *diabetes insipidus* results. Because of the loss of antidiuretic hormone, large quantities of urine, amounting to many liters, are eliminated by the kidney each day. In order to maintain water balance, large amounts of water must be drunk.

In mammals, including humans, oxytocin acts chiefly on the smooth muscle of the uterus and also on certain smooth muscle cells of the mammary gland known as *myo-epithelial cells.* The hormone is particularly effective in inducing uterine contractions during the later stages of pregnancy, and especially during parturition. It is often used as an aid in labor. In the mammary gland, it activates the special smooth muscle cells that cause the ejection of milk (the formation of milk is regulated by *prolactin* from the adenohypophysis). The release of oxytocin from the neurohypophysis is triggered by the act of suckling; the nerve impulses ini-

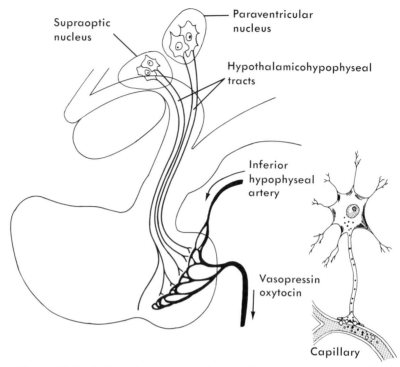

Figure 15-9. Schematic representation of the neurohypophysis and the hypothalamicohypophysial tract. The figure at the lower right indicates that the brain hormone is transported by way of the axon to axon terminals, where the hormone may be stored before being released into the circulation. (Based on Guillemin, R., and Burgus, R., in Sci. Amer., 227:24–33, 1972, by permission of the authors and publisher. Copyright 1972 by Scientific American, Inc. All rights reserved.)

tiated in sensory endings in the nipple reach the spinal cord and ascend in the brain stem to the paraventricular nuclei.

PINEAL BODY

The pineal body is located at the posterior end of the third ventricle. In lower vertebrates, such as the frog, it is a photoreceptor organ that is similar to the retina in development and structure. Its photoreceptive cells can generate nerve impulses in direct response to light. In mammals, the pineal cells lack an outer segment and have no direct connections with the brain. However, the pineal body is heavily supplied by postganglionic sympathetic fibers that form the end of a complicated indirect connection between the brain and the pineal body. The varicosities of these fibers are closely related to the pineal cells.

There is as yet no complete agreement on the functions of the pineal body. (Species differences are marked.) Nevertheless, certain features have been clarified. The sympathetic pathway mentioned above is involved in the effect of light upon the output of a gonad-inhibiting substance which is synthesized by the pineal cells. (Many consider this substance to be *melatonin.*) The pathway begins in the retina and involves the medial forebrain bundle, the hypothalamus, projections to the spinal cord, preganglionic outflow to the superior cervical ganglia, and postganglionic fibers coursing along blood vessels to reach the pineal body. The release of norepinephrine initiates the processes that lead to the synthesis of the gonad-inhibiting substance (GIS).

The output of GIS varies in a circadian rhythm that is regulated by the hypothalamus, and which is modulated by an inhibition that is produced by exposure to light. The circadian rhythm exhibits increased release of GIS at night, and less during the day. In experimental animals, prolonged exposure to light can abolish the output of GIS. Also, in many experimental animals, GIS inhibits the gonads. Hence, in blinded animals a resulting overproduction of GIS may cause the gonads to atrophy. Conversely, gonadal hypertrophy may follow prolonged exposure to light. In humans, tumors of the pineal body may be accompanied by various changes in the gonads.

The pars intermedia of the hypophysis produces a melanin-stimulating hormone. The functional relationship, if any, between this hormone and GIS is still obscure.

SUPRARENAL GLANDS AND CHROMAFFIN CELLS

The suprarenal glands are small, paired endocrine glands that, in humans, lie above the kidneys. In most animals the glands are termed adrenal because they are near the kidneys but not necessarily above them. Each gland comprises two endocrine glands, the *cortex* and the *medulla*. The cortex produces steroid hormones that are essential to life. The cells of the medulla are chromaffin cells (so-called because early staining methods employed chrome salts). These cells are supplied by preganglionic sympathetic fibers and are therefore analagous to sympathetic ganglion cells; they produce norepinephrine and epinephrine. The epinephrine is discharged into the blood stream and, by acting upon effectors, tends to enhance the effects of sympathetic stimulation.

Cells similar to those of the suprarenal medulla are commonly found in front of the vertebrae, especially along the aorta. These *paraganglia* or *para-aortic bodies* may be fairly large and constant in position, especially in the fetus. Chromaffin cells are also present in sympathetic ganglia, where they appear to act as interneurons (p. 342).

JUXTAGLOMERULAR CELLS OF THE KIDNEY

The renin-angiotensin system is an important mechanism in the regulation of arterial pressure and sodium and water retention. *Renin* is a highly specific proteolytic enzyme that is produced by the juxtaglomerular cells of the kidney (these are specialized cells adjacent to the arterioles leading into the glomeruli). Renin is released into the circulation where it leads, by a series of enzymatic reactions, to the generation of an active polypeptide hormone, *angiotensin II*. This hormone is a potent direct vasoconstrictor, and it also stimulates the production of aldosterone. (Aldosterone is the principal electrolyte-regulating steroid secreted by the suprarenal cortex.)

The release of renin is under autonomic and humoral control. One of the important humoral factors is the antidiuretic hormone. Angiotensin II plays a major role in maintaining circulation, especially during depletion of blood and tissue fluid volume. It is probably not necessary for the acute maintenance of blood pressure if volume and salt concentration are normal. As angiotensin circulates in the blood, it can activate renin release. It is also a potent *dipsogen,* acting chiefly on the septum and on the anterior portion of the hypothalamus, thereby bringing about the synthesis and release of antidiuretic hormone. Thus, this stimulus to drinking triggers the mechanisms that maintain blood and fluid volume.

ALPHA AND BETA CELLS OF PANCREATIC ISLETS

The islets are the endocrine portions of the pancreas. The *alpha* cells of the islets secrete *glucagon,* a polypeptide that brings about a breakdown of liver glycogen, thereby elevating the concentration of blood sugar. The *beta* cells of the islets secrete *insulin,* which, like glucagon, is a polypeptide hormone that is involved in carbohydrate metabolism. Insulin stimulates the conversion of glucose to glycogen, and increases the cellular uptake of glucose. One of the effects is a lowering of blood sugar concentration. Both hormones are also involved in fat and protein metabolism.

The secretion of both hormones is under neural and humoral control. Stimulation of the parasympathetic system increases insulin secretion; sympathetic stimulation inhibits insulin secretion. The converse is true for glucagon secretion. The humoral control of insulin secretion is varied. It is increased when the brain is exposed to increased glucose uptake, and also by food-related stimuli (sight, taste, smell). Circulating growth hormone may also serve as a humoral control. Somatostatin, which inhibits the release of growth hormone, also inhibits glucagon secretion by acting directly upon *alpha* islet cells.

SUMMARY

Visceral activities are controlled, directly or indirectly, by the autonomic nervous system, which is one of the three effector mechanisms of the nervous system and which supplies smooth muscle, cardiac muscle, and glands. The levels of nervous control are the cerebral hemispheres, hypothalamus, brain stem, spinal cord, and peripheral autonomic ganglia. The higher the level, the more general, widespread, and nonspecific are the connections and functions. The fibers that leave the central nervous system do so as preganglionic fibers, synapsing with peripherally located ganglion cells and reaching viscera as postganglionic fibers. Axons leaving by way of the oculomotor, facial, glossopharyngeal, vagus, and accessory nerves and by way of ventral roots of the second and third sacral nerves form the craniosacral or parasympathetic division. The ganglia are in or near the organs innervated. The axons leaving by way of the ventral roots of the thoracic and first three lumbar roots form the thoracolumbar or sympathetic system. The peripheral synapses occur in the ganglia of the sympathetic trunks and in the prevertebral ganglia. Most organs are supplied by both divisions of the autonomic system.

The autonomic functions of the cerebral hemispheres are mediated through the limbic system and hypothalamus. The hypothalamus is involved in a number of visceral and metabolic functions, and carries out its functions by means of projections to the brain stem and to the hypophysis. Thus, it acts both upon the endocrine system and upon other nervous levels. The brain stem is concerned with a number of visceral activities, each rather specific, such as the reflex control of respiration and blood pressure. The brain stem and spinal cord contain still lower and functionally more specific levels which project to peripheral autonomic ganglia. The latter constitute the lowest and most specific autonomic level.

Both systems are critically important elements of homeostatic mechanisms. In addition, the parasympathetic system as a whole is concerned with rather specific functions, such as digestion and excretion, each of which is initiated by fairly definite stimuli. The sympathetic system is particularly concerned in responses to stress, and its pattern of activity may be initiated by a wide variety of situations and agents.

The neuroendocrine system is one of the three effector mechanisms of the nervous system. The effectors, which are cells that convert neural impulses into hormonal output, include the following: hypothalamic releasing factor cells, the paraventricular and supraoptic nuclei, suprarenal medulla, pineal body, juxtaglomerular cells of the kidney, and alpha and beta cells of the pancreatic islets. This neuroendocrine system is the means by which the brain and endocrine glands are integrated in the total spectrum of bodily functions and behavior.

NAMES IN NEUROLOGY

CLAUDE BERNARD (1813–1878)

Bernard was one of the greatest of experimental physiologists, the founder of experimental medicine. Born near Lyons, he studied medicine in Paris, where he became an assistant to Magendie at the Collège de France. In 1854 he was appointed professor of general physiology. To him we owe much of our knowledge of the digestive and vasomotor systems. In 1843, he discovered that cane sugar appeared in the urine after being injected into the veins, but not if it had been first treated with gastric juice. This observation was the beginning of a long series of investigations of digestive processes. In 1849 he discovered that a puncture of the floor of the fourth ventricle produced a temporary diabetes. Shortly after this, he investigated the factors controlling blood vessels and demonstrated the mechanisms of constriction and dilatation. Later he studied carbon monoxide poisoning. One of the most fundamental concepts in physiology results from his statement that all the vital processes maintain the constancy of the milieu intérieur or internal environment. His book, *Introduction à l'étude de la médicine expérimentale* (Paris, Baillière, 1865), is a classic discussion of the experimental method. Even if his work on the nervous system were all that he had done, his name would still go down in scientific history.

REFERENCES

See the references cited on pages 113 and 159.
The following are classic reviews by investigators who pioneered in studies of autonomic and neuroendocrinological functions.

Cannon, W. B.: The Wisdom of the Body. New York, W. W. Norton and Company, 1939.
Harris, G. W.: Neural Control of the Pituitary Gland. London, Edward Arnold (Publisher) Ltd., 1955.
von Euler, U. S.: Noradrenaline. Springfield, Ill., C. C Thomas, 1956.
Scharrer, E., and Scharrer, B.: Neuroendocrinology. New York, Columbia University Press, 1963.

The following are major source texts.

Appenzeller, O.: The Autonomic Nervous System. New York, American Elsevier Publishing Company, 1970.
Bligh, J.: Temperature Regulation in Mammals and Other Vertebrates. Vol. 30 of Frontiers of Biology. Neuberger, A., and Tatum, E. L. (editors). New York, American Elsevier Publishing Company, 1973.
Donovan, B. T.: Mammalian Neuroendocrinology. London, McGraw-Hill, 1970.
Goodman, I., and Gilman, A.: Pharmacological Basis of Therapeutics, 4th ed., New York, The Macmillan Company, 1970.
Haymaker, W., Anderson, E., and Nauta, E. J. H. (editors): The Hypothalamus. Springfield, Ill., C. C Thomas, 1969.
Martini, L., Motta, M., and Fraschini, F.: The Hypothalamus. New York, Academic Press, 1970.
Pick, J.: The Autonomic Nervous System. Philadelphia, J. B. Lippincott Company, 1970.
Szentágothai, J., Flerkó, B., Mess, B., and Halász, B.: Hypothalamic Control of the Anterior Pituitary. 3rd ed. Budapest, Akadémiai Kiadó, 1972.
Turner, C. D., and Bagnara, J. T.: General Endocrinology. 5th ed., Philadelphia, W. B. Saunders Company, 1971.
Wolstenholme, G. E. W., and Knight, J. (editors): The Pineal Gland. A CIBA Foundation Symposium. Edinburgh, Churchill Livingstone, 1971.
Wurtman, R. J., Axelrod, J., and Kelly, D. E.: The Pineal. New York, Academic Press, 1968.

The following are valuable reviews.

Axelrod, J.: The pineal gland: a neurochemical transducer. Science, *184*:1341-1348, 1974.
Guillemin, R., and Burgus, R.: The hormones of the hypothalamus. Sci. Amer., *227*:24–33, 1972.

Knigge, K. M.: Role of the ventricular system in neuroendocrine processes. pp. 40–47, in Frontiers in Neurology and Neuroscience Research. Seeman, P. and Brown, G. M., (editors). Toronto, The University of Toronto Press, 1974.

Knigge, K. M., Scott, D. E., and Weindl, A. (editors): Brain-Endocrine Interaction. Basel, S. Karger, 1972.

Martin, J. B.: Neural regulation of growth hormone secretion. New Engl. J. Med., *288*:1384–1393, 1973.

Mason, J. W.: The integrative approach in medicine—implications of neuroendocrine mechanisms. Perspectives Biol. Med., *17*:333–347, 1974.

Mason, J. W.: Specificity in the organization of neuroendocrine response profiles. pp. 68–80 in Frontiers in Neurology and Neuroscience Research. Seeman, P. and Brown, G. M. (editors). Toronto, The University of Toronto Press, 1974.

Oparil, S., and Haber, E.: The renin-angiotensin system. New Engl. J. Med., *291*:389–401, 1974.

Sawyer, C. H. (chairman, Symposium): "Brain-Endocrine Interactions", Amer. J. Anat., *129*: 193–246, 1970.

Schmid, P. G., and Abboud, F. M.: Neurohumoral control of vascular resistance. Arch. Int. Med., *133*:935–945, 1974.

Woods, S. C., and Porte, D., Jr.: Neural control of the endocrine pancreas. Physiol. Rev., *54*: 596–619, 1974.

Wurtman, R. M.: Biogenic amines and endocrine function. Fed. Proc., *32*:1769–1771, 1973.

Chapter 16

THE CEREBELLUM

The cerebral cortex, the basal ganglia, and the cerebellum are inextricably interrelated in the control of muscular activity. Each, nevertheless, has certain characteristic intrinsic functions. Those of the cerebellum have been compared to a computer that is programmed for rapid, repetitive analyses and whose output, based on these analyses, brings about smooth, coordinated movement. In order to carry out these functions, the cerebellum requires information about the position of the body, the degree of bending and twisting at joints, tension in muscles and tendons, frequency of muscular contraction, states of autonomic functions, stimulation of skin, subcutaneous and special sense organs, and ongoing activity in the cerebral cortex and basal ganglia.

GENERAL ARRANGEMENT AND INTERNAL STRUCTURE

The cerebellum is connected to the brain stem by three pairs of peduncles and is grossly divisible into two hemispheres and a connecting portion termed the *vermis* (Fig. 16–1). The hemispheres and vermis are partitioned by fissures of varying depth into *folia* and *lobules.* These in turn are often grouped into *anterior, posterior,* and *flocculonodular* lobes (Fig. 16–2). Another grouping in common use is also shown in Figure 16–2; the three groups are *archicerebellum* (flocculonodular lobe), *paleocerebellum,* and *neocerebellum.* Both subdivisions, which are based on comparative anatomy, sequence of prenatal development, and various functional aspects, are arbitrary but nevertheless indicate a certain degree of topographic and functional localization. The archicerebellum is closely associated with the vestibular nerve and its connections, it is the first part of the cerebellum to develop embryo-

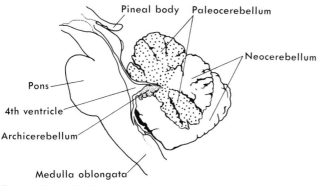

Figure 16-1. Outline sketch of a median section of the brain stem and vermis of the cerebellum, after Figure 7-9, p. 134. The neocerebellum, which forms the bulk of the cerebellar hemispheres, is only partially visible.

logically, and it is separated from the rest of the cerebellum by the *posterolateral fissure* (Fig. 16-2, Table 16-1). The paleocerebellum is chiefly associated with the limbs. The neocerebellum is associated with the neocortex; it is best developed in primates where it forms the bulk of the cerebellum.

The foregoing are crude subdivisions that reflect our lack of understanding of many aspects of cerebellar organization and functions. Nevertheless, they are useful in considering certain

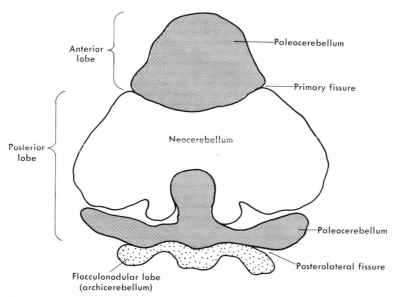

Figure 16-2. Generalized scheme of mammalian cerebellum, viewed from behind, as if the cerebellum were flat rather than curved. The vermis (not labeled) is the portion of the cerebellum in the median plane; there is no anatomical mark that clearly separates it from the hemispheres on either side.

Table 16-1. The subdivisions of the human cerebellum in sequence (folia and fissures) from above, posteriorly, and downward. The names are from the *Nomina anatomica.* A portion of the inferior semilunar lobule is also known as the *gracile lobule,* and a bit of tissue between the tonsil and the flocculus is known as the *paraflocculus.*

Within the *Corpus cerebelli,* the paleocerebellum includes the anterior lobe and, in the posterior lobe, the pyramis and uvula, with biventer and tonsil. The remainder of the corpus cerebelli is neocerebellum.

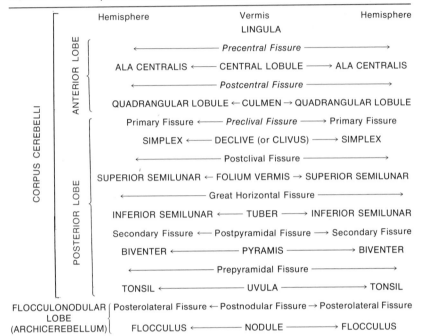

	Hemisphere	Vermis	Hemisphere
		LINGULA	
	←————————	Precentral Fissure	————————→
	ALA CENTRALIS ←——	CENTRAL LOBULE	——→ ALA CENTRALIS
	←————————	Postcentral Fissure	————————→
	QUADRANGULAR LOBULE ←	CULMEN	→ QUADRANGULAR LOBULE
	Primary Fissure ←——	Preclival Fissure	——→ Primary Fissure
	SIMPLEX ←——	DECLIVE (or CLIVUS)	——→ SIMPLEX
	←————————	Postclival Fissure	————————→
	SUPERIOR SEMILUNAR ←	FOLIUM VERMIS	→ SUPERIOR SEMILUNAR
	←————————	Great Horizontal Fissure	————————→
	INFERIOR SEMILUNAR ←——	TUBER	——→ INFERIOR SEMILUNAR
	Secondary Fissure ←	Postpyramidal Fissure	→ Secondary Fissure
	BIVENTER ←——————	PYRAMIS	——————→ BIVENTER
	←————————	Prepyramidal Fissure	————————→
	TONSIL ←——————	UVULA	——————→ TONSIL
	Posterolateral Fissure ←	Postnodular Fissure	→ Posterolateral Fissure
	FLOCCULUS ←——————	NODULE	——————→ FLOCCULUS

(Row labels on left: CORPUS CEREBELLI — ANTERIOR LOBE, POSTERIOR LOBE; FLOCCULONODULAR LOBE (ARCHICEREBELLUM))

functional aspects, and they permit one to manage what can only be described as an appalling terminology. Table 16–1, which is intended only as guide, lists the names given by the *Nomina anatomica* to the various portions of the human cerebellum. However, differences in terminology still exist, and in comparative neurology entirely different terms are often used.

The cerebellum, like the cerebral hemispheres, has a cortex of gray matter and an interior of both white and gray matter. There are four distinct cellular masses in the white matter of each half of the cerebellum; these are termed the *deep cerebellar nuclei.* Most medial is the *nucleus fastigii.* More laterally are two minor nuclei, the *globose* and *emboliform nuclei.* Most lateral is a large, wrinkled nucleus, the *dentate nucleus.* The two nuclei fastigii lie in the roof of the fourth ventricle and are sometimes known as the *roof nuclei.* The cells of the deep cerebellar nuclei receive afferents from various sources; their axons all leave the cerebellum.

The characteristic surface appearance of the cerebellum results from the deep fissures that separate a large number of narrow folia. The folia in turn are folded into secondary and tertiary folia, each with a core of white matter and a surface of cortex. In median sections, the complex branching of white matter and cortex resembles the branching of a tree and is termed the *arbor vitae.*

Microscopic Structure.   Unlike the cerebral cortex, the cerebellar cortex is uniform in thickness and synaptic arrangement. It is divided into an outer *molecular layer,* the deepest part of which contains a row of *Purkinje cells,* and an inner *granular layer* (Fig. 16-3). The molecular layer contains neuronal processes, a few small nerve cells (*basket cells, Golgi cells,* and *stellate cells*), and neuroglial cells that are intimately related to Purkinje cell dendrites. The granular layer contains billions of *granule cells,* the smallest of all neurons.

The Purkinje cells are the most conspicuous cellular elements in the cerebellum (Fig. 16-4). Their dendritic trees spread out in the molecular layer, in one plane only, perpendicular to the long axis of the folium. Their axons pass into the white matter and then to the cerebellar nuclei or to vestibular nuclei. As they do so, they give off recurrent collaterals that synapse with several different neurons, including Golgi cells and other Purkinje cells.

Two types of afferent fibers enter the cerebellum by way of the peduncles. *Mossy fibers,* which are derived from many different

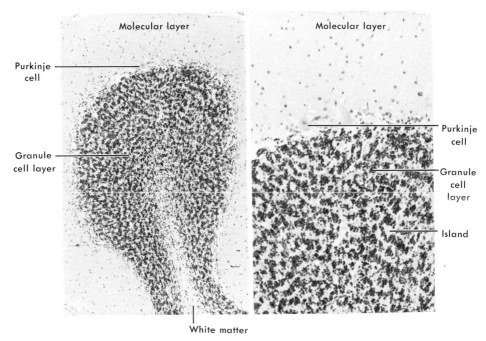

Figure 16-3.   Photomicrographs of cerebellar cortex, hematoxylin and eosin stain. Note the clear area or "island." Ordinary stains fail to show the complex synaptic glomerulus that occupies this island (see Figure 16-5). Note also that this histological stain fails to show the details of the Purkinje cells (see Figure 16-4). Magnifications about 100 × (left section) and 250 × (right section).

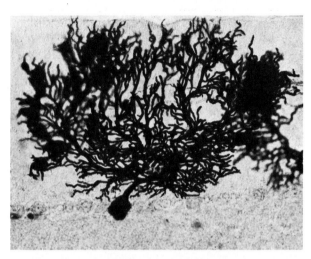

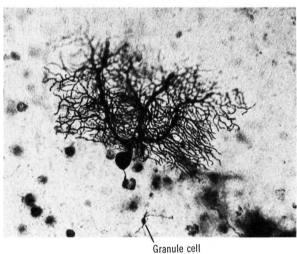

Figure 16-4. Photomicrographs of Purkinje cells, Golgi stain. In the lower photograph a thin axon is seen extending downward from the cell body. This cell is incompletely impregnated. Hence the larger dendrites are less obscured than in the upper cell.

Granule cell

sources, synapse with *granule cells* in the granular layer. The synaptic arrangement is complicated; it is termed a *synaptic glomerulus* (Fig. 3–24, p. 49), and each one occupies an island in the granular layer (Fig. 16–3). The axons of granule cells enter the molecular layer where they bifurcate; the two branches, called *parallel fibers,* run along the longitudinal extent of folia, synapsing with the dendrites of many Purkinje cells. This remarkable anatomical arrangement provides a mechanism for input from one mossy fiber to huge numbers of Purkinje cells; it also provides a mechanism for the sequential activation of successive Purkinje cells. *Climbing fibers,* the second type of afferent fiber, are thought to arise chiefly (some think entirely) from the inferior olives in the medulla oblongata. Each one traverses the granular layer and synapses chiefly with the dendrites of one or but a few Purkinje cells. It has been estimated that a given Purkinje cell may have two hundred thousand synapses from parallel fibers, and a few hundred from a single climbing fiber.

Figure 16–5 shows the general arrangement of the cerebellar cortex, with some of the synaptic connections. Figure 16–6 presents certain principles of cortical organization and function. The granule cells are excitatory; all others are inhibitory. The Purkinje cells are the output of the cortex and they inhibit the cells of the deep cerebellar nuclei. Purkinje cells may be activated (by granule cells and climbing fibers) or inhibited (by basket cells or by a decrease in granule cell activity resulting from their relationship with Golgi cells). These examples illustrate that impulses entering the cerebellum activate both inhibitory and excitatory circuits. These two types of inputs and their circuits may, therefore, represent delicately balanced systems that act in rapid on-off sequential fashion, with their ultimate effects (stopping or starting, depressing or enhancing, muscular activity) being directed by way of the deep cerebellar nuclei to other parts of the nervous system and thereby to muscles. Such a rapid, on-off sequential mechanism could enable the cerebellum to engage in a continuous ongoing correction of movements, much as occurs for a target-finding missile.

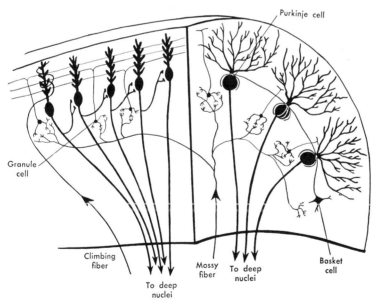

Figure 16–5. Diagram of cells in a folium of the cerebellum. The Purkinje cells have a large dendritic tree across the plane of the folium, hence in this view are much more extensive than in the plane parallel to the length of the folium. Mossy fibers synapse with many granule cells in the cerebellar glomeruli. The axons of granule cells enter the molecular layer and divide, each branch running lengthwise in the folium as a "parallel" fiber, synapsing with Purkinje cells and basket cells. Climbing fibers synapse directly with Purkinje cells. Axons of Purkinje cells have recurrent branches to adjacent Purkinje cells and to other cells (not shown).

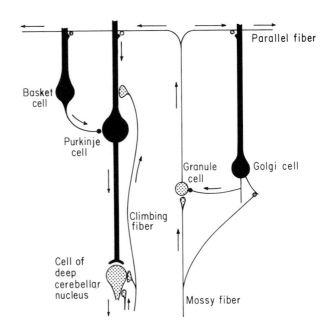

Figure 16-6. Schematic representation of some of the principal synaptic connections within
the cerebellum. Inhibitory cells
shown in black; excitatory cells
and synapses are stippled. (Based
on Eccles, J. C., in J. Physiol.
299:1–3, 1973.)

Figure 16–6 also illustrates that collaterals of cerebellar
afferents are given to cells of the deep cerebellar nuclei. Less is
known about the synaptic organization of these nuclei. It is
likely that they possess intrinsic activity that is controlled or
modified by the Purkinje cells which project to them.

CEREBELLAR CONNECTIONS

If the pathways that convey information to the cerebellum
are compared to the various cerebellar outputs, it is evident that
the major input-output mechanisms of the cerebellum may be
regarded as "loops." For example, the portions of the cerebellum
that receive information from the limbs project to the motor
systems controlling limb movements. This is a highly simplistic
view, but nevertheless a useful one in presenting some of the basic
features of the major cerebellar connections. The anatomical
features of these loops are outlined in a highly schematic fashion
in the following paragraphs.

It should be emphasized that in contrast to the crossed control
so characteristic of the pyramidal system, cerebellar control is
largely ipsilateral. That is, each cerebellar hemisphere is related
to the corresponding half of the body (Fig. 16–7). This means that
if, for example, the right half of the cerebellum is damaged, the
resulting movement disorders will be present chiefly on the right

side of the body. It may be that the anatomical relationship is even more specific, that is, that a specific area of a cerebellar subdivision may have highly specific input-out relationships with a specific part of the body, such as a limb, but the evidence for this in humans is incomplete.

Vestibular loop. The cerebellar portion of this loop is the flocculonodular lobe, that is, the archicerebellum. The loop is activated by the stimulation of receptors in the vestibule and semicircular canals, that is, by changes in the position of the head, including linear and rotational movements. Some of the nerve impulses reach the archicerebellum directly by vestibular nerve fibers, whereas others are relayed by vestibular nuclei. Both the direct and the secondary fibers are carried by the inferior cerebellar peduncles. Some of the Purkinje cells of the archicerebellum project directly to the brain stem, whereas others project to the nuclei fastigii. In both instances, the destinations are those portions of the vestibular nuclei and reticular formation of the brain stem that control the muscles of the head, neck, and trunk.

Spinal cord loop (Figs. 16–8, 16–9). The cerebellar portion of this loop is the paleocerebellum. The input is chiefly from the limbs by a number of ascending pathways whose exact origins and topographical relations in humans are still uncertain. The following outline is a simplified statement of current views.

Impulses arising from skin, muscles, tendons, and joints reach the cerebellum by *spinocerebellar, spino-olivary,* and *spinoreticular tracts.* The spinocerebellar tracts are *anterior* and *posterior* (also known as ventral and dorsal). Each anterior tract arises from spinal gray matter (layers 5 to 7), crosses and ascends in the

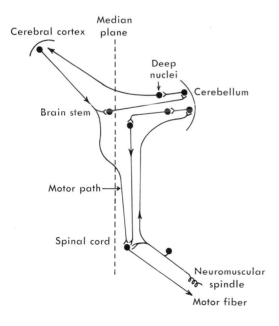

Figure 16–7. Schematic representation of the principles of cerebellar connections (vestibular connections omitted). Three features are emphasized: (1) loop arrangements; (2) relationship to motor pathways; and (3) ipsilateral control of muscles.

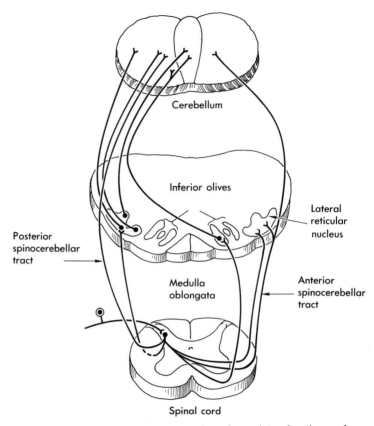

Figure 16–8. Schematic representation of a variety of pathways from the spinal cord to the cerebellum (anterior and posterior spinocerebellar tracts), including relays through the inferior olive and lateral reticular nucleus. (Modified from Gardner, E.: CIBA Foundation Symposium on Myotatic, Kinesthetic and Vestibular Mechanisms. London, J. and A. Churchill Ltd., 1967.)

opposite anterolateral funiculus, together with the spinothalamic tracts, and enters the cerebellum by way of the superior cerebellar peduncle. Each posterior tract arises from the nucleus thoracicus (layer 7), ascends ipsilaterally in the lateral funiculus, adjacent to the pyramidal tract, enters the medulla oblongata, and projects to the cerebellum by way of the inferior cerebellar peduncle. The anterior and posterior tracts are concerned chiefly with the lower limbs. Impulses from the upper limbs use·two main routes. One is by way of the posterior funiculus to the *lateral cuneate nucleus* (a small nucleus immediately lateral to the nucleus cuneatus of the medulla) and thence to the cerebellum. The other is by way of a "rostral spinocerebellar tract" whose precise location in humans is unknown.

A large number of afferent fibers to the inferior olives and lateral reticular nuclei of the medulla oblongata arises throughout the spinal cord. They are activated by many modalities, and they are relayed to the cerebellum by way of the inferior cerebellar peduncles.

The Purkinje cells of the paleocerebellum project to the deep nuclei (chiefly the nuclei fastigii), and these nuclei in turn project to those portions of the vestibular nuclei and the reticular formation that control the motor neurons supplying the limb musculature.

Finally, there are projections to the cerebellum from central trigeminal connections, carrying information from the skin, mucous membrane, teeth, muscles, and joints and muscles of the head, including the muscles of the eyes.

Cerebrocerebellar loop (Fig. 16–10). The neocerebellum, which comprises most of the cerebellar hemisphere, receives a massive input from the neocortex. Arising from all parts of the neocortex, *corticopontine fibers* descend in the internal capsules

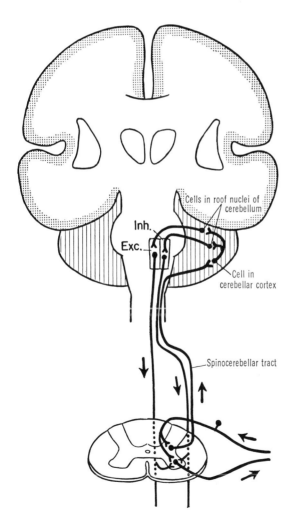

Figure 16–9. Connections of the cerebellum and spinal cord showing possible links to descending paths.

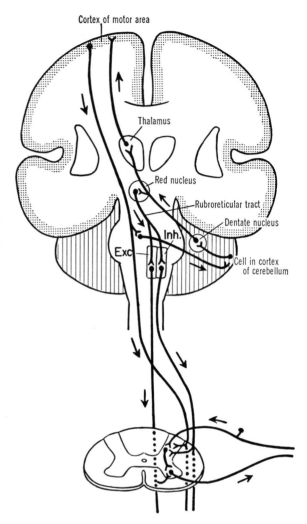

Figure 16-10. Diagram of some of the connections between cerebral cortex and cerebellum. Corticospinal fibers are represented as giving off collaterals in the' pons. The cells with which they synapse give rise to the middle cerebellar peduncle. The path ascending from the dentate nucleus is the superior cerebellar peduncle. In humans impulses from the red nucleus reach the spinal cord directly and by way of relays at brain stem levels.

and cerebral peduncles to pontine nuclei. Here they synapse with cells whose axons cross the median plane, form the middle cerebellar peduncles, and are distributed throughout the neocerebellum. (Since the neocortex and neocerebellum are well developed in primates, the anterior portion of the pons is correspondingly large.) The Purkinje cells of the neocerebellum project to the deep nuclei, chiefly the dentate nuclei, whose axons form the bulk of the superior cerebellar peduncles. The fibers in each peduncle ascend and cross to the opposite side while traversing the midbrain. After crossing, most of the fibers pass through the red nucleus and reach the thalamus, where they end chiefly in the *nucleus ventralis lateralis* (the projection to the thalamus is sometimes known as the *dentatorubrothalamic path*). From the thalamus they project to the cerebral cortex, especially to the motor areas. While traversing the red nucleus, collaterals may be given to the constituent neurons. (Some fibers end in the nucleus.) These connections to the red nucleus provide for control of brain stem and spinal mechanisms, and represent coordination with paleocerebellar functions.

Although many anatomical and functional details are still quite uncertain in humans, there is little doubt that the neocerebellum exerts its influence on all muscular activity by way of its projections to the cerebral cortex, brain stem, and spinal cord.

Other Connections. The cerebellum receives a significant input from the visual and auditory systems by way of *tectocerebellar fibers*. Moreover, there appears to be a major projection from the visual cortex to the neocerebellum by way of corticopontine fibers. These inputs reflect the important role of the cerebellum in the regulation and coordination of eye movements; that from the visual cortex might well be a pathway concerned with saccadic eye movements (p. 209).

Experimental evidence indicates that the cerebellum has connections with various autonomic centers of the brain stem. The precise functions of these connections are still uncertain, but may well consist of coordinating muscular activity and certain autonomic functions.

There is also evidence in experimental animals that the monoaminergic cells that project to the cerebellum (p. 319) synapse directly with Purkinje cells throughout the cerebellar cortex, and that some of these (e. g., locus ceruleus) inhibit the Purkinje cells. The functions of these connections are unknown.

FUNCTIONS OF THE CEREBELLUM

In the chapter on the control of muscular activity, it was pointed out that smoothly coordinated muscular activity requires perfect timing. If a muscle group does not contract (or relax) at the proper time with respect to other muscle groups, movement will be jerky and awkward. It has been difficult to analyze cerebellar functions in humans, and experimental studies have been largely confined to other mammals and lower vertebrates. Nevertheless, from these studies and from clinical experience with cerebellar disorders, it seems clear that the cerebellum is largely responsible for coordinating the timing of activity in various groups of muscles, both in static or postural and phasic or locomotor mechanisms. In so doing, the cerebellum seems to enhance muscle tone, especially through excitatory effects upon muscle spindles. The functions of the cerebellum are not subject to voluntary control; we are not directly conscious of the functions of the cerebellum and defects resulting from cerebellar disorders cannot be voluntarily controlled or modified to any extent.

In carrying out its functions the cerebellum analyzes information derived from all available sources about position and movement, including angles and torsion at joints, degree of tension in muscles, frequency of contraction, etc. The cerebellum acts like a computer, performing successions of almost instantaneous analyses of the information it receives and initiating the actions dictated by the analyses. The information is received over many pathways, from the cerebral cortex and peripheral receptors—retinal, labyrinthine, cutaneous, muscle, tendon, and joint. The microscopic structure of the cerebellum reflects the computer-like structure, and the output of the cerebellum is directed to the cerebral cortex and to the motor centers of the brain stem. Here, the cerebellum probably affects the excitability of cortical and brain stem neurons.

It should be noted that if the cerebellum is a computer for the continuous analysis of position and movement, such analysis takes time, especially if it depends upon feedback over the cerebellar loops. The time may be shortened, if the information already on hand is used in a "feedforward" mechanism to establish appropriate timing and coordination from the moment that movement starts. However, neither feedback or feedforward mechanisms are satisfactory for very fast ballistic movements, such as saccadic eye movements. Hence, some argue that the necessary timing and coordinating mechanisms for very rapid movements are programmed ("preset") in the cerebellar cortex and are put into operation without the necessity of input information.

It is often stated that the paleocerebellum is primarily concerned in the coordination of postural activity, and the neocerebellum in locomotor activity. This is based on the fact that in animals, such as the cat, it has been demonstrated experimentally that electrical stimulation of the anterior part of the cerebellum (paleocerebellum) may be followed by relaxation of antigravity muscles. Whether there is actually such a sharp distinction is open to question. For example, it is possible to obtain opposite effects by changing the frequency of the stimulating current.

Little is known of the functions of the archicerebellum in humans. There is a malignant tumor termed a *medulloblastoma,* which is composed of undifferentiated, rapidly growing cells. It occurs in children and frequently starts in the archicerebellum. The earliest signs may be incoordination in trunk musculature. It has been deduced, therefore, that this part of the cerebellum is concerned in the coordination of the musculature of the trunk. The validity of these deductions is still uncertain, because the symptoms also resemble those that result from disturbances of balance in vestibular disorders. On the basis of the connections of the archicerebellum, it is more likely that it, together with the other portions of the cerebellum, plays a major role in the coordination of head and eye movements.

DISORDERS OF THE CEREBELLUM

In general, cerebellar disorders are characterized by difficulties in timing, coordination, and balance, and by *ataxia.* The disruption of timing and coordination may result in jerky movements (*intention tremors*). These may be especially noticeable at the end of movement (*terminal tremor*). These disruptions may be elicited by asking the patient to put his finger to his nose. He may do so, but is often unable to stop his finger at his nose, or he may point much to one side of it. Ataxia is evident as a stumbling, incoordinated gait. Rapid alternating movements may be difficult or impossible to perform. If the patient puts his feet close together, he may sway severely and fall over. Cerebellar signs may be compensated for if the lesion is not progressive. That is, symptoms may partially or completely disappear after several weeks or months. Perhaps vision is used to tell when muscular contractions reach the proper point, thus compensating for the loss of the more automatic mechanisms.

Another common cerebellar sign is *hypotonia.* This may be so great that the muscles are limp or flaccid, and the deep reflexes are decreased or absent. Hypotonia is thought to result from decreased muscle spindle activity, due to decreased excitability of neurons in the cerebral cortex following loss of impulses from the cerebellum, and also to decreased discharge from the red nucleus.

It is known that interference with the input can produce cerebellar disturbances, including limb ataxia. However, the multiplicity of ascending paths provides a wide margin of safety. In fact, fairly widespread involvement of ascending tracts is necessary before significant or permanent cerebellar signs result. For example, section of the lateral spinothalamic tract for relief of pain also severs spinocerebellar fibers, chiefly those of the anterior tract. Yet the resulting ataxia, if any, may be temporary.

Finally, it is of clinical importance that cerebellar effects are chiefly ipsilateral (Fig. 16–7). This means that a lesion in the *left* cerebellum will cause signs on the *left* side of the body, in contrast to a lesion in the *left* internal capsule which can cause a *right* hemiplegia. A confusing situation results when there is a lesion in a superior cerebellar peduncle after it has crossed in its ascent, in which case there are cerebellar signs contralateral to the side of the lesion. Thus, it is not unknown for cerebellar signs to follow lesions in the frontal lobe, so that with a left-sided frontal lobe lesion the signs would be on the right side.

SUMMARY

The cerebellum is a fissured structure attached to the brain stem by three pairs of peduncles. It has a cortex, composed of an inner granular and an outer molecular layer; the deep portion of the latter contains a row of Purkinje cells. The input to the cerebellum is by way of mossy and climbing fibers, which activate excitatory and inhibitory circuits. The output of the cortex is by way of Purkinje cell axons to deep cerebellar nuclei. These cells in turn project to other parts of the nervous system.

The cerebellum has widespread reciprocal connections with the cerebral cortex, particularly the motor and sensory areas. It has many connections with the spinal cord, chiefly with paths derived from peripheral receptors, and there are many connections with cranial nerves, particularly the vestibular, auditory, trigeminal, and optic nerves. These reciprocal connections form pathways that can be described as loops. The vestibular loop associates the vestibular system and the archicerebellum. The spinal loop involves the paleocerebellum. The cortical loop is a massive connection of neocortex and neocerebellum.

The cerebellum is involved in timing or coordination of muscular activity. It receives information from peripheral receptors and from motor and sensory regions of the cerebral cortex. It carries out its functions primarily through brain stem inhibitory and excitatory mechanisms, which it modifies, and also the motor cortex. The anatomical connections are such that each cerebellar hemisphere is concerned mainly with muscles on the ipsilateral or same side of the body.

Disorders of the cerebellum are manifested chiefly as hypotonia and as defects in coordination of muscular activity.

NAMES IN NEUROLOGY

JAN EVANGLISTA PURKYNĚ (JOHANNES PURKINJE) (1787–1869)
See the biographical sketch on p. 285.

REFERENCES

See the references cited on pages 159 and 219.
The following are major texts and reference sources.

Eccles, J. C., Ito, M., and Szentágothai, J.: The Cerebellum as a Neuronal Machine. New York, Springer-Verlag, 1967.
Larsell, O., and Jansen, J.: The Comparative Anatomy and Histology of the Cerebellum. Minneapolis, The University of Minnesota Press, 1972. This volume deals with the human cerebellum, its development, connections, and cortex.
Llinás, R. (editor): Neurobiology of Cerebellar Evolution and Development. Chicago, American Medical Association, 1969.
Palay, D. L., and Chan-Palay, V.: Cerebellar Cortex. Berlin, Springer-Verlag, 1974. A major treatise on cytology and organization.

The following reviews and papers provide a comprehensive coverage of cerebellar structure, organization and function.

Bloedel, J.: Cerebellar afferent systems: a review. Progress Neurobiol., Vol.2 (1). Kerkut, G. A., and Phillis, J. W., editors. Oxford, Pergamon Press, 1973.

Eccles, J. C.: The cerebellum as a computer: patterns in space and time. J. Physiol., 229:1–32, 1973.

Evarts, E. V., and Thach, W. T.: Motor mechanisms of the CNS: cerebrocerebellar interactions. Ann. Rev. Physiol., 32:451–498, 1969.

Fox, C. A., Hillman, D. E., Siegesmund, K. A., and Dutta, C. R.: The primate cerebellar cortex: a Golgi and electron microscopic study. In The Cerebellum, vol. 25, pp. 174–225. Fox, C. A., and Snider, R. S. editors. Amsterdam, Elsevier Publishing Company, 1967.

Ito, M.: The control mechanisms of cerebellar motor systems, pp. 293–303, in The Neurosciences: Third Study Program. Schmitt, F. O., and Worden, F. G. (editors-in-chief). Cambridge, Mass., The MIT Press, 1974.

Kornhuber, H. H.: Cerebral Cortex, cerebellum, and basal ganglia: an introduction to their motor functions, pp. 267–280, in The Neurosciences: Third Study Program. Schmitt, F. O., and Worden, F. G., (editors-in-chief). Cambridge, Mass., The MIT Press, 1974.

Llinás, R.: Neuronal operations in cerebellar transactions. Pp. 409–426. In The Neurosciences: Second Study Program. Schmitt, F. O. (editor-in-chief). New York, Rockefeller University Press, 1969.

Llinás, R.: Motor aspects of cerebellar control. The Physiologist, 17:19–46, 1974.

Mann, M. D.: Clarke's column and the dorsal spinocerebellar tract: a review. Brain, Behav., Evol., 7:34–83, 1973.

Chapter **17**

THE FOREBRAIN: CEREBRAL CORTEX AND SUBCORTICAL STRUCTURES

In the embryo, the forebrain or prosencephalon is the rostral portion of the neural tube from which the telencephalon and diencephalon differentiate. In this and the next two chapters, the term forebrain refers to the adult derivatives, that is, the cerebral hemispheres and the diencephalon. The term *cerebrum* (Latin, *brain*) refers to the two cerebral hemispheres and the diencephalon; it has also been used to refer to the forebrain and midbrain, and even to the entire brain. The adjective *cerebral* is derived from it. By contrast, the term *encephalon* is of Greek origin (*enkephalos,* brain). Terms such as *encephalitis,* which means inflammation of the brain, are derived from it.

CEREBRAL HEMISPHERES

The human cerebral hemispheres include an enormous volume of cortex and masses of subcortical gray matter, which can be categorized as follows: neocortex, basal ganglia (corpus striatum), olfactory structures (including paleocortex), and portions of the limbic system (including archicortex). There is substantial overlap between these groups.

Human behavior is correlated to a large extent with the relatively massive size of the forebrain. Here reside most of the mechanisms governing learning, memory, intelligence, language, emotion, and behavior. Moreover, the volume of neocortex can be correlated not only with higher level functions (e.g., speech mechanisms, various perceptive mechanisms and motor skills, and upright posture), but also with hemisphere specialization. Hemisphere specialization, in which the right hemisphere differs significantly from the left in function (Chapter 19), is a uniquely human feature.

NEOCORTEX

The earliest anatomical studies of the brain led to the naming of various parts, for example, lobes, gyri, and sulci. Subsequently, microscopic studies led to the conclusion that the neurons of the cerebral cortex are arranged in layers and that the organization of the layers is similar in all mammals. In Nissl-stained microscopic sections it is apparent that the neuronal cell bodies form layers that are tangential to the surface. The limits and subdivisions of the individual layers are not always clear, and many different schemes for identifying the layers have been proposed. Investigators of cortical lamination based on Nissl and Weigert sections developed systems of numbering or lettering, each number or letter supposedly representing a portion of the cortex with distinctive cytoarchitectonic features. Several hundred such areas have been described and diagrammed, giving the impression of a clear-cut parcellation of the cerebral cortex. Actually, none of the studies established objective criteria for critical distinctions between cortical areas and individual variations were seldom taken into account. Except in a few instances, sharp parcellation cannot be substantiated. This does not mean that there are no structural or functional differences between different regions of the cerebral cortex. There are, but Nissl stains do not often demonstrate them satisfactorily. The synaptic arrangements demonstrated by silver and Golgi staining, electron microscopy, and experimental studies indicate an enormous complexity that defies simple analysis.

It is now generally recognized that the *neocortex (isocortex)* has six layers. It is also recognized that individual layers may vary in thickness in different regions of the cortex, and that layers may be subdivided in some regions or merge in others. Table 17–1 outlines the basic arrangement of six-layered or *homotypical* cortex; the scheme is based on the shapes and sizes of the predominant neurons in the various layers. The table also includes information based on silver and Golgi stains. It should be emphasized that most layers contain more than one kind of cell; stellate cells for example, are present in layers 2 and 3, as well as in 4.

In certain regions six layers cannot be identified. Examples of this *heterotypical* cortex are shown in Figure 17–1, in which the fifth layer, with small and giant pyramidal cells, is prominent in the motor cortex. Indeed, the number of pyramidal neurons in

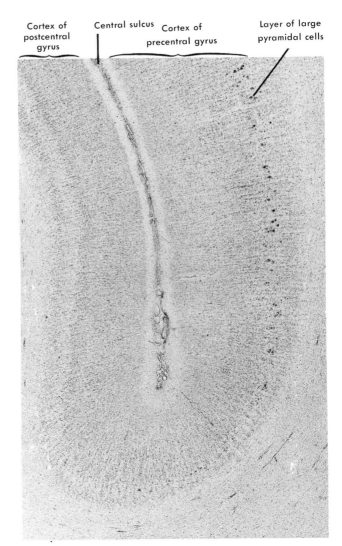

Cortex of postcentral gyrus

Central sulcus

Cortex of precentral gyrus

Layer of large pyramidal cells

Figure 17-1. Photomicrograph of Nissl-stained section of central sulcus with the motor cortex (postcentral gyrus) on the left. Note large pyramidal cells in the motor cortex. The central fissure between the two is filled with a pia mater and blood vessels.

the motor cortex is so great that layers 2 to 5 tend to merge and to obscure the granular layers. Hence, motor cortex is sometimes termed *agranular cortex.* In the sensory cortex the number of stellate cells is so great in layers 2, 3, and 5, as well as in 4, that layers 2 to 5 tend to merge. This conglomerate layer, which is characteristic of heterotypical sensory cortex (also known as *granular cortex),* is evident as a lighter staining band in the postcentral gyrus of Figure 17-1. Weigert-stained sections indicate that myelinated fibers entering sensory cortex over specific afferent paths form a prominent myelinated stripe in the inner granular layer (Fig. 17-2).

Many different kinds of neurons have been described in the neocortex. On the basis of cell shape, size, dendritic arborization, and axonal distribution, there are two basic types, *pyramidal* and

Table 17-1. The layers of homotypical neocortex.

Layer	Chief Type of Cell	Other Features	Axonal Distribution of Predominant Cell
1. Molecular layer (plexiform layer)	Occasional horizontal and stellate cells	Cell poor; it is an important synaptic field	Throughout layer 1.
2. Outer granular layer	Small and medium-sized pyramidal cells	Also contains stellate cells	Intracortical and to white matter
3. Pyramidal cell layer (outer pyramidal layer)	Medium and large pyramidal cells	Also contains stellate cells	To white matter
4. Inner granular layer	Stellate cells (granule cells)	Main termination of specific afferent fibers	Intracortical
5. Ganglionic layer (inner pyramidal layer)	Small to giant pyramidal cells	Giant cells mostly limited to precentral gyrus	To white matter
6. Fusiform cell layer (layer of polymorphic cells)	Fusiform cell	Other cells of different shapes and sizes (hence the term polymorphic)	To white matter

stellate, as indicated in Table 17-1 (Figs. 3-5 and 3-6, pp. 30 and 31). A number of subtypes can be distinguished.

Pyramidal cells have a conical-shaped body from which a large apical dendrite extends toward the surface, reaching layer 1. This apical dendrite is characterized by a large number of short processes termed *spines.* In addition, short thick dendrites arise from the base of the cell. The axons of pyramidal cells leave the cortex and enter the white matter. Those in layers 5 and 6 often have recurrent collateral branches that ramify in the cortical layers, especially in layer 1.

Stellate cells are small oval or spindle-shaped cells with thin,

White matter   Cortex (gray matter)

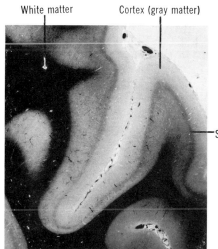

Stripe of myelinated fibers

Figure 17-2. Photomicrograph of a section of occipital cortex. The entering visual fibers form a band or stripe as they end in the fourth cell layer. Weigert stain.

short, branching dendrites, some of which may possess spines. The axons of some stellate cells may enter the white matter. Many, however, ramify throughout the cortex, reaching layer 1, and still others ramify within their own dendritic field. Some stellate cells have remarkable characteristics. One type is a cell in layers 2 to 4 which has a double bouquet of dendrites arising from the upper and lower poles of the soma; each bouquet consists of arborizing beaded dendrites. The axon has an extraordinarily marked vertical arborization throughout the whole thickness of the cortex. There are great numbers of such stellate cells. Still another important type of stellate cell is present in layers 3 and 4. It has a star-shaped dendritic tree, and an ascending or descending axon that immediately divides into many horizontal or oblique branches of great length. Fusiform cells are spindle-shaped, with dendrites arising from each pole. The lower dendrites ramify within the layer, whereas the upper dendrites may reach the surface. The axons enter the white matter.

Other axons present in the cortex are those that enter from the white matter. The specific afferents to the primary sensory cortex end chiefly in layer 4, where they form a myelinated stripe (Fig. 17–2). Fibers derived from other cortical regions (association and commissural fibers) end in all layers of the cortex except the uppermost. The various afferent fibers tend to synapse chiefly on the spines and dendritic trees of the pyramidal cells, whereas axons of intracortical neurons end mostly on the somas and dendritic trunks.

It is clear from the foregoing anatomical evidence that the neocortex is characterized by a vertical organization that reaches as far as the surface, where layer 1 consists chiefly of recurrent collateral axons, axons of stellate cells, and apical dendrites. Physiological studies support this concept of vertical organization, to the extent that the neocortex may be considered as a mosaic of overlapping columns of cells. Each column would have a functional specificity based on incoming fibers, and an internal processing carried out by interneurons (stellate cells; Fig. 17–3). Horizontal connections with adjacent columns might well be chiefly inhibitory, serving to sharpen the specificity of the column. The pyramidal cells serve as the output for each column, with their axons entering white matter and descending to subcortical structures, brain stem, or spinal cord (*projection neurons*), or crossing to the opposite hemisphere (*commissural neurons*), or connecting portions of the cortex in the same hemisphere (*association neurons*).

The functions of the neocortex are considered during discussion of the limbic system and in also in Chapters 18 and 19. Of pertinence here, however, are the spontaneous electrical activity of the brain, which is brought about by synaptic field potentials in the neocortex, and the potential changes that are evoked by peripheral stimulation.

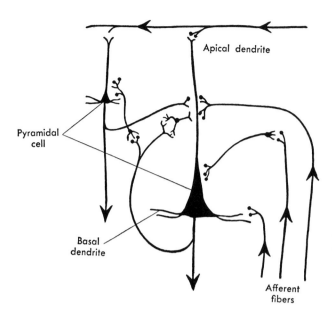

Apical dendrite

Pyramidal cell

Basal dendrite

Afferent fibers

Figure 17–3. Schematic representation of some cortical neurons and a few of their connections, based on Golgi staining. Microscopic studies using Nissl stains (thus showing only cell bodies) do not reveal the connections of nerve cells. Note that pyramidal cells can be activated directly by afferent fibers and interneurons and indirectly by recurrent collaterals. This diagram does not reveal vertical organization, nor does it distinguish the various types of synapses.

Electroencephalogram. The spontaneous electrical activity of the brain can be detected and recorded by methods similar to those used for other electrically active structures. In the method most commonly employed in humans, electrodes are placed on the scalp, with the subject at rest in a darkened room, and the potential differences between pairs of electrodes are amplified and recorded. The record obtained is an *electroencephalogram* (EEG; popularly known as "brain waves"). It represents the changes that occur in the voltage field distribution on the head as a function of time. With appropriate recording, almost any frequency can be observed. These range from frequencies as slow as 1 cycle per second to frequencies in excess of 50 cycles per second. The most common frequencies have been grouped and identified by Greek letters. These, however, are general notations and are presented chiefly to serve as a guide, especially in connection with the older literature. The common frequencies are as follows: The *alpha* frequency ranges from 8 to 13 cycles per second, the *beta* from 13 and faster, the *theta* from 4 to 7 cycles per second, and the *delta* 3 cycles per second or less.

Although the electroencephalographic pattern varies from one person to another, certain rhythmical activity is usually present. The *alpha rhythm (Berger rhythm;* Fig. 17–4) is a rhythmic activity in the posterior quadrants of the head which ranges in frequency from 8 to 13 cycles per second. The *alpha* rhythm is characteristically responsive to arousal, eye opening and closing (Fig. 17–4), and mental activities; there is evidence that *alpha* activity is associated with a feeling of calm or well-being. It is interesting that one may learn to control the amount of *alpha* rhythm if the rhythm

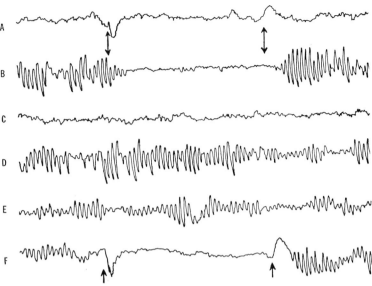

Figure 17-4. Normal electroencephalograms of a medical student. *A,* Record from right and left frontal regions and, *B,* from right and left occipital regions, taken simultaneously. The first arrow indicates opening the eyes. Note the subsequent deflection in the frontal record. This is an artifact due to the movement. Note that the activity in the occipital leads is suppressed. The second arrow indicates eye closing, again followed by an artifact, with a reappearance of occipital activity. *C* and *D,* Continuations of *A* and *B* to give an idea of variations in activity. The frontal records are mainly low voltage, relatively fast *beta* activity. The occipital records are mainly higher voltage *alpha* rhythm. *E,* Record between right occipital and right frontal, continued in *F,* in which the opening and closing of the eyes, indicated by arrows and blinking artifacts, is accompanied again by suppression of *alpha* activity.

is fed back through another sensory system (e.g., if the *alpha* rhythm is used to trigger an oscillator that produces a tone that the subject listens to). This feedback control may be a form of operant conditioning.

The *alpha* rhythm is in contradistinction to wave forms of a similar frequency (*alpha frequency*) which may be recorded from the central parts of the head and which are attenuated on one side by movement of the contralateral limbs. This rhythmic activity at an *alpha* frequency is called the *mu rhythm.*

Beta activity is present chiefly in the anterior quadrants of the head (Fig. 17–4). It may sometimes be recorded from the occipital regions, but in such instances is masked by the *alpha* rhythm and is therefore evident only when the eyes are open or the subject is mentally active.

The electrical activity that is recorded from the scalp originates only from the cerebral cortex. No activity occurring in subcortical structures is seen. The potential changes are almost certainly due to synaptic field potentials, especially those due to cells oriented at right angles to the surface of the cortex. (The most prominent ones are the large pyramidal cells with their apical dendrites, which form great numbers of more or less parallel active elements of relatively low internal resistance and relatively large intracellular and extracellular current flow). Rhythmic cortical activity, at least that which occurs in the frontal areas (e.g., spindle activity; see below), is triggered by rhythmic activity occurring in the specific projection nuclei of the thalamus (p. 388). The phasic character of these wave forms (i.e., the rhythmic characteristic) is probably due to recurrent inhibition in these specific thalamic nuclei. The nonspecific thalamic nuclei (p. 390), which "desynchronize" the cortical activity and which are involved in arousal, influence or modulate the mechanisms of recurrent inhibition.

The magnitude of the recorded potential changes is approximately 50 microvolts. However, certain wave forms, even in normal individuals, may be as high as 1 millivolt. No particular frequency or combination of frequencies is specifically normal or specifically abnormal. They are evaluated according to the context within which they occur, depending upon age, clinical state, and state of arousal or consciousness of the subject or patient. An important example of a specific state of consciousness is sleep, in which there are characteristic electroencephalographic patterns, as outlined below (see also p. 323).

In stage 1 of non-REM sleep, the electroencephalogram is of relatively low voltage. It consists mainly of fast activity mixed with some slower rhythms in the range of 4 to 7 cycles per second. With increasing drowsiness and light sleep (stage 2), the slower activity becomes somewhat more prominent and *K-complexes* are seen. These are high voltage sharp waves, maximal at the central vertex, which are occasionally associated with slow waves. The K-complexes are auditory evoked potentials and are similar to vertex sharp waves or *V waves* that can sometimes be recorded, especially in children. Also appearing during stage 2 is rhythmic, fast activity occurring for short periods of time at a frequency of 12 to 14 cycles per second in the anterior quadrants of the head. These wave forms are termed *sleep spindles.* In stages 3 and 4 (moderate to deep sleep), the slow waves increase in amount and the spindles gradually disappear. K-complexes may continue to be present. Throughout stages 1 to 4, some slow eye movements may be present.

In REM sleep, the electrical activity resembles that of stage 1, but rapid eye movements are present.

Provided that certain limitations are recognized, the electroencephalogram is an important procedure for evaluation and diagnosis. The limitations include a lack of full understanding of the neurophysiological basis of the electroencephalogram, individual variations, age differences (the electroencephalogram in infancy and childhood is more difficult to obtain and interpret), and susceptibility to drugs and to such physiological variables as blood sugar levels, acid-base equilibrium, and level of attention or awareness.

The clinical conditions in which the electroencephalogram is of particular value include epilepsy (an example is given in Figure 17–5), intracranial space-occupying lesions (e.g., tumors), head injuries, and cerebral infections. Finally, the electroencephalogram can be employed to assess states of unconsciousness (e.g., sleep, levels of anesthesia, coma) and brain death. In the latter instance, determination of brain death is critical in certifying the availability of organs for transplant.

Evoked Potentials. *Evoked potentials* are surface waves that are elicited by peripheral stimulation. For example, in a subject who actively looks at something, a large, long-lasting (100 to 200 milliseconds in duration) *lambda wave* may be recorded from the occipital regions. *Lambda* waves are visual evoked potentials that are probably related to the eye movements that are involved in the scanning of objects being looked at. Similar wave forms during sleep are called *positive occipital sharp waves of sleep,* and may also be related in some way to eye movements. Auditory evoked potentials (K-complexes and V waves) associated with the electroencephalogram have already been mentioned. Controllable evoked potentials can be elicited by means of a precisely controlled peripheral stimulus, for example, a flash of light of known intensity and duration, a sound of known intensity and frequency, or an electrical stimulus of known voltage and duration applied to a peripheral nerve. The cortical potential resulting from the arrival of a volley of synchronous afferent impulses is easily recorded from the surface of the brain, but when recorded from the scalp is usually so small that averaging of successive responses must be employed. Evoked sensory potentials may be useful in assessing the integrity of receptors and their pathways (e.g., in determining the extent of deafness). They may also be useful when the cooperation of the patient is difficult or impossible to obtain.

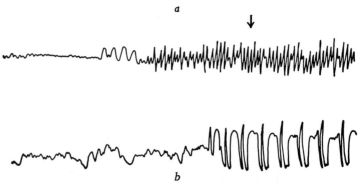

a

b

Figure 17–5. *a,* Electroencephalogram of a nine-year-old boy. Tonic-clonic seizure with fast, high voltage waves. Arrow indicates appearance of clinical evidence of seizure. *b,* Petit mal attack, with staring, blinking, and loss of consciousness. Characteristic wave and spike discharge in electroencephalogram.

Another kind of evoked phenomenon is the *contingent negative variation*. If a subject is presented with a warning stimulus that is followed by a stimulus to which the subject must respond, a small (20-microvolt) negative potential can be recorded from the frontal portions of the head at some time between the first stimulus and the operant response. This wave represents a kind of attention or expectancy and is therefore occasionally termed the *expectancy wave* or *E wave*.

OLFACTORY CORTEX

The olfactory cortex, or *paleocortex,* consists, in humans, of a strip of cortex that extends from the uncus of the temporal lobe, across the anterior perforated substance (Fig. 12–26, p. 283), to the septal area (p. 394). This is a three-layered cortex (*molecular, pyramidal,* and *polymorphic layers*) whose constituent cells include projection and intrinsic neurons. The lateral portion of the olfactory cortex is the primary receptive area for smell (p. 415).

HIPPOCAMPUS

The hippocampus and the dentate gyrus are a part of the limbic system, which is described later (p. 390). The cortex of the hippocampus has a three-layered arrangement (*molecular, pyramidal,* and *polymorphic layers*), as does that of the dentate gyrus (*molecular, granular,* and *polymorphic layers*). The cortex of each is also known as *archicortex* or *allocortex*.

TRANSITIONAL CORTEX

Transitional cortex is present where paleocortex and archicortex merge into neocortex. In addition, most of the cingulate gyrus, which is a part of the limbic system, is intermediate histologically between three and six layers and is sometimes known as *mesocortex.*

BASAL GANGLIA

The term basal ganglia is used loosely and inconsistently to refer to some or all of the masses of gray matter within the cerebral hemispheres. The major basal ganglia are the *corpus striatum (caudate nucleus, putamen,* and *globus pallidus)* and *subthalamic nucleus* (Figs. 17–6 to 17–9). On the basis of anatomical and functional connections, the *substantia nigra* and *red nucleus* are often included. (The subthalamic nucleus and globus pallidus, together

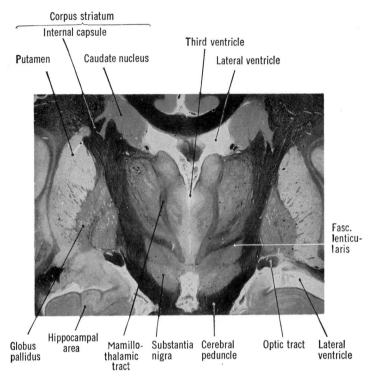

Figure 17–6.   Photograph of a coronal section of the cerebrum. Weigert stain.

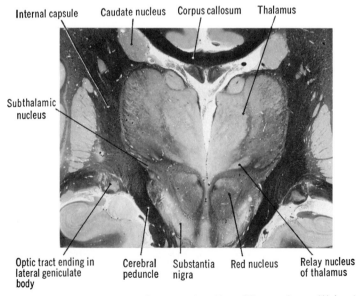

Figure 17–7.   Photograph of a coronal section of the cerebrum. Weigert stain.

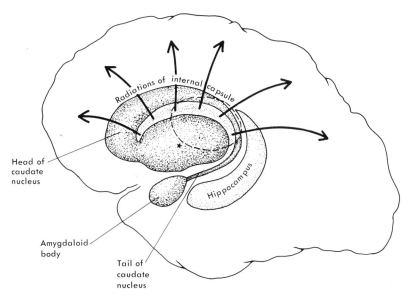

Figure 17-8. Diagrammatic representation of the basal ganglia viewed from the lateral aspect of the brain. The ★ marks the putamen as shown in Figure 7-11. p. 136. The thalamus is shown in broken outline; it is medial to the internal capsule, which is represented by arrows.

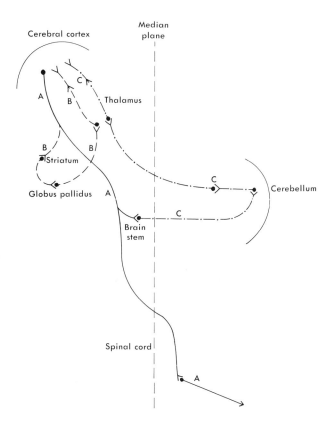

Figure 17-9. Schematic representation of the basic relationships of the cerebral cortex, basal ganglia, cerebellum, brain stem, and spinal cord.

with a portion of the substantia nigra, develop from the diencephalon. The caudate nucleus and putamen are of telencephalic origin and are sometimes referred to collectively as the *striatum*.) Because of topographical relationships, the amygdaloid bodies are often listed with the basal ganglia, but they belong to the olfactory and limbic systems. The thalami are subcortical masses of gray matter and are closely linked with the basal ganglia, but have many other functions and are considered separately.

Some of the terminology has arisen because the internal capsule lies between the thalamus and head of the caudate nucleus medially and the globus pallidus and putamen laterally. Myelinated fibers passing between the caudate nucleus and putamen give the region a striated appearance, hence the terms corpus striatum and striatum. Adding more terminological confusion is the fact that the putamen and globus pallidus together are sometimes referred to collectively as the *lenticular nucleus* or *lentiform nucleus*. Finally, the striatum is also known as the *neostriatum*, the globus pallidus has been called the *paleostriatum*, and the amygdaloid body has been termed the *archistriatum*. The above listing is intended to serve as a guide to terms that are encountered in textbooks and papers.

Connections (Figs. 17–10, 17–11).   The main afferent inflow to the striatum is from at least three sources: (1) a massive, widespread projection from nearly all parts of the cerebral cortex, but especially from the motor areas; (2) certain intralaminar thalamic nuclei that project to the striatum; (3) many afferents that arise from the dopamine-synthesizing cells of the substantia nigra and

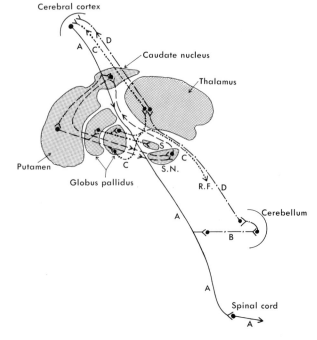

Figure 17–10. Some details of connections of the basal ganglia. Motor fibers (solid line) descending from the cerebral cortex give branches to the striatum. Neurons in the striatum project to globus pallidus and substantia nigra (S.N.). The globus pallidus is the chief motor outflow of the corpus striatum, projecting to thalamus (to the same nuclei receiving cerebellar projections, and thereby back to cortex, to subthalamic nucleus (S), and to reticular formation (R.F.). Note that the substantia nigra projects to striatum; this is a dopaminergic pathway. (Based on Nauta, W. J. H., and Mehler, W. R.: Fiber connections of the basal ganglia. *In* Crane, G. E., and Gardner, R., Jr., editors: Psychotic Drugs and Dysfunctions of the Basal Ganglia. A Multidisciplinary Workshop. Workshop Series of Pharmacology Section, N.J.M.H., 1969.)

Cerebral cortex

Caudate nucleus

Thalamus

Putamen

Globus pallidus

S.N.

R.F.

Cerebellum

Spinal cord

project to dopamine-sensitive cells in the striatum. (Many other cells in the striatum are acetylcholine-sensitive, but their afferents have not yet been established.)

The efferent fibers from the striatum enter the globus pallidus. Some end there, but many project through the globus pallidus to the substantia nigra, giving collateral branches during their passage. The globus pallidus is the chief motor outflow of the corpus striatum. It sends massive bundles of fibers: (1) to the subthalamic nucleus; (2) to the reticular formation of the brain stem; and (3) through and around the internal capsule to the ventrolateral, ventral anterior, and certain intralaminar nuclei of the thalamus. (One of the projections is the *fasciculus lenticularis* shown in Figure 17–6.) The first two of these thalamic nuclei project to the cerebral cortex.

Thus, the basal ganglia receive major inputs from the cerebral cortex, project back to the cortex, and also send major extrapyramidal projections to the brain stem.

Functions. The basal ganglia are important functional components in complex, supporting muscular activities, including posture, balance, locomotion, and associated movements (such as arm swinging during walking). They seem to be especially important in inhibitory mechanisms, in the "suppression" of muscle tone, and in the coordination of muscular activity (the "selection" of the appropriate muscle groups). Diseases of the basal ganglia are common and often disabling. Signs of these diseases include increased muscle tone, rigidity, and various dyskinesias or abnormal involuntary movements. Some of these signs occur in the disease known as parkinsonism, which results from destruction of the dopaminergic nigrostriatal pathway. One of the treatments is the administration of L-dopa, a precursor of dopamine.

It must be emphasized, however, that the ways in which the functions of the basal ganglia are mediated and, indeed, just what they are, remain largely unknown. Moreover, many of the connections of the basal ganglia in humans remain to be determined.

DIENCEPHALON

The diencephalon, which is often regarded as the rostral portion of the brain stem, is the median unpaired portion of the forebrain. It consists of four parts, each of which is represented bilaterally. These four parts are: (1) the *thalamus* (see below); (2) the *epithalamus,* which is situated at the posterior end of the third ventricle, and which consists of the pineal body (p. 352) and the habenular nuclei (p. 394); (3) the *hypothalamus* (p. 333); and (4) the *subthalamus,* which includes the subthalamic nucleus, various bundles of fibers entering and leaving the thalamus, and the rostral extensions of the red nucleus, substantia nigra, and reticular formation.

THALAMUS

The thalami are the largest constituents of the diencephalon. Each is a mass of gray matter that is subdivided by a vertical sheet of myelinated fibers, the *internal medullary lamina*, into three smaller masses of gray matter, the *lateral, medial,* and *anterior nuclei.* The internal medullary lamina consists mainly of fibers that interconnect the thalamic nuclei; its anterior part is formed by the *mamillothalamic tract* (Fig. 17–6). Each of the three nuclear masses listed above consists of a number of nuclei. These can be grouped according to their connections, and from these connections, as well as from experimental studies and clinical evidence, certain functions can be inferred.

Sensory Relay Nuclei. The lower or ventral portion of the lateral nucleus is sometimes known as the *ventrobasal complex.* The posterior part of this complex, together with the medial and lateral geniculate bodies, are the sensory portions of the thalamus. (All of the sensory pathways, except that for smell, relay in the thalamus.) The spinothalamic tracts, the medial lemniscus, the trigeminothalamic projections, and the taste pathway end in this posterior portion. The topographical representation is such that the opposite lower limb projects to the lateral part of the posterior portion (*nucleus ventralis posterolateralis*), the opposite upper limb is medial in this nucleus, and the opposite side of the head is most medial, in the *nucleus ventralis posteromedialis.* (The relay nucleus indicated in Figure 17–7 is the nucleus ventralis postero-medialis). The cells of these nuclei include principal or relay cells, which project to the primary receptive areas of the parietal lobe (p. 408), and intrinsic neurons (interneurons) that probably comprise a recurrent inhibitory mechanism. All thalamic nuclei that project to the cerebral cortex receive corticothalamic fibers from the cortical areas to which they project. Hence, thalamic and cortical functions can scarcely be separated. The available evidence indicates that the sensory relay nuclei are integral parts of perceptive and discriminative functions. It seems likely that the thalamic cells are organized in groups that correspond to columns in the cerebral cortex.

The medial geniculate body is a part of the auditory pathway; each one receives fibers from both ascending auditory pathways and projects to the temporal lobe (p. 413). The lateral geniculate body, which receives most of the axons of ganglion cells of the retina (some continue to the superior colliculus), consists of six layers. The optic nerve fibers that arise from the retina of the same side end in layers 2, 3, and 5, whereas the crossed optic nerve fibers end in layers 1, 4, and 6. Thus, each lateral geniculate body receives impulses related to the opposite fields of vision (Fig. 12–13, p. 265). Moreover, there is a point-to-point representation of the retina in the lateral geniculate body. The geniculate neurons include principal cells, which relay to the occipital cortex, and interneurons, which probably serve as inhibitory mechanisms that enhance contrast. The geniculate bodies, like the other relay nuclei, receive corticothalamic fibers.

Motor Relay Nuclei. The anterior portion of the ventrobasal complex consists of the ventrolateral and anterior ventral nuclei (often lumped as *nucleus ventralis anterolateralis*). These nuclei receive projections from the cerebellum (p. 368) and from the globus pallidus (p. 386), and in turn project to the motor areas of the frontal lobe.

Association Nuclei. The bulk of the thalamus has reciprocal connections with the association cortex. This cortex accounts for much of the volume of the human cortex, hence the thalamus is correspondingly large in humans.

The medial thalamic nucleus receives fibers from the other thalamic nuclei and is reciprocally connected with the cortex of most of the anterior half of the frontal lobe, with the inferolateral temporal cortex, with the olfactory cortex, and with the limbic midbrain area. The large size and widespread connections of this nucleus indicate that it plays a major role in limbic system functions. The exact role, however, is still unknown. Clinical evidence suggests that it may be important in memory.

The dorsal portion of the lateral thalamic nucleus comprises several nuclei that receive fibers from other thalamic nuclei, and which have extensive reciprocal connections with the parietal, occipital, and temporal association cortex. They undoubtedly function in high-level, integrative mechanisms, but again the precise nature of these functions is unknown. One of these dorsal nuclei is termed the *pulvinar.* It is posterior in position, overhangs the midbrain, and is reciprocally connected with the visual cortex. It is the largest of the thalamic nuclei in humans and may well function as a visual integrating center.

Limbic Relay Nucleus. The anterior nucleus of the thalamus is also a part of the limbic system. It receives a massive projection from the mamillary body of the hypothalamus and projects to the cingulate cortex.

Intralaminar and Reticular Nuclei. The central portion of the internal medullary lamina contains several *intralaminar nuclei.* One, the *centromedian nucleus (nucleus medialis centralis),* is especially prominent in humans. The major input to the intralaminar nuclei is from the reticular formation, although the centromedian nucleus also has prominent connections with the basal ganglia. In turn, they project to other thalamic nuclei.

The *reticular nucleus* consists of a thin sheet of cells on the lateral aspect of the thalamus, adjacent to the internal capsule. This sheet is continuous with the reticular formation of the brain stem and its cells have widespread connections to the cerebral cortex. These cells, together with those of the intralaminar nuclei, are probably the thalamic portions of the reticular activating system and are also known as *nonspecific thalamic nuclei.* Their role in electrical activity has already been mentioned. It should be noted that their tendency to rhythmic activity may be a factor in convulsive disorders.

Functions of the Thalamus. In spite of its large size, widespread connections, reciprocal relationships with the cerebral cortex, and obvious importance, most of the functions of the thalamus are still unknown. Much attention has been paid to the sensory relay nuclei, which in many respects are organized like gray matter at lower levels. Destruction of the somatosensory nuclei of the thalamus of one side leads to diminished sensation on the opposite side of the body. Characteristically, however, stimuli above a certain intensity may be perceived as exaggerated disagreeable sensations, and patients may also experience spontaneous pain in the areas where sensation is diminished. These abnormal sensations may well represent uncontrolled actions of a portion of the limbic system (see discussion of pain, p. 236). The motor relay nuclei of the thalamus are known to be important elements in the control of muscular activity by the cerebellum and the basal ganglia. Beyond this, one can only surmise functions, basing the assumptions on anatomical connections, some clinical evidence, and experimental studies.

LIMBIC SYSTEM

The *limbic system,* a major portion of which is the *limbic lobe* (Broca's lobe), includes portions of the cerebral hemispheres and the diencephalon which are central elements in the neural mechanisms that govern emotion and behavior. Because of the marked autonomic and endocrinological features of many aspects of emotion and behavior, the limbic system is also known as the *visceral brain.* Today it is known that the limbic system has other important functions, including a major role in memory. The limbic system is also implicated in a number of neurological and psychiatric disorders.

LIMBIC LOBE

The limbic lobe (Broca's lobe) is a group of structures on the medial aspect of the cerebral hemisphere. The most prominent of these structures are the cingulate gyrus, septal area, and hippocampal formation; they develop as a margin or limbus around the evaginating cerebral hemispheres. In many respects the limbic lobe is a synthetic lobe; its cortex includes neocortex, paleocortex, and archicortex. Traditionally, the limbic lobe was assigned an olfactory function. Within the last few decades, however, it has become clear that these medial limbic structures are chiefly involved in emotion and behavior, although they possess significant olfactory connections. In addition, the concept of a limbic system,

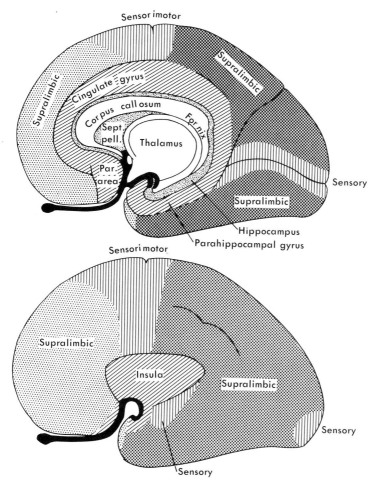

Figure 17-11. Schematic representation of the extent of the major cortical regions. *Upper:* Medial aspect. *Lower:* Lateral aspect, represented as if the lateral sulcus were opened to expose the insula. *Solid black:* Olfactory structures. (Based on Yakovley, P. I., in Hockman, C. H. By permission of the author and publisher.)

which is broader in scope than the limbic lobe, has developed by the inclusion of important basolateral and neocortical elements. The extent of limbic cortex is indicated in Figure 17-11, and the major connections of the limbic system are shown in Figure 17-12.

The internal connections of the limbic lobe form a medial circuit that begins in the cingulate gyrus, projects to the hippocampal formation, reaches the hypothalamus by way of the fornix, and is projected back to the cingulate gyrus from the mamillary body by way of the anterior nucleus of the thalamus.

The medial circuit overlaps substantially with the basolateral structures; it has strong connections with the olfactory system and a powerful projection to the limbic midbrain area by way of the mamillary bodies.

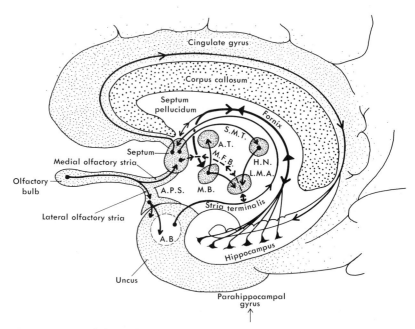

Figure 17–12. Schematic representation of some of the connections of the limbic system. Arrows indicate direction of conduction, and some structures carry fibers conducting in different directions. S.M.T., stria medullaris thalami; H.N., habenular nucleus; A.T., anterior thalamic nucleus (its projection to the cingulate cortex is omitted); M.F.B., medial forebrain bundle; L.M.A., limbic midbrain area; M.B., mamillary body; A.P.S., anterior perforated substance; A .B., amygdaloid body. The arrow below indicates the plane of section through the hippocampus in Figure 17–13.

Cingulate gyrus.   This gyrus, whose cortex is a mesocortex (p. 383), overlies the corpus callosum and becomes continuous anteroinferiorly with the septal area. Posteriorly, the gyrus turns around the corpus callosum and becomes continuous with the parahippocampal gyrus. The white matter of the gyrus contains a bundle of fibers which is termed the *cingulum.* These fibers interconnect different portions of the gyrus and provide its major efferent and afferent connections.

Hippocampal Formation.   The hippocampal formation consists of the *hippocampus,* the *dentate gyrus,* and portions of the *parahippocampal gyrus* (the last is shown in Figure 7–8, p. 133).

The hippocampus derives its name from its supposed resemblance to a sea horse. In humans, it extends folded inward along the floor of the temporal horn of the lateral ventricle and along the hippocampal fissure (Fig. 17–13). Its anterior end falls short of the temporal pole and is expanded. Posteriorly it tapers, and extends almost to the corpus callosum. The dentate gyrus is a narrower band of cortex lying along the medial aspect of the hippocampus (Fig. 17–13). Grossly it presents a notched or dentate appearance. Its cortex is also arranged in a folded manner but opposite to that of the hippocampus. In transverse section, the

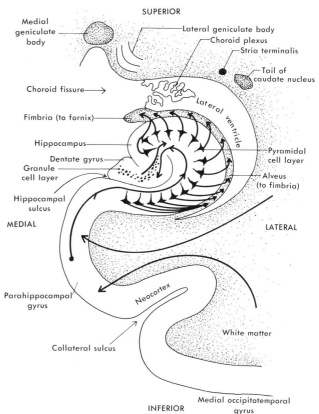

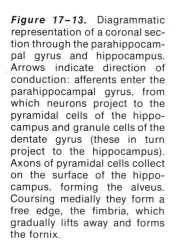

Figure 17-13. Diagrammatic representation of a coronal section through the parahippocampal gyrus and hippocampus. Arrows indicate direction of conduction: afferents enter the parahippocampal gyrus, from which neurons project to the pyramidal cells of the hippocampus and granule cells of the dentate gyrus (these in turn project to the hippocampus). Axons of pyramidal cells collect on the surface of the hippocampus, forming the alveus. Coursing medially they form a free edge, the fimbria, which gradually lifts away and forms the fornix.

cells of the hippocampus are arranged like the letter C, which interlocks with the C-shaped cellular layers of the dentate gyrus.

An additional part of the hippocampal formation is formed by a long strip of gray matter, the *induseum griseum,* on the upper surface of the corpus callosum. This gray matter, which extends from the septal area to the dentate gyrus (Fig. 17–13), is the earliest portion of the hippocampal formation to develop embryologically. It decreases in size, both relatively and absolutely, as the hemispheres increase in size and the corpus callosum forms.

The cortex of the hippocampus is three-layered. The layers, from the ventricular surface outwards, are polymorphic, pyramidal, and molecular. The most characteristic feature of hippocampal cortex is the presence of large and small pyramidal cells. The dentate gyrus also consists of three layers: molecular, granular, and polymorphic. The granule cells are the principal neurons of the dentate gyrus and send their axons to the molecular layer of the hippocampus.

Axons of the pyramidal cells emerge on the ventricular surface of the hippocampus and form a thin sheet of fibers called the *alveus.* The fibers then converge on the medial surface of the hippocampus and form a flattened band, the *fimbria.* Each fimbria (from the right and left hippocampi) gradually becomes free and is then termed the *fornix.* The two fornices, which are the major outflow from the hippocampi, are first connected by the *hippocampal commissure (commissure of the fornix)* and then become contiguous. The two contiguous structures, which occupy the median plane under the corpus callosum, together comprise the *body of the fornix,* which runs forward to the rostral end of the thalamus. Here the two fornices separate. Each one arches in front of the interventricular foramina, behind the anterior commissure. Some of the fibers of the fornix end in the septal region and hypothalamus, but many of them continue downward and backward and end in the corresponding mamillary body. (The fornix also contains fibers that begin in the septal nuclei and end in the parahippocampal gyrus.) The mamillary bodies contain the mamillary nuclei, which belong to the posterior hypothalamic group (p. 333). They provide major connections back to the cingulate gyrus (by way of the *mamillothalamic tract* and *anterior nucleus of the thalamus*), thereby completing the circuit. Each mamillary body also sends axons caudally to the limbic midbrain area by way of the *mamillotegmental tract.*

The parahippocampal gyrus is the most medial convolution on the inferior surface of the temporal lobe and is limited medially by the hippocampal fissure. Anteriorly, it continues into the *uncus,* the interior of which contains the amygdaloid body. The uncus and the anterior portion of the parahippocampal gyrus are olfactory association cortex (p. 415). The remainder of the parahippocampal gyrus is a portion of the hippocampal formation. The major input to the hippocampus is from widespread areas of the cerebral cortex, including the cingulate gyrus. These areas project first to the parahippocampal gyrus and then to the dentate gyrus and hippocampus (Fig. 17–13). In addition, the hippocampus has an indirect input from the olfactory system and amygdaloid bodies.

Septal Area. The septal area (known also as the *medial olfactory area*) receives the medial olfactory stria; it is an integral part of the limbic system. It consists of scattered cells in the *septum pellucidum,* together with the *paraterminal gyrus,* which lies immediately below the anterior end of the corpus callosum and immediately adjacent to the *lamina terminalis.* (The lamina terminalis is a thin membrane that forms the anterior limit of the third ventricle.)

The septal area has widespread connections, as shown in Figure 17–12. It is the major source of the *medial forebrain bundle,* which traverses the lateral portion of the hypothalamus and which provides the chief pathway for reciprocal connections with the biogenic amine systems of the brain stem (p. 319). The septal area also contributes to the *stria medullaris thalami,* which projects to the brain stem by way of the *habenular nucleus.* The two habenular nuclei, which are located adjacent to the pineal body, have extensive projections to the brain stem and thereby provide for olfactory reflexes.

BASOLATERAL LIMBIC SYSTEM

The chief basolateral structures and regions are the amygdaloid bodies and the cortex of the orbital aspect of the frontal lobes, the insulae, and the anterior portions of the temporal lobes. The overlap with the olfactory system and the limbic lobe is substantial.

Amygdaloid Body. The amygdaloid body is a mass of gray matter situated in the dorsomedial portion of the tip of the temporal lobe, between the putamen and the end of the temporal horn of the lateral ventricle. Behind, it is in contact with the tail of the caudate nucleus (Fig. 17–8). The uncus lies below it.

The amygdaloid body consists of a number of nuclei, which form a *corticomedial* (or *dorsomedial*) and a *basolateral* (or *ventrolateral*) group. The corticomedial group is usually included with the lateral olfactory area (p. 415). The larger basolateral group has major connections with (1) the cortex of the adjacent temporal convexity (which in turn is connected with the hippocampal formation), (2) the medial thalamic nucleus (and thereby with the neocortex of the frontal and temporal lobes and insulae), (3) the hippocampus by way of the adjacent parahippocampal gyrus, and (4) the septal area and hypothalamus by means of ventrally coursing fibers and the *stria terminalis.* The stria terminalis (Fig. 17–12) follows the tail of the caudate nucleus and reaches the septal area. Some fibers continue to the hypothalamus, and others reach the habenular nuclei by way of the stria medullaris thalami. Thus, by these hippocampal and diencephalic connections, the basolateral limbic system converges with the limbic lobe upon the hypothalamus and the limbic midbrain area.

Limbic neocortex. It is now recognized that the cortex of the anterior frontal lobe, especially of its orbital aspect, of the insula, and of the inferolateral aspect of the temporal lobe each have extensive connections, directly and indirectly, with the amygdaloid bodies, with the medial thalamic nuclei, and with the limbic lobe. Nevertheless, the precise nature and extent of these connections are still unknown in humans.

FUNCTIONS OF THE LIMBIC SYSTEM

It should be emphasized that the functions of the different portions of the limbic system are still mostly unknown. Moreover, there are significant species differences, and extrapolation from animal experimentation to humans demands extreme caution. Nevertheless, the widespread connections of the limbic system with the neocortex and with the autonomic and neuroendocrinological systems, coupled with clinical evidence, indicate that the limbic system is a central mechanism that governs emotion and behavior and that takes part in the integration of internal and external environments.

In humans, bilateral lesions of the anterior portions of the temporal lobes produce severe disturbances in emotional and discriminative behavior and in sexual and dietary habits. The emotional disturbances may include hallucinations, disordered recognition and memory, disturbances of reality, dream states, clouding of consciousness, and sensory fits. Bilateral surgical removal of the anterior temporal lobes may result in the complete absence of emotion, a procedure that has succeeded in taming wild or unmanageable animals. If the hippocampi are included in the removal in humans, severe and sometimes permanent loss of memory results. (Removal of one hippocampus may have no readily apparent effect upon memory, but see p. 427).

The management of aggressive behavior in animals, which has been related to the amygdaloid bodies, has led to widely expressed views that disorders of these structures are responsible for aggressive, violent behavior in humans. This, however, has not been substantiated. The increasing evidence of the enormous complexity of the limbic system indicates the unlikelihood that violent, aggressive human behavior can be pinpointed to defects in any one structure, if, indeed, it results from any organic disorder.

In general terms, one can view the limbic lobe and the basolateral limbic system as counterbalanced systems. Consequently, many types of emotional and behavioral disturbances may represent hypoactive or hyperactive imbalances, that is, a lessening or an enhancement of central activation. Hypoactivity may bring apathy, akinesia, or mutism, whereas hyperactivity may bring exaggerated or aggressive behavioral and motor changes. Likewise, hypoactivity or hyperactivity may be expressed in the internal mood, feeling, or affect related to perceptual phenomena (see discussion of pain, p. 236).

An additional feature of clinical importance is the marked tendency of hippocampal neurons to fire rhythmically. Damage to the hippocampus may disrupt hippocampal activity and is known to be a major cause of epilepsy.

SUMMARY

The adult forebrain includes the paired cerebral hemispheres and the diencephalon. The cerebral hemispheres are characterized by a massive volume of cortex and by masses of gray matter in their interior.

The cerebral cortex consists of neocortex, paleocortex, and archicortex. The homotypical neocortex is arranged into six layers in which the cells form vertically organized columns. The basic cortical neurons are stellate cells, which are intracortical in distribution, and pyramidal cells, whose axons leave the cortex as projection, commissural, or association fibers. In heterotypical neocortex, lamination is obscured by the increase in pyramidal cells in the motor cortex and stellate cells in the sensory cortex. Paleocortex (olfactory) and archicortex (hippocampus and dendate gyrus) are characterized by a three-layered arrangement.

The brain exhibits spontaneous electrical activity that is generated by synaptic potentials in neuronal precesses oriented at right angles to the cortical surface. This electrical activity, which is termed the electroencephalogram, is modulated by subcortical structures and generally exhibits patterns that are designated as *alpha* rhythm (8 to 13 cycles per second) and *beta* activity (13 cycles per second and faster). Slower waves, *theta* and *delta,* may also be recorded under certain conditions. The electroencephalogram varies with age, attention, and physiological status, and shows characteristic patterns during sleep. An analysis of the EEG is a useful diagnostic procedure in many clinical conditions.

The basal ganglia are certain masses of gray matter within the cerebral hemispheres. The major ones are the corpus striatum and subthalamic nucleus. On the basis of functional connections, the red nucleus and substantia nigra are often included. The basal ganglia have extensive connections with the neocortex, certain thalamic nuclei, the biogenic amine systems, and the brain stem reticular formation. They are important elements in the control of muscular activity, being involved in inhibitory mechanisms, the suppression of muscle tone, and in the coordination of groups of muscles. Disorders of the basal ganglia may be characterized by increased muscle tone, rigidity, and dyskinesias.

The diencephalon includes the thalamus, epithalamus, hypothalamus, and subthalamus. The thalamus is a large mass of gray matter which is subdivided into anterior, medial, and lateral nuclei. These are further subdivided into smaller nuclei that can be grouped according to their connections. The groups are: sensory relay nuclei, motor relay nuclei, association nuclei, limbic relay nuclei, and intralaminar and reticular nuclei. All except the last group are reciprocally connected with the cerebral cortex. The grouping and cortical connections suggest the functions that the thalamus carries out, but knowledge of function is still limited. Thalamic lesions may interfere with or distort sensation and may be a factor in epileptic disorders.

The limbic system includes the limbic lobe and certain basolateral and neocortical structures and regions. The limbic lobe is a group of structures on the medial aspect of the cerebral hemisphere. The chief ones are the cingulate gyrus, septal area, and hippocampal formation. They have widespread interconnections and connections with the neocortex, certain thalamic nuclei, and the autonomic-neuroendocrine systems. The chief basolateral limbic structures are the amygdaloid bodies and the orbital frontal, insular, and anterior temporal cortex. They have widespread interconnections with the whole extent of neocortex, with certain thalamic nuclei, and with the autonomic-neuroendocrine systems. The overlap between the limbic lobe and basolateral system is considerable and both converge upon the hypothalamus and the limbic midbrain area. The two systems act as counterbalancing mechanisms in the neural control of emotion, behavior, and integration of internal and external environments. Clinical disorders involve disorders in emotional and discriminative behavior and in sexual and dietary habits. Destruction of a portion of a hippocampus may be followed by epileptic disorders; destruction of both hippocampi is followed by severe, even permanent, memory loss.

NAMES IN NEUROLOGY

PIERRE-PAUL BROCA (1824–1880)

Broca is considered to be the founder of brain surgery in France. Born near Bordeaux, he was educated at Bordeaux and Paris. He received his M.D. in 1848, served as a professor in the faculty of medicine in Paris, and was appointed to the chair of "pathologie externe" in 1867. He held several hospital appointments and was the first to trephine the skull for a cerebral abscess that he located by symptoms relating to his theory of localization of brain function. He was a renowned anthropologist and anatomist, and in 1861 in a famous case study he postulated that the posterior part of the inferior frontal gyrus of the left hemisphere was involved in speech mechanisms. In 1878, Broca published his concept of the limbic lobe (Anatomie comparée circonvolutions cérébrales: Le grand lobe limbique et al scissure limbique dans la série des mammifères. Rev. Anthropol., 1:384–498, 1878).

HANS BERGER (1873–1941)

Berger, a neurologist in Jena, was the first to record the electrical activity of the brain in humans. He studied the electroencephalogram extensively, and the *alpha* rhythm bears his name.

REFERENCES

See also references cited on pp. 67, 159, 219, and 244.
The following are excellent texts, monographs, and reports of symposia.

Brain, Behav., Evol., 6:1972. This entire volume is devoted to Basic Thalamic Structure and Function.
Denny-Brown, D.: The Basal Ganglia. New York, Oxford University Press, 1962.
Hockman, C. H. (editor): Limbic System Mechanisms and Autonomic Functions. Springfield, Ill., Charles C Thomas, 1972.
Kiloh, L. G., McComas, A. J., and Osselton, J. W.: Clinical Electroencephalography. 3rd ed. London, Butterworths, and New York, Appleton-Century-Crofts, 1972.
Martin, J. P.: The Basal Ganglia and Posture. Philadelphia, J. B. Lippincott Company, 1967.
Purpura, D. P. and Yahr, M. D. (editors): The Thalamus. New York, Columbia University Press, 1966.
Shepherd, G. M.: The Synaptic Organization of the Brain. New York, Oxford University Press, 1974.

Sholl, D. A.: The Organization of the Cerebral Cortex. New York, John Wiley and Sons, Inc., 1956.

Smythies, J. R.: Brain Mechanisms and Behavior. New York, Academic Press, 1970.

The following references include original papers, reviews of important topics and concepts, and analyses of clinical disorders.

Altmann, J., Brunner, R. L., and Bayer, S. A.: The hippocampus and behavioral maturation. Behav. Biol., 8:557–596, 1973.

Andersen, P. O.: Correlation of structural design with function in the archicortex. In Eccles, J. C. (editor): Brain and Conscious Experience, New York, Springer-Verlag, 1966.

Brutkowski, S.: Functions of the prefrontal cortex in animals. Physiol. Rev., 45:721–746, 1965.

Colonnier, M. L.: The structural design of the neocortex. In Eccles, J. C. (editor): Brain and Conscious Experience. New York, Springer-Verlag, 1966.

Falconer, M. A.: Reversibility by temporal-lobe resection of the behavioral abnormalities of temporal-lobe epilepsy. New Engl. J. Med., 289:451–455, 1973. Mesial temporal (Ammon's horn) sclerosis as a common cause of epilepsy. Lancet, 2:767–770, 1974.

Fox, C. A., Hillman, D. E., Siegesmund, K. A., and Sether, L. A.: The primate globus pallidus and its feline and avian homologues: a Golgi and electron microscopic study. In Evolution of the Forebrain. Hassler, R., and Stephan, H. (editors): Stuttgart, Georg Thieme Verlag, 1966.

Gerebtzoff, M. A., Ziegels, J., and Duchesne, P. Y.: Le thalamus des Mammifères et de l'Homme. Organization structurale. fonctionnelle et cytochemique. Bull. Assoc. Anat., 57:727–828, 1973.

Goldstein, M.: Brain research and violent behavior. Arch. Neurol., 30:1–35, 1974.

Green, J. D.: The Hippocampus. Physiol. Rev., 44:561–608, 1964.

Hamburg, D. A.: Psychological studies of aggressive behavior. Nature, 230:19–23, 1971.

Kemp, J. M., and Powell, T. P. S.: The cortico-striate projection in the monkey. Brain, 93:525–546, 1970.

Lashley, K. S., and Clark, G.: The cytoarchitecture of the cerebral cortex of Ateles: a critical examination of architectonic studies. J. Comp. Neurol., 85:223–305, 1946. This is a classic paper on the objective criteria that need to be established in cytoarchitectonic studies.

Livingstone, K. E., and Escobar, A.: Anatomical bias of the limbic system concept. Arch. Neurol., 24:17–21, 1971.

Nauta, W. J. H.: Hippocampal projections and related neural pathways to the mid-brain in the cat. Brain, 81:319–340, 1958.

Nauta, W. J. H., and Mehler, W. R.: Fiber connections of the basal ganglia. In Crane, G. E., and Gardner, R., Jr. (editors): Psychotropic Drugs and Dysfunctions of the Basal Ganglia. A Multidisciplinary Workshop. Workshop Series of Pharmacology Section, N.I.M.H., 1969.

Papez, J. W.: A proposed mechanism of emotion. Arch. Neurol. Psychiat., 38:725–734, 1937. This is a classic paper in which it is proposed that the structures comprising the limbic lobe play a major role in emotion.

Passingham, R. E.: Anatomical differences between the neocortex of man and other primates. Brain, Behav. Evol., 7:337–359, 1973.

Penfield, W., and Mathieson, G.: Memory. Arch. Neurol., 31:145–154, 1974.

Spencer, W. A., and Kandel, E. R.: Cellular and integrative properties of the hippocampal pyramidal cell and the comparative electrophysiology of cortical neurons. Intern. J. Neurol., 6:266–296, 1968.

Welker, W. I.: Principles of organization of the ventrobasal complex in mammals. Brain, Behav. Evol., 7:253–336, 1973.

Williams, D.: Temporal lobe epilepsy. Brit. Med. J., 1:1439–1442, 1966.

Chapter **18**

THE FOREBRAIN: MOTOR AND SENSORY FUNCTIONS

The motor areas of the cerebral cortex, together with the cerebellum, basal ganglia, and brain stem, carry out coordinated muscular activity. The cortical sensory functions are the initial responsibility of primary receptive areas to which the sensory paths project. These motor and sensory functions, however, are inseparable from those of the so-called association cortex, hence there is substantial overlap of this chapter with the next.

MOTOR AREAS

The motor areas are often defined as those areas of the cerebral cortex from which motor paths arise and which are electrically excitable (that is, muscles contract when the areas are electrically stimulated). These areas are found mostly in the posterior portions of the frontal lobes. (Certain paths for eye movements originate in the occipital lobes [p. 209].) The following terminology is in common use: *Motor cortex* is the cortex of the precentral gyrus and its extension to the paracentral lobule on the medial aspect of the hemisphere. This cortex is also termed *area 4* (Figs. 18–1 and 18–4); it is heterotypical cortex of the agranular type (Fig. 17–1, p. 376). *Premotor cortex* is the term applied to *areas 6* and *8*, which lie immediately in front of area 4; area 8 is also known as the *frontal eye field.* The cortex of the remainder of the frontal lobe, exclusive of the cingulate gyrus and the septal area, is often termed *prefrontal cortex.* The basal aspect of the frontal lobe rests on the orbital plate of the frontal bone. Its cortex is often referred to separately as the *orbital cortex;* it is an integral part of the limbic system (p. 390).

400

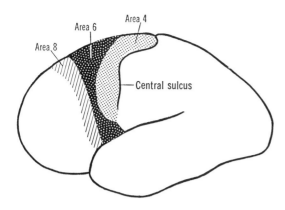

Figure 18-1. Diagram indicating the approximate locations of the motor areas on the lateral surface of the frontal lobe.

Area 4 is a major source of pyramidal fibers (corticospinal and corticobulbar); it is reciprocally connected with the postcentral gyrus, and it receives a major input from the cerebellum and basal ganglia by way of the thalamus (pp. 367 and 386). The pyramidal cells of area 4 are largest and most numerous in the portion that projects to the lumbosacral part of the spinal cord. Their size reflects the distance that their axons travel. Area 6 appears to have a major extrapyramidal function, and, like area 4, has an input from the cerebellum and basal ganglia. It also has a significant input from association cortex. It probably projects chiefly to subcortical structures. Area 8 is concerned with head, neck, and eye movements, especially smooth pursuit movements.

It should be emphasized that Figures 18–1, 18–3, and 18–4 illustrate only the approximate locations of the various areas. There are no sharp lines of demarcation between them, either grossly or microscopically. In a brain exposed at operation it is very nearly impossible to identify precisely the areas in the operating field. The arachnoid, pia mater, and blood vessels obscure surface landmarks, and there is great individual variation in the relation of surface landmarks to bony landmarks. Consequently, electrical stimulation may be employed to identify motor areas.

The division of the motor areas into areas 4, 6, and 8 has been made chiefly on the basis of studies employing electrical stimulation, and to some extent on microscopic studies and the results of extirpations. In addition, clinical studies have provided valuable information.

If the motor cortex is explored with a stimulating electrode, an inverted representation of movements is found: movements in the lower limb (mostly the contralateral limb) result from stimulation of the upper portion of the gyrus and the medial aspect of the hemisphere; movements in the upper limb occur when the middle of the region is stimulated; and the movements in the head and neck occur following stimulation of the lower portion of the gyrus. The pattern of response, however, is not precise. Figure 18–2 illustrates what might be called overlap. For example, if one stimulates a small portion of the motor cortex with a single electrical

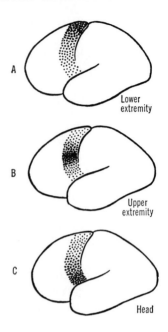

Figure 18–2. Diagram of the manner in which movements are represented in the cerebral cortex. *A,* Stimulation of the heavily shaded area usually, or most easily, elicits movements in the lower limb. Stimulation anywhere else in the motor cortex can also elicit movements in the lower limb, but less easily, and the degree of shading is some indication of the degree of response. *B,* Similar situation for upper limb and, *C,* for head and neck. If these three drawings were superimposed so as to represent the actual situation, then in any one region (even a very small region) of motor cortex, all types of movements would be represented, but some one type much more so than any other. Conversely, destruction of a part of the motor cortex would have its greatest effect on one type of movement, so that there might be weakness or paralysis of a muscle or group of muscles in this particular movement, but the same muscles might be used effectively in other movements.

pulse, a muscle or a few muscles on the opposite side of the body will twitch. If the strength of the stimulus is increased, other muscles will also respond. By varying the frequency, strength, and wave form of the stimulating current, it can be shown that in the arm region of area 4, the nerve cells producing movements of the arm are the most easily excited, but that with appropriate stimulation, movements of the leg (or head) may be produced. One might suppose that contraction of a leg muscle when the arm area is stimulated is due to the intracortical spread of the stimulus. However, it is possible to isolate the stimulated region surgically and leave only the projections into the white matter. Stimulation of the isolated region may still yield multiple patterns of response. The results indicate, therefore, that many types of movements are represented in even small portions of area 4, and that some of them are predominantly represented, that is, more easily elicited by stimulation. However, it is also possible that portions of area 4 are interconnected by short association bundles coursing in the white matter, and that these connections play a role in multiple representation.

It must be emphasized that electrical stimulation is an artificial procedure, and that only by the merest chance would such a procedure activate a pattern of cells in the same manner as would a physiological stimulus. The results depend not only upon the strength of the stimulus, but also upon the frequency. Contraction may occur in one group of muscles during stimulation at one frequency and in another group during stimulation at another frequency. Conscious human subjects on whom stimulation experiments are carried out report that any movements that result seem quite beyond their control and without any sense of being willed or initiated. It is interesting that stimulation of the precentral gyrus sometimes causes tingling or some other sensation rather than movement.

The results of electrical stimulation also depend upon posture. That is, if a muscle or a group of muscles is placed in a particular position, the results of stimulation may be different than if the muscles had been placed in another position. This means that impulses from skin, muscles, and joints have an effect upon the result of cortical stimulation. It should be noted that the interpretation of cortical stimulation may be complicated by secondary movement. If one observes a pattern of activity in response to stimulation, one cannot assume that the entire pattern was a direct result of the stimulus. It is possible for cortically induced contractions to initiate activity in other muscles through spinal reflexes independent of the cerebral cortex.

Multiplicity of representation is encountered clinically. A tumor of the motor cortex may stimulate the neurons and thereby cause involuntary movements or convulsions on the opposite side of the body. The convulsions start in those muscles that are predominantly represented in the affected area and then rapidly involve other muscles. These spreading seizures, without loss of consciousness, are often called *jacksonian convulsions.*

Stimulation of area 6 is frequently without obvious or positive effect. It has been concluded that inhibitory mechanisms are characteristic of this area, and that they are probably mediated by projections to the basal ganglia and to the brain stem centers. Thus, area 6 may be considered a part of the extrapyramidal system. Stimulation of area 8, the frontal eye field, is often followed by conjugate eye movements as well as by various head and neck movements. The extent of area 8 in humans is uncertain. The existence of this area, together with the head portion of area 4, indicates the enormous importance of cortical representation of head, neck, and eye movements, including the motor aspects of speech.

Visceral as well as somatic responses may follow cortical stimulation. Thus there is increased blood flow through muscles active in cortically induced movements, and the impulses mediating this vasomotor reaction probably originate in the cortex. Changes in systolic blood pressure and heart rate may also occur. Strong stimulation of area 8 may be followed, not only by conjugate eye movements, but also by the formation and flow of tears, and by changes in pupillary diameter.

Considering the total actions of the motor areas in each half of the brain in terms of control of movements, full control appears to be exerted by each hemisphere over contralateral forearm, hand, and finger movements. Control of arm movements, however, is mainly ipsilateral and trunk musculature is bilaterally controlled.

Secondary and Supplementary Motor Areas. A *secondary*

motor area is located in the cortex overlying the lateral sulcus at the foot of area 4. Electrical stimulation indicates that the entire body is represented here. Its functional significance is unknown. *There is also a supplementary motor area* on the medial aspect of the hemisphere, in front of the leg portion of area 4. The entire body appears to be represented here. It may be an extension of area 6, and some consider it to be a second speech area.

Results of Extirpation.   Many of the functions of the motor areas have been deduced by studying the loss of function following cortical lesions. If a part of the motor cortex is damaged, either experimentally or by disease, upper motor neuron types of disorders occur. In general, the more widespread the destruction, the more pronounced and enduring is the weakness or paralysis. The degree to which functions can be assessed, however, is limited, because it is difficult to destroy one area precisely without affecting neighboring ones. This is especially true of pathological processes, which rarely limit themselves to one region.

The chief sign of area 4 involvement is weakness in the opposite side of the body. The weakness may be limited to a limb or to a part of a limb, depending upon the amount of cortex destroyed. (Spasticity may be present if the adjacent portion of area 6 is also involved.) A Babinski reflex (p. 214) will generally be present if the leg portion of area 4 is affected. Complete paralysis is rare, unless the cortical destruction is extremely widespread. Moreover, weakness following cortical lesions is only relative, and this is clearly shown when the lesions are small. In such instances, a muscle may seem to be paralyzed when attempts are made to use it in one type of movement pattern but appear normal at other times. For example, with a loss of a part of the arm area, a patient may be unable to extend his wrist on command. Yet the wrist may extend when making a fist. This illustrates again the multiplicity of representation, that any one small part of the motor cortex deals with many movements, and that any one movement is represented in many parts of the motor cortex.

Weakness and even paralysis are also relative as to time, because with time and proper training and practice, motor deficits from cortical lesions (and even subcortical ones) may diminish substantially. Recovery may be much more complete in children.

Certain types of pathological responses appear to be characteristic of large frontal lobe lesions. For example, the *grasp reflex* and *groping response* seem to follow damage to large areas, especially when area 6 or the supplemental motor area on the medial surface of the hemisphere are involved. The grasp reflex, seen normally in infants, is the reflex grasping of an object placed in the hand; it is dependent upon the cerebral cortex. It has been postulated that area 4 is responsible for carrying out this reflex and that area 6 inhibits it in the adult. The groping response is more complex. Contact with an object by the fingers is followed by reflex reach toward and grasping of the object. Tactile, pressure, and proprioceptive afferents are necessary for the initiation of the response, which, like the grasp, is carried out by the cerebral cortex and it probably represents the onset of lemniscal functions in exploratory movements (p. 232) and in the development of stereognosis.

Removal of the motor cortex in man, either partially or completely, does not cause any memory loss. The patient still knows how to carry out even the most complex maneuvers he has ever learned and, if he has a usable limb left, can attempt learned patterns with that limb. In other words, the "desire" to move remains; the defects are in the execution of motor activity.

Relation to Sensory Areas. Experimental work has shown that the motor and sensory cortices are interconnected (*sensorimotor cortex*), and clinical evidence indicates that this is also true in humans. As was pointed out previously, discharges from, or results of, stimulation of the motor cortex are modified, or even determined, by the state of contraction or activity in the muscle group supplied by the stimulated region. Even passive alteration of the position of a muscle may alter its subsequent response, or even abolish it. In other words, the proprioceptive impulses reaching the cerebral cortex condition the motor cortex.

Motor Areas at Birth. The motor areas appear to have little function at birth. The neurons are not fully matured and the pyramidal tracts are not fully myelinated. The newborn infant shows little voluntary or coordinated activity, although eye movements are soon prominent, especially during REM sleep, which is proportionately greater in infants (p. 324). Infants show reflex patterns that are usually not present in adults. For example, a grasp reflex is easily demonstrated by placing one's finger in a baby's hand. A Babinski reflex is present and only gradually disappears when walking begins. One can argue that the withdrawal that a Babinski reflex represents would conflict with walking and that it is therefore inhibited when the cortex begins to function. At least it disappears and in an adult is elicited only in upper motor neuron disorders, in fatigue, or in deep sleep. The newborn infant also shows static and dynamic responses, reflex patterns much like those of a thalamic animal. Not until the child begins to walk does the fine coordination characteristic of more complete cortical functioning begin its development. Experimental evidence, obtained from studies on animals, indicates that many basic movement patterns are genetically determined and do not depend upon sensory input for their appearance and development. Whether or to what degree this is true in humans is quite uncertain.

LEARNING, MUSCULAR ACTIVITY, AND CEREBRAL SPECIALIZATION

The mechanisms by which one learns complex motor sequences are unknown, and the reasons for individual differences in motor skills are equally unknown (aside from factors of weight, skeletal construction, etc.). There are *willed* or *purposeful movements,* but what the *will* is, how we generate a movement, is unknown. What is known is that for any meaningful or purposeful motor sequence there is a period during which the component movements are learned until there is a total pattern with usually no conscious awareness of component movements. In fact, if asked to describe just how all the necessary actions are carried out (for example, in fastening buttons), one might be hard put to do so. What has been learned and retained is a total pattern.

Learned motor sequences, regardless of the parts of the body involved, are controlled by one cerebral hemisphere, which is usually the left. The control appears to reside in association cortex; such control is not a function of the motor cortex. The role of this hemisphere is shown by apraxias. An *apraxia* is the inability to perform a familiar act, that is, a purposeful or "voluntary" movement, when there is no paralysis. Apraxias result when association cortex of the dominant hemisphere is destroyed. (Similar lesions in the other hemisphere may have no effect upon motor activity.) There is no one specific part of association cortex which has to be involved in order to cause an apraxia. For example, destruction of the major supramarginal gyrus in one patient may cause an apraxia characterized by inability to play the piano (when such an ability had been present before), as well as difficulties with other movement patterns. Yet in other patients similar apraxias may follow lesions elsewhere, or lesions in this gyrus may cause other types of disorders, for example, an aphasia (p. 424). Some patients lose their concept of how to carry out a movement pattern. Others may remember quite well, but be unable to perform it properly. It must be emphasized that these patients are *not* paralyzed unless the lesion has also involved motor cortex or pathways. The muscles that cannot be used to light a cigaret properly may be used to thread a needle. The tongue which cannot be protruded on command may be used in talking.

SENSORY AREAS

The primary receptive area for the general senses is the postcentral gyrus (areas 3, 1, and 2). That for vision is area 17 in the occipital lobe, and that for hearing is area 41 on the upper surface of the superior temporal gyrus; this area is mostly buried in the lateral sulcus. The primary areas are shown in Figures 18–3 and 18–4. The primary cortex for smell is in the piriform lobe, that for taste is probably in the postcentral gyrus, and that for balance (vestibular system) is thought to be in the superior temporal gyrus. All of the afferent pathways except that for smell are relayed by the thalamus to the primary cortex.

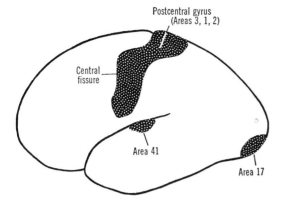

Postcentral gyrus
(Areas 3, 1, 2)

Central
fissure

Area 41

Area 17

Figure 18–3. Diagram indicating the approximate locations of primary receptive areas. Secondary sensory areas not shown.

The cortex of the somatic, visual, and auditory areas is generally thinner than that of the motor areas; it is heterotypical cortex of the granular type (Fig. 17–1, p. 376). The afferent fibers that enter these areas form bands that are often visible to the naked eye, especially in the occipital cortex where the fibers form a stripe so definite that this cortex is often called the *striate cortex* (Fig. 17–2, p. 377) (the immediately adjacent visual association cortex, areas 18 and 19, form the *peristriate* or *circumstriate cortex*).

The primary areas have been artificially stimulated, but the resulting sensations are not those normally experienced. Electrical stimulation of the visual cortex gives rise to sensations of flashes of light. One would not expect it to be otherwise, unless by chance the stimulation affected a group of neurons which would normally be activated by objects in the visual fields. Such stimulation is just as artificial as that which simultaneously activates all the fibers of a peripheral nerve.

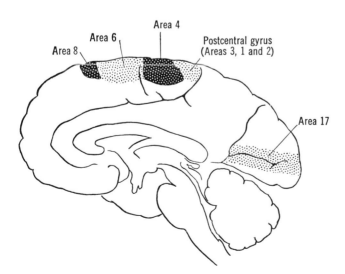

Area 4

Area 6

Area 8

Postcentral gyrus
(Areas 3, 1 and 2)

Area 17

Figure 18–4. The motor and sensory areas on the medial surface of the cerebral hemisphere. Supplementary motor area not shown.

Stimulation may also result from the actions of certain drugs. If, for example, strychnine is applied to the somatic cortex of cats, the resulting excitation evidently is accompanied by subjective sensations, because the animal scratches, bites, or licks those parts of the body which are represented in the stimulated part of the cortex. From studies of human patients, it is clear that the sensations resulting from stimulation are projected sensations, perceived by the patient as if they were in some part of the body, and without any sensation directly referable to the surface of the brain. Stimulation may also result from pathological processes. Tumors may stimulate sensory cortex much as they do motor cortex, and the patient may experience subjective sensations. These may take the form of a "sensory fit," which is a form of epilepsy.

It is possible to record the electrical activity of sensory cortex in a manner that gives a clue to representation of different parts of the body. If brain waves are suppressed with a drug, such as a barbiturate, and a sense organ or a nerve is then stimulated, the arrival at the cerebral cortex of the resulting impulses is indicated by a well-defined potential change (evoked potential). This method has been used to map the primary receptive areas, and is one of the methods that has been used to locate these areas in humans.

PRIMARY SOMATIC, VISUAL, AND AUDITORY AREAS

These are considered together because of the way in which projections from these areas ultimately converge and because of their functional interrelationships. It should also be emphasized that the functions of these areas and, indeed, those of any portion of the neocortex, are inseparable from those of the thalamus. If a part of the neocortex is destroyed, the thalamic fibers that project to the destroyed area are injured and undergo retrograde degeneration. Their cells of origin suffer severe chromatolysis and often die, being replaced by glial cells. Thus, there is no "pure" neocortical lesion. This characteristic loss of a thalamic nucleus or nuclei following cortical injury has been the basis of many studies of thalamo-cortical relationships.

Primary Somatic Areas. The postcentral gyrus is the primary receptive area for the general senses. It receives projections from the sensory relay nuclei of the thalamus by way of the posterior part of the internal capsule. As in the motor cortex, the body is represented upside down and mostly contralaterally. That is, impulses from the leg project to the opposite postcentral gyrus, to its upper portion (and to its extension to the medial aspect of the hemisphere), whereas the arm projects to the intermediate portion, and the head and neck to the lower portion, above the lateral sulcus. This topographical representation by region, rather than by dermatome or peripheral nerve, indicates that the somatic pathways sort out and regroup the different modalities, according to body region. Moreover, the gray matter at each level "processes" information in a way that brings about enhancement and suppression that is associated, for example, with the recognition and discrimination of two points that simultaneously touch the skin (see later discussion).

Recent studies indicate that there is a secondary somatic area, and the postcentral gyrus is therefore known as *Somatic Area 1* (S1) and the secondary somatic area as *Somatic Area 2* (S2). Impulses from the entire body reach S2 bilaterally. The location of S2 varies according to species, and it seems likely that the one in humans is above the lateral fissure, near the lower end of the central sulcus. The significance of the secondary area is unknown.

It is generally stated that the postcentral gyrus, acting together with the thalamus, is concerned with initial perception. For example, if the skin is touched, the recognition (perception) of touch is said to be a function of the postcentral gyrus, whereas the location of the stimulus and determination of its intensity is said to be a function of association cortex (in the parietal lobe immediately behind the postcentral gyrus) to which the postcentral gyrus projects. To what degree this separation exists is quite uncertain. Lesions of the postcentral gyrus are not followed by marked sensory losses. Position sense is severely affected, touch less so, and pain and temperature relatively little. But in such cases, a patient may recognize that he has been touched and yet have difficulty in distinguishing degrees or intensities of stimulation. Furthermore, there is clinical evidence that a considerable degree of recovery from such defects is possible. The role of the postcentral gyrus in pain mechanisms is still an enigma. Pain mechanisms in general, and in particular the role of the limbic system, were discussed in Chapter 12. In Chapter 17 (p. 390), it was pointed out that spontaneous pain may occur with thalamic lesions, as if the limbic system were released from control. It is likely that the discriminative aspects of cutaneous pain (for example, the precise localization of a pin prick) are a function of the postcentral gyrus.

The difficulties inherent in determining sensory and perceptual functions are illustrated by the fact that the postcentral gyrus is clearly not uniform in structure or function. The lemniscal system projects to it, principally from the distal parts of the limbs. This topographical representation fits the concept that the lemniscal system is important in guiding the manipulation of objects and exploration by the limbs (p. 232). Other sensory projections are concerned with a variety of stimulus features and patterns, that is, they subserve more stationary discriminative functions. The complexity of these types of functions may be illustrated by a discussion of two-point discrimination.

The conventional diagrams of receptors and their afferent

paths are useful in indicating anatomical configuration and location, but they are too schematic to enable one to correlate the structural and functional properties that are involved in two-point
discrimination. For example, a dorsal root fiber that enters an
area of skin does not end by forming only a single group of tactile
receptors. If this were true, the simultaneous stimulation of adjacent touch spots could not be differentiated, for there would be
no unstimulated spot in between to form a neutral background.
Perception involves the recognition of a figure against a background. The background may represent stimulation, but if its
activity is generally less (because of inhibitory mechanisms at
higher levels as well as less stimulation peripherally) than that of
the stimulated point or area, then a comparison is possible and
configuration appears. A dorsal root fiber branches over a relatively wide area, probably hundreds of square millimeters or
more, and may give rise to many groups of endings. If this were the
only fiber supplying this area of skin, one could detect differences
in intensity of stimulation, because an increase in intensity causes
an increase in frequency of impulses traversing the afferent path
and reaching the cerebral cortex. Localization, however, would not
be possible, because the impulses resulting from stimulation of
one side of the area and traveling in the parent fiber would be
similar to those resulting from excitation on the other side. So far
as the brain is concerned, the impulses might be arising anywhere
in the area.

The actual situation is that any one skin area is supplied by
several fibers, and in a single touch spot there are receptors
derived from several parent fibers. The simplest possible arrangement that accounts for tactile localization is shown in Figure
18–5. Stimulation of a single touch spot results in impulses traversing two different fibers, thus allowing a comparison between
these and impulses from other parts of the area. But this arrangement does not correlate with the electrical activity recorded at
the cortex under such conditions. Such activity is found over a
relatively wide expanse and is of greater magnitude in the center
of what might be called a field of activity. When even a small skin
area is touched, there is not true point stimulation. The skin is
bent or depressed, and the receptors in the center of the depression are more intensely stimulated than those at the periphery.
Impulses starting here are therefore of a higher frequency. If, as
shown in Figure 18–5, one fiber gives more receptors to a touch
spot than another fiber, the result is a higher frequency of impulses following stimulation. Consequently, there arrives at the
cerebral cortex a group of impulses which activates a field or
region of cortex (probably a number of cortical columns). Impulses
to the central part of this group are more frequent; the resulting
activity of the central part of the cortical field is therefore more
intense. Localization of a stimulated spot is therefore a matter of
intensity discrimination.

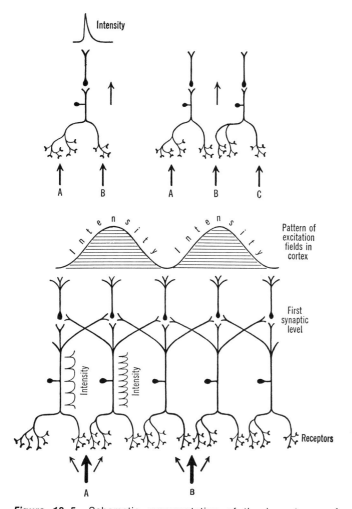

Figure 18-5. Schematic representation of the importance of interrelationships of peripheral receptors and their central connections. *Upper left:* The conventional scheme. Stimulation of a touch spot at *A* is not distinguishable from stimulation at *B,* since the impulses traverse the same fiber. The electrical activity recorded on arrival at the cortex is represented as a spike of activity in a restricted field. *Upper right:* The touch spot at *B* is derived from two dorsal root fibers. Stimulation here is localizable, but not distinguishable from simultaneous stimulation of either *A* or *C.* In either case there would be a single field of cortical activity. *Lower:* The simplest arrangement for two-point discrimination. Stimulation at *A* results in a higher frequency of impulses over the second neuron, since it contributes more endings to the touch spot and is therefore more intensely stimulated. The same situation obtains for the fourth neuron giving endings to *B.* The interconnections at the first and subsequent synaptic layers (omitted from the diagram) allow a spread of excitation. The recorded cortical response is over a wide area and is a field of algebraic summation of many spikes, more pronounced in the center because of the higher frequency of entering impulses. With two such fields, two-point discrimination is possible. Discrimination is sharpened because central inhibition suppresses impulses from areas around the stimulated points (surround inhibition).

With a two-neuron arrangement, however, two-point discrimination is not possible. At least five neurons are necessary, as indicated in Figure 18–5. Stimulation of two separate spots in their receptor pattern results in two fields of cortical activity. The differences between the two fields are enhanced by the inhibitory processes that occur at the various levels of gray matter. Regional variations in sensitivity (two-point discrimination is much more exact in the skin of the hand than in that of the back) appear then to be at least partially explained by differences in pattern and zonal distribution of fibers and receptors.

How may subjective interpretations be related to these facts? Can any correlation be made or law derived? There is a certain relationship between subjective sensation and intensity of stimulation. Suppose that to an object of a certain weight the arbitrary unit of 100 is assigned, and the same unit to the subjective sensation of weight. Then it is found that an object just enough heavier to be subjectively detected (101) has the weight of 110. The next subjective increase (to 102) necessitates an object of weight 121. These arbitrarily selected units indicate that the stimulus increases logarithmically while the sensation increases arithmetically—the *Weber-Fechner law.* So far as peripheral receptors and afferent paths are concerned, increasing intensity of stimulation results in higher frequency of impulses. Frequency of impulses entering the cerebral cortex must therefore be of great importance in perception. The Weber-Fechner law, however, holds mainly for moderate intensities of stimulation.

Primary Visual Area. The optic pathway from the retina (p. 264) is organized so that the left fields of vision project to the right occipital lobe, and vice versa. Thus, functionally, the visual pathways are crossed. Area 17 lies mostly on the medial aspect of the occipital lobe, immediately above and below the calcarine sulcus. It projects to areas 18 and 19, which are immediately adjacent and which constitute the visual association cortex, and it sends fibers to the lateral geniculate body. The optic projections are arranged so that there is a precise, almost point-to-point representation of the retina in the visual cortex. The receptive fields of the retina are represented over and over again in the cellular columns of the striate, peristriate, and association cortex, with increasingly complex responses to stimulation. Broadly speaking, the columns of the visual cortex are organized for the localization of stimuli and for the identification of patterns, as well as for the initiation of movement of the head, neck, and eyes. Integration into more complex phenomena and with other senses appears to be a function of association cortex, to which the primary cortex projects. If an optic radiation (the path from lateral geniculate body to area 17 by way of the most posterior part of the internal capsule) or area 17 are destroyed, the patient is blind in the opposite halves of the visual fields. If both areas 17 are destroyed, the patient is totally blind. If, however, area 17 is left intact when adjacent cortex is damaged, higher perceptual phenomena are impaired while perception of light remains (see p. 415).

Primary Auditory Cortex. The auditory pathway (p. 271) projects to the medial geniculate body, and this in turn to the auditory cortex, area 41, which is a transverse strip of the superior temporal gyrus mostly hidden in the lateral sulcus. Area 41 projects to the auditory association cortex, which is immediately behind and below and which, in the left hemisphere, is known as Wernicke's area (p. 424). Although each ascending auditory pathway carries impulses from both cochleae, the contralateral projection is the more pronounced. That is, the left auditory cortex receives chiefly from the right ear, and vice versa.

It seems likely that the auditory pathway, from cochlear nuclei to primary cortex, is organized, like the visual system, to localize stimuli and to identify patterns. Moreover, a striking feature is the ability to "extract" biologically significant sounds while rejecting coexisting unnecessary sounds.

Projections of Primary Receptive Areas. The primary receptive areas are not directly connected with each other. Rather, there exists a complicated system whereby each primary area projects to a portion of adjacent association cortex, where convergence with one other primary system may occur, and also to a portion of the premotor cortex. (In addition, S1 and S2 are reciprocally connected and S1 and the motor cortex are strongly interconnected.) The association and premotor areas in turn exhibit a complicated pattern of projection to still other portions of the association cortex, and it is within these tertiary patterns that the three sensory systems begin to converge. The convergence of projections probably takes place chiefly in the cortex of the frontal pole, in the orbital portion of the frontal lobe, and in the depths of the superior temporal sulcus. This convergence is preceded and followed by powerful projections to the limbic system.

It seems likely that a considerable amount of "processing" occurs before the sensory systems converge. For example, the portion of the parietal lobe above and behind the end of the lateral sulcus receives the projections from the postcentral gyrus in front and from the visual cortex behind. Damage to this region in the dominant hemisphere for spatial and body relationships (usually the right hemisphere) will result in defects of certain complex somatic and visual functions. For example, route finding by maps is impaired whether the maps are presented visually or are handled (tactile-kinesthetic perception). Further examples are given below.

Functional Integration of Sensory Modalities. A familiar object or tool is familiar because it has been seen and used. But it is not necessary to see the object or tool in order to identify it. For example, the sound of a typewriter in another room is sufficient to identify it as a typewriter. If one is blindfolded, it can be recognized by handling it. By watching a typewriter in use, one might learn to operate it, though certainly not skillfully at first. The sensory phenomena involved are extremely complex. Although nearly all of the senses may be involved in any one of the examples cited, the final result or experience is not a group of separately recognized senses, but a holistic experience, the component factors of which are not consciously distinguished. One does not say, "Here is something which feels like this, looks like this, sounds like this, and is named a typewriter." It is simply a typewriter. Moreover, the process of recognition is often accompanied by a complex motor sequence.

So it is with most sensory phenomena. Although it is true that the various senses may be individually detected or experienced under certain conditions, more complex perceptual phenomena nevertheless depend upon the integration of several modalities. Even the simpler phenomena involve several modalities. When the base of a vibrating tuning fork is placed over a bony prominence, the resulting sensation is probably due to the stimulation of tactile receptors as well as Pacinian corpuscles. Sensations of weight, shape, texture, etc., clearly involve the projection of several modalities to association cortex. The synthesis of modalities and their further integration into more complex perceptual phenomena is given the general term *eugnosia,* and appears to be a function of association cortex, especially of the hemisphere specialized for spatial and holistic functions. This is usually the right hemisphere.

Manual examination of a lead pencil with the eyes closed illustrates such processes for the general senses. The individual modalities are integrated into factors of size, weight, shape, texture, and temperature. Past experience relates these qualities to a lead pencil. This *stereognosis* usually proceeds rapidly and, for familiar objects, is completed almost immediately without the conscious intervention of the component qualities.

The quality of rapid synthesis is especially marked in visual phenomena. If the picture of an airplane is flashed upon a screen, a certain time is necessary to determine its type, purpose, and nationality. If the time upon the screen is gradually reduced, it is not long before a fraction of a second suffices for identification. This is recognition of a total pattern and not a sequential recognition of individual qualities.

Similar functions obtain in regard to hearing. Dropping a lead pencil might or might not produce a characteristic sound, but dropping a coin on a hard surface certainly would. A subject could not only recognize that a coin produced the sound, but might very well be able to tell its denomination.

Agnosias may follow lesions of the association areas of the dominant hemisphere. Agnosia literally means "without knowledge." Here it is used in the sense that knowledge or recognition of objects is impaired or impossible. There are many grades and types of agnosias, and many of them cannot be related to specific cortical areas.

One type is *visual agnosia,* which often follows a lesion of the occipital or parieto-occipital cortex on the lateral surface of the dominant hemisphere. Previously familiar objects are seen but not recognized. A lead pencil may mean nothing unless the patient is allowed to handle it. A bunch of keys is not recognized until they are shaken; their characteristic sounds are then the determining qualities. Loss of visual recognition and visual memory may also follow destructive lesions of the cortex of the inferior aspect of the temporal lobe. It has been shown in nonhuman primates that this cortex, which is connected with the peristriate cortex and the pulvinar, contains neurons that respond to complex visual stimuli.

Lesions of the parietal lobe behind the postcentral gyrus may be followed by *astereognosis,* the loss of the normal quality of stereognosis. If the lead pencil is held in the hand opposite to the involved lobe, it is not identified even though the primary modalities are relatively intact. Identification may also be impaired if the pencil is examined by the ipsilateral or "normal" hand. If the eyes are open, recognition is possible because of visualization.

OLFACTORY AREAS

The axons of the mitral cells in the olfactory bulb project posteriorly in the olfactory tract and end in several different regions (pp. 282 and 394). Those that turn into the lateral olfactory stria end in cortex on either side of and immediately above the stria. This olfactory cortex (paleocortex, p. 383) is known as the *lateral olfactory area* or *prepiriform cortex;* it lies at the edge of the insula (*limen insulae*), it includes the corticomedial amygdaloid group, and it appears to be the primary receptive area for smell. Thus, the pathway to perception is uncrossed and does not involve the thalamus.

The primary olfactory cortex projects to olfactory association cortex, namely, the uncus (periamygdaloid area), and the anterior portion of the parahippocampal gyrus. This anterior portion is transitional cortex and is also known as the *entorhinal cortex.* The entorhinal cortex, the uncus, and the lateral olfactory area together comprise the *piriform lobe* or *area.*

The olfactory cortex of each hemisphere is connected by the *anterior commissure,* a small bundle of fibers which crosses the median plane in the lamina terminalis. The commissure also contains fibers that connect the neocortices of the temporal lobes.

TASTE

Little is known about the taste pathways in humans. The secondary fibers from the nucleus of the tractus solitarius probably ascend near or within the medial lemniscus to the ventrobasal portion of the thalamus. The primary receptive area is probably the head portion of the postcentral gyrus. The projections to association cortex, and thereby to integration with smell, are unknown.

BALANCE OR EQUILIBRIUM

The pathway to perception for impulses from the vestibule and semicircular canals is thought to be similar to that for hearing, namely to a primary receptive area in the temporal lobe. An equally good argument could be made for a projection to the postcentral and integration into kinesthetic mechanisms and body image.

SUMMARY

The motor areas of the brain project to subcortical centers, the brain stem, and the spinal cord. They include the motor cortex (precentral gyrus; area 4) and the premotor cortex (areas 6 and 8). Area 4 is a major source of pyramidal fibers; it is reciprocally connected to the postcentral gyrus. Its projections to the brain stem are mostly bilateral, as are its projections to the spinal cord for trunk muscles. Its projections to limb musculature are mostly contralateral. Electrical stimulation of area 4, as well as clinical studies, indicate that the body is represented upside down in area 4. There is also multiple representation of movements in each topographical subdivision of area 4. The type and extent of movement produced by electrical stimulation depend upon the strength, frequency, and wave form of the stimulus. Multiplicity of movement representation may also be evident during pathological stimulation, for example, by a tumor, when jacksonian convulsions may occur.

Stimulation of area 6 may be without positive effect, and it is thought that this area, which projects to subcortical centers of the extrapyramidal system, is chiefly inhibitory in function. Area 8, which is also known as the frontal eye field, is concerned with movements of the head, neck, and eyes.

A secondary motor area is present at the foot of area 4, and a supplementary area is present on the medial aspect of the hemisphere.

Destructive lesions of the motor cortex are characterized chiefly by weakness, generally on the opposite side of the body. The severity of the weakness and the presence of other signs depends upon the location and extent of destruction. When area 6 is involved in adults, the grasp reflex and groping response may be present.

The mechanisms by which willed movements are generated are unknown. The learning and control of complex purposeful movements are controlled by one hemisphere, usually the left. A destructive lesion of the association cortex of this hemisphere may result in an apraxia, which is the inability to perform a familiar act or voluntary movement, even though there may be no paralysis.

The primary receptive areas are those to which the afferent paths project. Except for smell, they are mostly crossed and relay in the thalamus. The primary receptive area for the general senses is the postcentral gyrus (areas 3, 1, 2), that for vision is mostly on the medial aspect of the occipital lobe (area 17), and that for hearing is mostly buried in the lateral sulcus (area 41). The primary receptive area for smell is the lateral olfactory area, whereas that for taste is probably in the lower part of the postcentral gyrus, and that for balance (vestibular system) is thought to be in the superior temporal gyrus. Stimulation of a primary receptive area gives rise to a relatively simple sensation, for example, tingling or flashes of light, depending upon the area stimulated. Potentials evoked by electrical stimulation have been used to map the receptive areas.

The body is represented upside down and mostly contralaterally in the postcentral gyrus. The body is also represented in a second somatic area near the lower end of the central sulcus. The postcentral gyrus and the thalamus are concerned in initial perception, as are the other primary areas. The optic pathway from the retina is organized so that the left fields of vision project to the right occipital lobe, and vice versa. The left auditory cortex receives chiefly from the right ear, and vice versa.

The primary receptive areas are not directly connected. Each projects to a portion of adjacent association cortex and also to a portion of the premotor cortex, and these in turn exhibit a comlicated pattern of projection to still other portions of association cortex, where the sensory systems begin to converge. The convergence is preceded and followed by projections to the limbic system. Functionally, the convergence is marked by the integration of the modalities into complex perceptual phenomena. The synthesis of the general senses is termed stereognosis and is a function chiefly of the right hemisphere. Agnosias, an impairment or loss of recognition of familiar objects, may follow destructive lesions of the association cortex of this hemisphere.

NAMES IN NEUROLOGY

GUSTAV THEODOR FECHNER (1801–1887)

Fechner was a professor of physics at Leipzig who wrote the first treatise on psychophysics. He carried out extended experiments on cutaneous and muscle senses and restated Weber's law in its logarithmic form.

JOHN HUGHLINGS JACKSON (1835–1911)

Jackson was an English physician and one of the world's outstanding clinical neurologists. He attended the York Medical School (no longer in existence), and then secured appointments to the London Hospital and the National Hospital for Paralysis and Epilepsy. For forty-five years (from 1862) he served as its most brilliant staff member. His remarkable powers of clinical observation and his deductive philosophic grasp led him to formulate neurological concepts that are still fundamental to our knowledge of the nervous system. From clinical and postmortem studies of epilepsy, aphasia, and paralysis, he concluded that certain cortical areas were concerned in motor activities, sensory mechanisms, and language, and he accurately located the regions concerned. He did not, however, suggest fixed centers, but rather cortical representation of function. He pointed out that positive signs in neurological disorders are often the result of release of lower centers from the control of higher centers.

ERNST HEINRICH WEBER (1795–1878)

Weber was a distinguished professor of anatomy and physiology at Leipzig (1821–1866) and professor of anatomy until 1871. In 1825, he collaborated with his brother, Eduard Friedrich Weber (1806-1871), in pioneer experiments on the hydrodynamics of wave motion and showed the velocity of the pulse wave. In 1846 they described the inhibitory effects of the vagus nerve. Ernst studied sensory phenomena and stated that the just detectable increment in the intensity of a sensation is some constant proportion of the stimulus intensity itself. A third brother, Wilhelm Eduard Weber (1804–1891), a professor of physics at Göttingen, collaborated with Eduard in a study of the mechanics of human locomotion.

REFERENCES

See also references on pp. 159, 219, and 244.
There are many excellent books on clinical neurology, a number of which are listed in the following introduction to clinical neurology.

Baker, A. B.: An Outline of Clinical Neurology. Dubuque, Kendall/Hunt Publishing Company, 1958. This useful guide, which is now in its sixth printing (1973), is organized according to clinical signs and symptoms rather than diseases, and provides a valuable list of supplementary reading.

The following texts deal with the psychological aspects of motor and sensory behavior and higher level functions.

Geldard, F. A.: The Human Senses. 2nd ed. John Wiley & Sons, Inc., New York, 1972.
Greenfield, N. S., and Sternbach, R. A. (editors): Handbook of Psychophysiology. New York, Holt, Rinehart and Winston, Inc., 1972.
Grossman, S. P.: A Textbook of Physiological Psychology. New York, John Wiley and Sons, Inc., 1967.
Hebb, D. O.: Textbook of Psychology. 3rd edition. Philadelphia, W. B. Saunders Company, 1972.
Kling, J. S., and Riggs, L. A.: Editors, Woodworth & Schlosberg's Experimental Psychology. 3rd ed. New York, Holt, Rinehart and Winston, Inc., 1971.
Morgan, C. T., and King, R. A.: Introduction to Psychology. 4th ed. New York, McGraw-Hill, Inc., 1971.

The following papers are to be found in Schmitt, F. O., and Worden, F. G.: (editors): The Neurosciences. Third Study Program, Cambridge, The MIT Press, 1974.

Graybiel, A. M.: Studies on the anatomical organization of posterior association cortex. Pp. 205–214.

Gross, C. G., Bender, D. B., and Rocha-Miranda, C. E.: Inferotemporal cortex: a single-unit analysis. Pp. 229–238.

Jones, E. G.: The anatomy of extrageniculostriate visual mechanisms. Pp. 215–227.

Werner, G.: Neural information processing with stimulus feature extractors. Pp. 171–183.

The following references include monographs, reviews, and original papers.

Békésy, G. von: Sensory Inhibition. Princeton, Princeton University Press, 1967.

Brinkman, J., and Kuypers, H. G. J. M.: Cerebral control of contralateral and ipsilateral arm, hand and finger movements in the split-brain rhesus monkey. Brain, 96:653–674, 1973. An important experimental study of cerebral motor functions.

Brodal, A.: Self-observations and neuro-anatomical considerations after a stroke. Brain, 96:675–694, 1973. A fascinating and important account by one of the world's outstanding neuroanatomists, who provides insight into this common and major neurological disorder from the viewpoint of both the patient and the neurologist.

Jones, E. G., and Powell, T. P. S.: An anatomical study of converging sensory pathways within the cerebral cortex of the monkey. Brain, 93:793–820, 1970.

Kimura, D., and Archibald, Y.: Motor functions of the left hemisphere. Brain, 97:337–350, 1974. A clinical study of hemisphere specialization in motor control.

Landau, W. M.: Spasticity: The fable of a neurological demon and the emperor's new therapy. Arch. Neurol., 31:217–219, 1974. An editorial on concepts of cause and therapy of spasticity.

Chapter 19

THE FOREBRAIN: CEREBRAL SPECIALIZATION

The purpose of this chapter is to present certain features of cerebral function and specialization which are important in intellectual and cognitive processes. The most striking of these features is specialization of the right and left cerebral hemispheres for different functions, a specialization that represents uniquely human attributes.

The psychological importance of these cerebral functions can scarcely be overestimated. Although their basic mechanisms remain unknown, it has been established that these functions are critically dependent upon areas of the cerebral cortex which are commonly termed association areas, and whose functional importance was introduced in the previous chapter. The extent to which human cerebral cortex is composed of association cortex is illustrated in Figure 19–1 and also in Figure 17–11, p. 390. Of major importance also are the *association fasciculi* and *commissures*. Association fasciculi are bundles of nerve fibers which course in the white matter and which provide for the transfer of information from one part of a hemisphere to another. Commissures, on the other hand, connect the two cerebral hemispheres and provide for the interhemispheric transfer of information. The largest and most important commissure is the *corpus callosum.* Another is the *anterior commissure* (p. 415).

A detailed presentation of the higher-level cerebral functions is beyond the scope of this text. Rather, what is intended is a brief discussion of certain classes of learned behavior, especially those that occur only in humans, and which are the special province of one of the hemispheres. The dominance of the left cerebral hemisphere for language is the most striking example of the phenomenon of cerebral dominance.

Specialized cerebral functions have been studied in a variety of ways, including psychological studies, the analyses of develop-

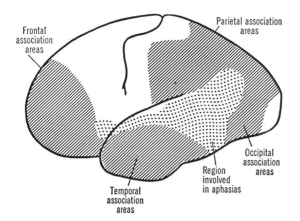

Figure 19–1. Diagram indicating the extent of supralimbic (association) cortex on the lateral surface of the dominant (left) hemisphere. See also Figure 17–11, p. 390. Within the supralimbic neocortex, the area indicated by stippling is important in language mechanisms; destruction of this area, or portions of it, results in aphasic disorders. The boundaries of this "language area" are not sharp.

mental stages during infancy and childhood, and psychobiological studies of language. To these must be added the analysis of the effects of unilateral lesions of the cerebral cortex, the study of defects that follow surgical division of the major commissures, and, in normal subjects, the study of hemisphere lateralization by a variety of experimental methods. In addition, studies of the temporary paralysis of one cerebral hemisphere produced by injecting sodium amytal into the common carotid artery supplying that hemisphere have been an important source of knowledge concerning lateralization of language mechanisms. Immediately after an injection, the patient shows a temporary contralateral hemiplegia, hemianesthesia, and hemianopia. The patient counts slowly as the injection is made, and if it is made on the dominant side, the patient usually becomes mute for about two minutes, and then makes many dysphasic errors, including the misnaming of common objects, and errors in repeating well-known series, such as days of the week forward and backward. If the injection is on the nondominant side, speech is rarely interrupted for more than a few seconds, and there are no dysphasic errors.

In normal individuals, the hemispheres are integrated in function owing chiefly to their commissural connections, and to the fact that the sensory pathways that convey information to the brain have some ipsilateral connections (e.g., some sensory impulses from the right side of the body reach the right cerebral hemisphere). Cerebral differences, however, can be detected by presenting competing stimuli. If, for example, two stimuli are presented simultaneously to each half of the body, the hemisphere dominant for that stimulus extinguishes the other stimulus, and only one stimulus is perceived. The extinction is probably carried out by the callosal fibers projecting from the dominant hemisphere. (It is likely that many fibers in the corpus callosum are inhibitory in function.)

Patients whose commissural fibers have been severed appear to be remarkably free of behavioral impairment in ordinary activity.

By one or two years after surgery, there is surprisingly little disruption. However, recent memory is affected, and, because there is no transfer of information, completely lateralized stimulation demonstrates hemisphere specialization. A person who is presented with an object in the visual fields of one side cannot remember the object when it is presented to the other visual fields. Objects identified by touch with one hand cannot be found and recognized with the other hand. The patient cannot describe objects in the left visual fields, objects felt with the left hand, or sounds heard by the right hemisphere.

It is now known from clinical studies that when all commissural fibers are severed, each cerebral hemisphere behaves as an independent brain. Each has its own independent perception, learning, memory, thoughts, and ideas, and neither is aware of what is experienced in the other. Furthermore, each half can independently generate emotional reactions.

LEFT CEREBRAL HEMISPHERE

In most individuals, the left cerebral hemisphere is specialized for hand control, language, analytical processes, and certain aspects of memory. Thus, most people are right-handed, and damage to the left cerebral hemisphere of right-handed individuals may cause severe defects in these functions.

Left hemisphere specialization is thought to be largely predetermined and present at birth. (Portions of the upper aspect of the left superior temporal gyrus are usually larger than the same region on the right side, and this difference is also present at birth. This region is a part of Wernicke's area; see later discussion.) Moreover, the left hemisphere tends to be dominant even in left-handed persons, but often to a lesser degree, that is, the right hemisphere tends to participate to a greater extent in the usual functions of the left hemisphere.

Figure 19–2 illustrates in a simplified way that the left hemisphere is the main language center; it is specialized for speech, writing, reading, and calculation. The right ear projects chiefly to the left hemisphere. (Musically experienced listeners are said to recognize melodies better with the right ear than with the left, whereas the reverse is said to be true for nonmusicians, who tend to listen to a melody as a whole.) The left hemisphere carries out stereognostic processes, but not to the same degree or for the same qualities as does the right hemisphere.

LANGUAGE

Although symbols may be learned and used by many animals, in nonhuman forms communication is confined to signaling and the expression of emotion. As a structural instrument of descrip-

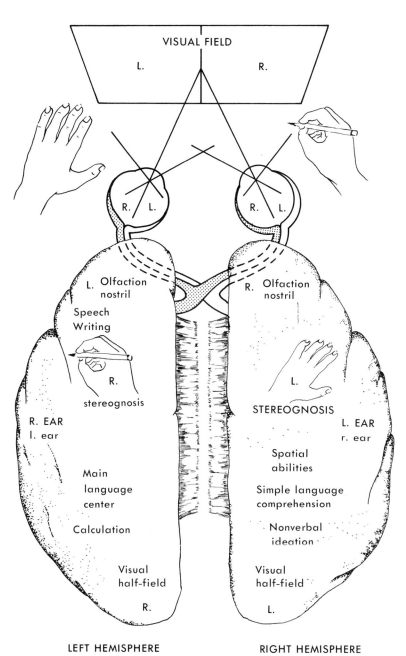

Figure 19-2. A simplified summary of cerebral specialization based on studies of patients whose major commissures have been surgically divided and patients with cortical lesions. (From R. W. Sperry, by permission of the author and publisher.)

tion and argument, language is uniquely human. The use of language is directly related to the intellectual development of an individual, so much so that it is difficult to estimate intelligence in the presence of illiteracy.

Studies of the acquisition of language in children suggest that the faculty of language includes an inborn knowledge of the formal principles of language structure, a knowledge that depends upon genetically determined portions of (usually) the left hemisphere. It should also be pointed out that the articulation of speech is dependent upon certain anatomical characteristics of the human larynx, pharynx, and oral cavity. In particular, the shape of the pharynx, the shape of the oral cavity, and the independent neural control of the shape of each of these cavities are critically important in speech mechanisms.

Although the specialization of the left hemisphere for language is well established, one cannot say that language is "located" in this or that part of the hemisphere. What is known is that disorders of language follow lesions in the general area indicated in Figure 19–1 or in the connections of this area. Disorders of language resulting from damage to the brain are called *aphasias*. Various kinds of aphasias have been described and classified, and, in each, certain symptoms appear to predominate.

The anterior portion of the "language area" shown in Figure 19–1 is termed Broca's area; it is located immediately in front of the cortical motor areas for the peripheral organs of speech. Lesions of this area (on the left side usually) interfere with the motor (articulatory) aspects of language. Speech is slow, labored, grammatically incorrect, and telegraphic, and may be impossible to carry out. Writing is likewise severely impaired. Comprehension of the spoken or written word, however, may be unimpaired or nearly so. (It is interesting that under the stress of emotion, a patient with Broca's aphasia may be temporarily fluent.) Because Broca's area is close to the motor cortex, the latter is often damaged simultaneously. Hence the patients often suffer from weakness or paralysis on the right side of the body. Similar lesions on the right side will cause a left-sided weakness or paralysis but will have no effect upon language.

In the posterior portion of the "language area" (near the auditory cortex) is Wernicke's area, which lies immediately below and behind the primary receptive area for hearing, and which constitutes the auditory association cortex. Damage to the posterior portion of the language area, especially to Wernicke's area, results in loss of comprehension of the spoken word, and often of the written word as well, just as if a foreign language were being used. In addition, the patient's own speech is rapid and well-articulated, but without content. Writing is defective, and words that are heard cannot be repeated. (Hearing itself is completely normal.) It is important to note that similar lesions in the right hemisphere usually have no effect upon language.

Broca's area and Wernicke's area are connected by a major association bundle, the *arcuate fasciculus,* and damage to this bundle in the white matter may also disrupt speech. The patient can understand words, both spoken and written, but cannot repeat them, although a fluent paraphasic speech may be carried on.

It seems, therefore, that information concerning the spoken and written word is conveyed to the posterior part of the "language area" for decoding or translation, and damage to this area consequently abolishes comprehension of the written and spoken word. Since this region relays information forward by the arcuate fasciculus to Broca's area for encoding and for the complex programming of the speech organs, language output is also disorganized when the decoding region and its connections are damaged, although not as severely or in the same way as when damage occurs to Broca's area.

It is to be noted that comprehension of the written language requires connections from the visual areas to the "language area." The angular gyrus, which lies immediately behind Wernicke's area, appears to be especially important for the correct understanding of the written word. If the left angular gyrus is damaged, the ability to read and write may be impaired or lost (*alexia* with *agraphia*), although the patient may still be able to speak and to understand the spoken word. Alexia without agraphia may follow destruction of the left visual cortex and the posterior portion of the corpus callosum. The explanation is that reading the written language can reach only the right hemisphere. In order to be dealt with as a language, there must be transmission to the language region of the left hemisphere, but this is impossible because of the destruction of the corpus callosum. Hence, what is seen is meaningless.

Damage to the "language area" in children results in severe aphasias, but often with an extraordinary degree of recovery, undoubtedly due to the development of language mechanisms in the right hemisphere. (This potential function is probably normally suppressed by the left hemisphere.) Aphasias from similar lesions in adults are often permanent. It is interesting that if one hemisphere is forced to combine both analytical and holistic processes, even very early in life, neither process may be done very well.

RIGHT CEREBRAL HEMISPHERE

The right cerebral hemisphere is said to look at matters in their entirety; it therefore deals with holistic processes, As indicated in Figure 19–2, it is specialized in stereognosis (see agnosias, p. 414), in spatial abilities, and in nonverbal ideation; it is therefore critical in the development and maintenance of body image. (Damage to the right parietal lobe may result in defects in body image; the patient may deny that the body part looked at is his.) As the perceptual hemisphere, the right hemisphere (especially the temporal lobe) is critical in judgments of familiarity (an aspect of memory) and in the interpretation of space.

The right hemisphere participates to a limited extent in simple language comprehension, but not in speaking or writing. Thus, it is much more difficult to investigate and, in spite of being clearly superior for all nonlinguistic, nonmathematical, spatial functions, it is still known as the minor or mute hemisphere.

LEARNING AND MEMORY

Learning and memory are inseparable. Learning is a general term used to indicate an attribute that is highly developed (relatively speaking) in humans. Learning includes, in the form of memory, relationships between neural processes which may last over scores of years. The time differential cannot be explained by any known physiological data or anatomical structure. Whether or not there are right and left hemispheric differences in learning is also unknown.

There appear to be two kinds of memory. One, which is known as "immediate" or "short-term" memory, is an active process in which a single experience results in neuronal activity. However, the memory trace of the experience is not laid down permanently except with time and repetition. The second type of memory involves some structural change in neurons, perhaps in synapses or postsynaptic structures; it is memory storage, or storage of *engrams*, and is known as "long-term" memory. It is, in fact, learning. The two kinds of memory are not sharply separated, they are much more complex than indicated here, and the first process undoubtedly initiates some of the processes that are necessary for the second. The two kinds of memory can be selectively affected by brain damage or disease. It is interesting that extensive bilateral lesions of the prefrontal cortex interfere with short-term memory. Experiments have shown that animals with such lesions cannot learn problems that demand a retention of facts for more than a few seconds, such as remembering in which of two cups food has been placed. Immediate memory is lost, but abilities that the animal has as a result of previous training are not. The latter are regained shortly after the operation producing the lesion has been performed. These findings indicate the distinction between short-term and long-term memory. Another symptom of interference with immediate memory in the learning of temporally arranged patterns is distractibility, which may be so pronounced that an animal can be deviated from any line of activity by extraneous stimuli. Humans with similar extensive prefrontal lesions have similar difficulties with memory and, therefore, they often have peculiar changes in personality as well.

A number of regions of the brain are known to be important in memory. Electrical stimulation of the lateral aspect of the temporal lobe in conscious patients may evoke a memory. Bilateral removal of the hippocampi causes a global amnesia. Removal of the left hippocampus results in defects of verbal memory, whereas removal of the right causes defects in spatial recognition. More extensive ablations, such as anterior temporal lobectomies, which remove temporal neocortex, amygdaloid bodies, and parts of the hippocampus and parahippocampal gyrus, cause severe defects. Left anterior lobectomy selectively impairs the learning and retention of verbal material regardless of whether it is heard or read, whereas the memory of perceptual details (places, faces, melodies) remains unimpaired. With a right anterior lobectomy, verbal memory is unimpaired, but there is impaired recognition and recall of visual and auditory patterns that cannot be coded verbally; tasks requiring spatial orientation, whether visually or through proprioceptive guidance, are learned with difficulty. To complicate the picture, section of the corpus callosum interferes with short-term memory, and lesions of the biogenic amine system may also interfere with learning and memory. In attempting to integrate these diverse findings, it has been suggested that engrams are stored in the upper portion of the brain stem, are interpreted by temporal neocortex, and are scanned and recalled by the hippocampi.

LEARNING AND CONDITIONED RESPONSES

The modification of behavior on the basis of past experience is an aspect of learning which is thought to be primarily a function of the cerebral cortex, especially of the limbic system, although obviously requiring the participation of many other neural structures and mechanisms. Such modification may involve visceral responses, and thus has important implications in understanding and treating psychosomatic disorders. How visceral responses may be modified or learned requires a brief description of conditioning.

We all know that the sight or smell of food may be as potent a stimulus for salivation as is taste. However, the objective response, salivation, which is an autonomic response activated by parasympathetic fibers to salivary glands, is present in newborn infants. Only later do sight and smell induce salivation. Salivation in response to taste is an *unconditioned reflex,* brought about by the stimulation by taste fibers of the cells of origin of the parasympathetic cells in the third cranial nerve.

Many unconditioned reflexes may be modified by, or adopted to, new stimuli. The sound of a bell is not ordinarily followed by salivation. Yet it is well-known that, if an animal is given food, or a mild acid placed in its mouth so that salivation occurs, and if this is accompanied or shortly preceded by another stimulus such as the sound of a bell, after repeated trials the sound alone may induce salivation. This is *conditioned response* — an increase in salivary gland activity in reaction to an auditory stimulus.

Conditioned responses generally have to be reinforced. In classical or Pavlovian conditioning, which is generally thought to be involuntary, the reinforcement must be by an unconditioned stimulus that already elicits the specific response to be learned. In the conditioning called *operant conditioning,* or instrumental learning, the reinforcement is a reward that has no natural relationship to the response. This reward can strengthen any immediately preceding response, which may be viewed as an anticipatory reaction, not a reflex.

It is now known that visceral and glandular responses can be learned, modified, and controlled through both classical and operant conditioning. An example is the psychogalvanic reflex, which is based on the fact that a reflex increase in sweating (mediated through sympathetic fibers to sweat glands, especially those of the hands) occurs during emotional states. If a mild direct current is passed through the hands, the flow of current increases as the sweating increases (because the increase in fluid lowers the resistance to the flow of current). Thus, the reflex response can be measured in a way that tends to furnish objective evidence of emotional reaction. In classical conditioning, this reflex can be tied to a stimulus that does not normally elicit it. In operant conditioning, this reflex and many other autonomic activities (heart rate, salivation, etc.) can be learned, that is, brought about by the subject in order to obtain a reward or some desired change.

The neurophysiological factors in conditioning are not definitely established. It has been shown, however, that responses resulting from electrical stimulation of motor pathways cannot be conditioned by simultaneous sensory stimuli of an auditory or visual type. On the other hand, conditioned responses result from electrical stimulation of afferent pathways. This indicates that there is a mechanism for forming the pattern or association of conditioning, and that it resides in the central nervous system elsewhere than in the longitudinal pathways. The association areas are the most likely locations.

Removal of part or all of the cortex does not abolish conditioned responses or the ability to form new ones, but these are never as precise as in a normal animal. Whereas flexion of a limb might be the normal conditioned response, general escape movements of a diffuse type constitute the response in a decorticate animal. Subcortical areas thus appear to be able to function in this regard, but for precise or discrete activity the association areas are indispensable. Conditioned responses, once established, are not invariable. They may gradually disappear if continually elicited without periodic reinforcement by the unconditioned stimulus, or if associated with extraneous stimuli.

The ultimate explanation of conditioning is lacking, just as it is in other types of learning, in memory, and in intelligent behavior. The fundamental difficulty is that the time scale is too great to be adequately explained.

SUMMARY

Human intellectual and cognitive processes depend in large part upon the association areas of neocortex, although the basic mechanisms of these processes remain unknown. The association areas of a given hemisphere are interconnected by association fasciculi, whereas commissures connect one hemisphere with the other.

In normal individuals, the right and left hemispheres are integrated in function, owing to their commissural connections. However, a variety of clinical, psychological, and experimental studies reveal that each hemisphere is highly specialized. In most individuals, the left cerebral hemisphere is specialized for hand control, language, analytical processes, and certain aspects of memory. This specialization is largely predetermined and is present at birth. Thus, most people are right-handed, and, in right-handed individuals, damage to the frontal-temporal association cortex of the left hemisphere causes language disorders known as aphasias.

The right cerebral hemisphere participates to a limited degree in simple language comprehension, but not in speaking or writing. It is, however, clearly superior in all nonlinguistic, nonmathematical, spatial functions, and in certain aspects of memory. It therefore deals with holistic, unitary processes.

Learning and memory include neural processes that may last for decades and which cannot yet be explained. Memory has a temporary or short-term component, and a long-term, permanent, or storage component, in which engrams are stored. Many regions of the brain are involved in memory, with the temporal lobes and upper brain stem being of special importance. It has been suggested that engrams are stored in the upper brain stem, that the temporal neocortex interprets them, and that the hippocampi scan and recall the engrams. Removal of the left temporal lobe results in defects of verbal memory, whereas removal of the right causes defects in spatial recognition.

Modification of behavior on the basis of past experience comprises a form of learning. Conditioned responses, both classical and operant, are examples of such modification. Visceral and glandular responses can be learned, modified, and controlled through both classical and operant conditioning.

NAMES IN NEUROLOGY

PIERRE-PAUL BROCA (1824–1880)

See the biographical sketch on p. 397.

CARL WERNICKE (1848–1905)

Wernicke was a German physician who, at the age of 26, published his classic monograph (Der aphasische Symptomenkomplex: Eine psychologische Studie auf anatomischer Basis. Breslau, Cohn and Weigert, 1874). He established the fact that there were linguistic differences between the aphasias produced by damage in the left temporal lobe (Wernicke's area), and those produced by lesions in the frontal lobe (Broca's area). Moreover, he provided a theoretical analysis of aphasia, one which was a major influence on modern studies in this field and which made it possible to predict the anatomical sites of syndromes not previously described and to predict the symptoms that would result from certain specific lesions.

REFERENCES

The following papers are contained in Schmitt, F. O., and Worden, F. B. (editors): The Neurosciences. Third Study Program. Cambridge, The MIT Press, 1974.

Broadbent, D. E.: Division of function and integration of behavior. Pp. 31–41.
Liberman, A. M.: The specialization of the language hemisphere. Pp. 43–56.
Darwin, C. J.: Ear differences and hemispheric specialization. Pp. 57–63.
Milner, B.: Hemispheric specialization: scope and limits. Pp. 75–89.
Sperry, R. W.: Lateral specialization in the surgically separated hemispheres. Pp. 5-19.
Teuber, H.-L.: Why two brains? Pp. 71–74.

The following are key papers, reviews, and texts.

Beuer, T. G., and Chiarello, R. J.: Cerebral dominance in musicians and nonmusicians. Science, *185*:537–539, 1974.
DiCara, L. V.: Learning in the autonomic nervous system. Sci. Amer., *222*:30–39, 1970.
Geschwind, N.: The organization of language and the brain. Science, *170*:940–944, 1970. Language and the brain. Sci. Amer., *226*:76–83, 1972.
Hilgard, E. R., and Marquis, D. G.: Conditioning and Learning. Revised by Kimble, G. A. 2nd ed. New York, Appleton-Century-Crofts, 1961.
Jakobson, R.: Verbal communication. Sci. Amer., *227*:72-80, 1972.
Kimura, D.: The asymmetry of the human brain. Sci. Amer., *228*:70–78, 1973.
Lenneberg, E. H.: Biological Foundations of Language. New York, Wiley, 1967. On explaining language. Science, *164*:635–643, 1969.
McGaugh, J. L.: Time-dependent processes in memory storage. Science, *153*:1351–1358, 1966.
Meyer, A.: The frontal lobe syndrome, the aphasias and related conditions. A contribution to the history of cortical localization. Brain, *97*:565–600, 1974. An important review with an extremely valuable bibliography.
Miller, N. E.: Learning of visceral and glandular responses. Sciences, *163*:434–445, 1969.
Penfield, W., and Mathieson, G.: Memory, Arch. Neurol., *31*:145–154, 1974.
Wolff, J. G.: Language, Brain and Hearing. London, Methuen and Co. Ltd., 1973.
Zaidel, D., and Sperry, R. W.: Memory impairment after commissurotomy in man. Brain, 97: 263–272, 1974.

The following symposium contains papers that will provide background and an introduction to the vast literature on aphasias. See also the references in the reviews by Geschwind and by Meyer, cited above.

de Reuck, A. V. S., and O'Connor, M. (editors): Disorders of Language. CIBA Foundation Symposium. Boston, Little, Brown and Company, 1964.

GLOSSARY OF TERMS

A number of medical and general scientific terms are listed here to show their Latin and Greek origins.

Abducent: L., *abducere,* to draw outward, away from the median plane. The muscle that the abducent nerve supplies turns the eyeball outward, that is, abducts it.

Acoustic: Gr., *akoustikos,* relating to hearing, from *akouein,* to hear.

Afferent: L., *ad,* to, plus *ferre,* to bear or to carry. In physiology, bearing or conducting inward to a part or organ.

Agnosia: Gr., ignorance, from *a,* without, plus *gnosis,* a knowing, denoting cognition or recognition. Loss of ability to recognize familiar objects.

Anatomy: Gr., *anatemnein,* to cut up. The science or branch of morphology which treats of the structure of animals.

Anesthesia: Gr., *an,* not, plus *aisthesis,* feeling. Loss of feeling or sensation.

Anterior: L., comparative of *ante,* before. Before or toward the front.

Aphasia: Gr., from *aphatos,* speechlessness, or not spoken, from *a,* not, plus *phanai,* to speak. A disorder of language.

Apraxia: Gr., *a,* without, plus *praxis,* a doing. Therefore, inactivity; inability to perform a familiar act.

Arachnoid: Gr., *arachnoeides,* like a cobweb, from *arachne,* spider or spider's web. One of the meninges is so called because the delicate network of the tissue resembles a spider's web.

Archicerebellum: Gr., *archein,* to be first, plus *cerebellum.* The oldest part of the cerebellum, that is, the part appearing first in the evolutionary scale.

Archipallium: Gr., *archein,* plus *pallium.* The first or oldest portion of the cerebral cortex.

Artery: Gr., *arteria,* air containing.

So called because the Greeks saw arteries after death when contractions had forced blood into the veins. Hence, they supposed them to contain air.

Astrocyte: Gr., *aster,* from *astron,* star, plus *kytos,* cell. A neuroglial cell so named because of its star shape.

Ataxia: Gr., *ataktos,* out of order, from *a,* not, plus *taktos,* ordered. Absence of arrangement or orderliness; ataxic movements are disordered.

Atrophy: Gr., *atrophia,* from *a,* not, plus *trephein,* to nourish. A wasting away from want of nourishment.

Autonomic: Gr., *autos,* self, plus *nomos,* law; acting independently. So named because that part of the nervous system is concerned with visceral (involuntary) processes.

Axon: Gr., *axon,* axis or vertebra. An axon is long, slender and relatively unbranched.

Brachial: L., *brachium,* from Gr., *brachion,* arm. The region between the shoulder and elbow.

Brachium conjunctivum: L., from Gr., *brachion,* plus L., *conjunctivus,* connective. A connecting arm. So called because the two peduncles cross each other.

Brachium pontis: L., from Gr., *brachion,* plus L., *pons,* a bridge. So called because these two peduncles resemble a bridge between the cerebellar hemispheres.

Capillary: L., *capillus,* a hair or minute tube. So called because of the minute size of these vessels.

Carotid: Gr., *karotides*, from *karos*, heavy sleep. Named because of the supposition that pressure and obliteration of the carotid arteries interfere with the blood supply of the brain and produce unconsciousness.

Cauda equina: L., *cauda*, tail, plus *equus*, horse. The lumbar and sacral spinal roots form a cluster in the lower spinal canal which resembles the tail of a horse.

Caudal: L., *cauda*, tail. Toward the tail or posterior end (in humans, inferior).

Cerebellum: L., diminutive of *cerebrum*, brain; therefore, little brain.

Cerebrum: L., *cerebrum*, from Gr., *kara*, head. The adult derivatives of the forebrain.

Chiasma: Gr., *chiasma.* Two lines placed crosswise, from *chiasein*, to make a mark with a *chi* or χ.

Choroid: Gr., *chorion*, a delicate membrane, plus *eidos*, form. Therefore, like or resembling a delicate membrane.

Chromatolysis: Gr., *chroma*, color, plus *lysis*, solution. To lose or dissolve color, and in neurology refers to the loss of Nissl substance.

Chronaxie: Gr., *chronos*, time, plus *axia*, value. A value of time.

Cochlea: L., *cochlea*, from Gr., *kochlias*, snail, from Gr., *kochlos*, a shellfish with a spiral shell. So named because of the coiled or spiral arrangement of the cochlea of the internal ear.

Colliculus: L., *colliculus*, mound, diminutive of *collis*, hill. Therefore, little hill. So called because each colliculus forms a small, rounded eminence or hill.

Congenital: L., *congenitus*, present at or dating from birth.

Conjugate: L., *conjugare*, to unite. In physiology, refers to muscles working in unison, as the eye muscles.

Coronal: L., *coronalis*, of or pertaining to the crown or corona. In the plane of the coronal suture of the skull, the coronal plane.

Corpus callosum: L., *corporis*, body, plus *callosum*, hard or indurated.

Cortex: L., *cortex*, bark of a tree, akin to *corium*, leather. Anatomically the term applies to the outer or superficial part of an organ, as the outer layer of gray matter of the cerebrum.

Cranial: Gr., *kranion*, the skull, akin to *kara*, head. Pertaining to or toward the skull or head.

Crista: L., *crista*, crest or cock's comb or ridge. So called because the crista of the semicircular canals are in the form of elevations or ridges.

Cuneatus: L., from *cuneus*, wedge. The fasciculus cuneatus is so named because it is short and wedge shaped.

Cytoplasm: Gr., *kytos*, a hollow (cell), plus *plasma*, thing formed.

Dendrite: Gr., *dendrites*, of a tree, from *dendron*, tree. Dendrites are nerve processes that are numerous and which branch repeatedly near the cell, forming a tree-like arrangement.

Diastole: Gr., *diastellein*, to put asunder, from *dia*, through, plus *stellein*, to set or place. The expansion or dilatation of the heart cavities as they fill with blood.

Diencephalon: Gr., *dia*, through or between, plus *enkephalos*, brain; the between-brain.

Distal: L., *distare*, be separate or distant from. Away from the center of the body.

Dorsal: L., *dorsum*, back. Pertaining to or situated near the back of an animal.

Dura mater: L., *durus*, hard, plus *mater*, mother. In ancient times the meninges were thought to give rise to all the membranes of the body; it is the tough, outer meningeal layer.

Ectoderm: Gr., *ektos*, outside, plus *derma*, skin. The outer, investing cellular membrane of multicellular animals; applies especially to the outer germ layer of embryos.

Efferent: L., *effere*, to bear or carry out or away from. In physiology, conveying outward or discharging.

Embryo: Gr., *embryon*, to swell in or teem in, from *en*, in, plus *bryein*, to swell, teem. In the human being, the period of development up to the third month *in utero.*

Encephalon: Gr., *enkephalos*, from *en*, in, plus *kephalos*, head. Refers to the brain.

Endocrine: Gr., *endon*, within, plus *krinein*, to separate. Secreting internally.

Endoderm: Gr., *endon*, within, plus *derma*, skin. The inner germ layer.

Ependyma: Gr., *ependyma*, an upper garment. Refers to the cloak or lining of the ventricles.

Epilepsy: Gr., *epilepsia,* a seizure, from *epi,* upon or beside, plus *lambanein,* to take.

Exteroceptive: L., *exterus,* outside, plus *capere,* to take. To receive from the outside.

Facial: L., *facies,* the face. Of or pertaining to the face or facial nerve (so called because of its distribution to the facial muscles).

Fasciculus: L., diminutive of *fascis,* bundle. Therefore, a little bundle. Commonly applied to a slender bundle of fibers, either nerve or muscle.

Fetus: L., *fetus,* fruitful, offspring. In the human being, the child in that period of development from the eighth week *in utero,* until birth.

Flaccid: L., *flaccidus,* flabby, from *flaccus,* lack of firmness or stiffness.

Foramen: L., *forare,* to bore or pierce. An aperture or opening.

Fovea: L., *fovea,* a small pit; probably akin to Gr., *cheie,* a hole.

Frontal: L., *frontale,* a forehead ornament. Of or pertaining to the forehead.

Funiculus: L., *funiculus,* diminutive of *funis,* cord. Therefore, a little cord, band or bundle of fibers. As applied to nerves, is less specific functionally than a fasciculus.

Ganglion: Gr., *ganglion,* swelling or enlargement. An enlargement or mass of nerve tissue containing nerve cells, usually outside the central nervous system.

Geniculate: L., *geniculum,* diminutive of *genu,* knee. Therefore, little knee or bend. So called because the lateral geniculate body is bent or angled like a knee.

Glossopharyngeal: Gr., *glossa,* tongue, plus *pharynx,* chasm or throat. The ninth cranial nerve, so called because of its distribution to these structures.

Gracilis: L., *gracilis,* slender, thin. The fasciculus gracilis is so named because it is long and slender, extending throughout the length of the spinal cord. Likewise, the gracilis muscle in the thigh is long and slender.

Gyrus: L., *gyrus,* from Gr., *gyros,* circle, circular or spiral form. On the surface of the brain, a convoluted ridge between grooves.

Hemiplegia: Gr., *hemi,* plus *plege,* stroke. Paralysis or weakness of one side of the body.

Hippocampus: Gr., *hippos,* horse, plus *kampos,* sea monster. A part of the brain next to the temporal horn of the lateral ventricle.

Histology: Gr., *histos,* web (denotes tissue), plus *logia,* discourse. The science which treats of the structure of tissues.

Homeostasis: Gr., *homoios,* like or similar, plus *stasis,* a standing still. A state of dynamic equilibrium in bodily processes.

Hydrocephalus: Gr., *hydor,* water, plus *kephalos,* head. Excessive amount of cerebrospinal fluid.

Hypoglossal: Gr., *hypo,* below, plus *glossa,* tongue. So named because the nerve courses below the tongue to reach the muscles it supplies.

Hypothalamus: Gr., *hypo,* below, plus *thalamos,* thalamus.

Incus: L., *incus,* anvil. The ear ossicle that resembles an anvil.

Inhibition: L., *inhibere,* to restrain or check.

Interoceptive: L., *inter,* between or within, plus *capere,* to take. To receive stimuli from within.

Labyrinth: Gr., *labyrinthos,* an intricate passageway or maze. Refers to the inner ear because of the intricacy of structure of this region.

Lateral: L., *lateris,* side or flank, akin to *latus,* broad or wide. In a direction or position opposed to medial.

Lemniscus: L., *lemniscus,* a ribbon hanging down, from Gr., *lemniskos,* fillet. A band of nerve fibers; usually applied to a collection of fibers of second order neurons.

Lesion: L., *laesus* or *laedere,* to hurt or injure. Any morbid change in tissues due to disease or injury.

Limbic: L., *limbus,* a border or hem. The limbic lobe forms a border or rim around the upper end of the brain stem.

Macula: L., *macula,* a spot or stain. Any structure forming a spot, as the macula of the utricle or of the retina.

Malleus: L., *malleus*, hammer. The ear ossicle whose shape resembles that of a hammer.

Median: L., *medius*, middle. Situated in the middle.

Medulla oblongata: L., *medulla*, marrow or essence, plus *oblongata*, oblong. The most caudal part of the brain stem.

Meninges: L., *meninges*, from Gr. *meninx*, membrane. A general term for any of the membranes covering the brain.

Mesencephalon: Gr., *mesos*, middle, plus *enkephalos*, brain. Therefore, midbrain.

Metencephalon: Gr., *meta*, after, plus *enkephalos*, brain. The afterbrain, part of the hindbrain.

Microglia: Gr., *mikros*, small, plus *glia*, glue. A small neuroglial cell.

Morphology: Gr., *morphe*, form, plus *logia*, science. Science of form and structure of animals.

Muscle: L., *musculus*, diminutive of *mus*, mouse. Therefore, little mouse. So called because of the fancied resemblance of movements of the biceps brachii to the movements of a mouse.

Myasthenia gravis: Gr., *mys* or *myos*, muscle, plus *aistheneia*, weakness, plus L., *gravis*, heavy. A disease of the muscles causing fatigue and eventually paralysis.

Myelencephalon: Gr., *myelos*, marrow, plus *enkephalos*, brain. The marrowbrain; refers especially to the medulla oblongata.

Myofibril: Gr., *mys*, muscle, plus L., *fibrilla*, a little fiber. Therefore, a little fiber within a muscle.

Myotatic: Gr., *mys*, muscle, plus *tasis*, stretching. Refers to stretch reflex.

Neocerebellum: Gr., *neos*, new, plus *cerebellum*, little brain. The newest portion of the cerebellum in evolutionary processes.

Neopallium: Gr., *neos*, plus L., *pallium*, cloak or mantle (refers to cortex). The newest portion of the cerebral cortex in evolutionary processes.

Nerve: L., *nervus*, akin to Gr., *neuron*, sinew or nerve.

Neurilemma: Gr., *neuron*, nerve, plus *lemma*, skin or peel. The outer skin or cell layer around a nerve fiber.

Neuroblast: Gr., *neuron*, nerve, plus *blastos*, germ. Means nerve forming and refers to embryonic cells that give rise to nerve cells.

Neuroglia: Gr., *neuron*, nerve, plus *glia*, glue. Means nerve glue and refers to the cells which support or hold nervous tissue together.

Neurology: Gr., *neuron*, nerve, plus *logia*, science. The science of the nervous system.

Nucleolus: L., diminutive of *nucleus*, from *nucis*, nut. Therefore, a little nut. A rounded, often conspicuous body within a nucleus.

Nucleus: L., *nucleus*, kernel, from *nucis*, nut. A central mass or point, as the nucleus of a cell.

Occipital: L., *occipitus*, back of head, as opposed to forehead.

Oculomotor: L., *oculus*, eye, plus *motor*, motion. Moving the eyeball. The nerve supplies muscles which move the eyeball.

Olfactory: L., *olfacere*, to smell. Refers to the sense of smell or to structures subserving this function.

Oligodendroglia: Gr., *oligos*, small or few, plus *dendron*, tree, plus *glia*, glue. A neuroglial cell with a few small branches.

Optic: Gr., *optikos*, akin to *opsis*, vision. Of or pertaining to vision and the structures subserving this function.

Orbital: L., *orbita*, track or circuit. Pertaining to the skull cavity in which the eye and appendages are located.

Ossicle: L., *ossiculum*, diminutive of *os*, bone. Therefore, little bone.

Paleocerebellum: Gr., *palaios*, old or ancient, plus cerebellum. A phylogenetically older portion of the cerebellum.

Paralysis: Gr., *para*, beside, plus *lyein*, to loosen, dissolve or disable. Hence, to disable on a side.

Peduncle: L., *pedunculus*, diminutive of *pes*, foot. Therefore, little foot. A stem or narrow part by which some part is attached to another, as the cerebellum to the brain stem.

Peristalsis: Gr., *peristaltikos*, clasping and compressing, as in the peculiar wavelike motions of the intestines.

Phagocyte: Gr., *phago*, I eat, plus *kytos*, cell. Phagocytic cells ingest and destroy other materials, including cells.

Physiology: Gr., *physis*, nature, plus *logia*. The branch of biology dealing with the processes and activities of living organisms.

Pia mater: L., *pius*, tender or kind, plus *mater*, mother. The more delicate and closely investing of the three meningeal layers.

Pineal: L., *pineus*, a pine cone. The pineal body in shape and attachment resembles a pine cone.

Plexus: L., *plexus*, a turning or braid. Refers to the interweaving of nerves as they form a plexus.

Pons: L., *pons*, a bridge. The pons consists of fibers that bridge across the brain stem to the cerebellum on either side.

Posterior: L., *posterus*, from *post*, behind or after. At or toward the hind end of the body; in a tailward or caudal direction (in humans, behind or dorsal rather than below).

Proprioceptive: L., *proprius*, one's own, plus *capere*, to take. Stimulation produced by inner structures, such as muscles, tendons, and joints.

Prosencephalon: Gr., *pos*, toward or near, plus *enkephalos*. The first or foremost of the primary brain vesicles.

Protoplasm: Gr., *protos*, first, plus *plasma*, thing formed. Originally designated formative material of young animal embryos. Now refers to the essential substance of cell body and nucleus.

Proximal: L., *proximare*, to come near. Next to or nearest, as to the point of attachment of a limb to the body.

Psychiatry: Gr., *psyche*, the mind, plus *iatreia*, healing. Although literally meaning mind-healing, it is really the science of behavior, including behavior disorders.

Pschology: Gr., *psyche*, mind, plus *logia*. The science which treats of mental and behavioral processes.

Reflex: L., *re*, back, plus *flectere*, to bend. To turn or refer back.

Restiform: L., *restis*, rope, plus *forma*, form. Ropelike; these peduncles are so named because of their ropelike or cordlike shape.

Retina: L., *rete*, a net. The light-sensitive membrane of the eye.

Rheobase: Gr., *rheos*, current, plus *basis*, base or foundation. The basic or minimal current required to excite.

Rhombencephalon: Gr., *rhombos*, equilateral parallelogram with o- blique angles, plus *enkephalos*. The hindbrain, so named because of its shape.

Saccule: L., diminutive of *saccus*, sac. Therefore, a little membranous bag in the inner ear.

Sagittal: L., *sagitta*, an arrow. Of or pertaining to the sagittal suture of the skull and any plane parallel to this suture.

Spastic: Gr., *spastikos*, from *span*, to draw. To cause convulsions.

Sphygmomanometer: Gr., *sphygmos*, pluse, plus *monometer*, an instrument for measuring pressure. An instrument for measuring blood pressure.

Substantia nigra: L., *substantis*, substance, plus *nigra*, black. So called because of the dark or black appearance of this area, resulting from the presence of melanin-containing cells.

Sulcus: L., *sulcus*, a groove or furrow.

Synapse: Gr., *synapsis*, a conjunction or union.

Systole: Gr., *systellein*, to contract. Refers to the contraction of the heart.

Tactile: L., *tactilis*, tangible, from *tactum*, to touch.

Telencephalon: Gr., *telos*, end, plus *enkephalos*. The far or endbrain.

Temporal: L., *temporalis*, or *temporal*, the temples. Of or pertaining to the region of the temples.

Thalamus: Gr., *thalos* or *thalamos*, inner chamber or anteroom.

Transverse: L., *transvertere*, to turn or direct across.

Trigeminal: L., *trigeminus*, born three together, from *tri*, three, plus *geminus*, twin. Pertaining to the trigeminal nerve with its three branches.

Trochlear: L., *trochlea*, block or pulley. So called because the muscle that this nerve supplies has a pulley for its tendon.

Tympanum: L., *tympanum*, drum. This membrane is stretched tightly across the end of the external ear canal, like the skin of a drum.

Utricle: L., *utriculus*, diminutive of *uter*, sac or vesicle; a skin bag.

Vagus: L., *vagari,* wandering. So called because of the long and extensive course of this nerve.

Vein: L., *vena,* akin to *vehere,* to convey.

Ventral: L., *ventralis,* from *venter,* belly. Anything pertaining to or toward this part of the body, as opposed to dorsal.

Ventricle: L., *ventriculus,* diminutive of *venter,* belly. A chamber or cavity.

Venule: L., diminutive of *vena,* vein. Therefore, a little vein.

Vermis: L., *vermis,* a worm. So called because of the narrow, wormlike appearance of the midpart of the cerebellum.

Vestibular: L., *vestibulum,* passage, hall or chanber.

Viscera: L., *viscus,* to turn or wind, as the internal organs.

INDEX